Movement Disorders

Editor

JOSEPH JANKOVIC

NEUROLOGIC CLINICS

www.neurologic.theclinics.com

Consulting Editor

RANDOLPH W. EVANS

February 2015 • Volume 33 • Number 1

ELSEVIER

1600 John F. Kennedy Boulevard • Suite 1800 • Philadelphia, Pennsylvania, 19103-2899

http://www.theclinics.com

NEUROLOGIC CLINICS Volume 33, Number 1
February 2015 ISSN 0733-8619, ISBN-13: 978-0-323-35446-2

Editor: Joanne Husovski
Developmental editor: Donald Mumford

Neurologic Clinics (ISSN 0733-8619) is published quarterly by Elsevier Inc., 360 Park Avenue South, New York, NY 10010–1710. Months of issue are February, May, August, and November. Periodicals postage paid at New York, NY, and additional mailing offices. Subscription prices are $300.00 per year for US individuals, $517.00 per year for US institutions, $145.00 per year for US students, $375.00 per year for Canadian individuals, $627.00 per year for Canadian institutions, $415.00 per year for international individuals, $627.00 per year for international institutions, and $210.00 for Canadian and foreign students/residents. To receive student/resident rate, orders must be accompanied by name of affiliated institution, date of term, and the *signature* of program/residency coordinator on institution letterhead. Orders will be billed at individual rate until proof of status is received. Foreign air speed delivery is included in all *Clinics* subscription prices. All prices are subject to change without notice. **POSTMASTER:** Send address changes to *Neurologic Clinics*, Elsevier Health Sciences Division, Subscription Customer Service, 3251 Riverport Lane, Maryland Heights, MO 63043. **Customer Service: Telephone: 1-800-654-2452 (U.S. and Canada); 314-447-8871 (outside U.S. and Canada). Fax: 314-447-8029. E-mail: journalscustomerservice-usa@elsevier.com (for print support); journalsonlinesupport-usa@elsevier.com (for online support).**

Reprints. For copies of 100 or more of articles in this publication, please contact the Commercial Reprints Department, Elsevier Inc., 360 Park Avenue South, New York, New York, 10010-1710; Tel.: +1-212-633-3874; Fax: +1-212-633-3820, and E-mail: reprints@elsevier.com.

Neurologic Clinics is also published in Spanish by Nueva Editorial Interamericana S.A., Mexico City, Mexico.

Neurologic Clinics is covered in *Current Contents/Clinical Medicine, MEDLINE/PubMed (Index Medicus), EMBASE/Excerpta Medica, and PsycINFO, and ISI/BIOMED.*

Contributors

CONSULTING EDITOR

RANDOLPH W. EVANS, MD
Clinical Professor of Neurology, Baylor College of Medicine, Houston, Texas

EDITOR

JOSEPH JANKOVIC, MD
Professor of Neurology, Department of Neurology, Distinguished Chair in Movement Disorders, Director, Parkinson's Disease Center and Movement Disorders Clinic, Baylor College of Medicine, Houston, Texas

AUTHORS

UMAR AKBAR, MD
Department of Neurology, Center for Movement Disorders and Neurorestoration College of Medicine, McKnight Brain Institute, University of Florida, Gainesville, Florida

ROGER L. ALBIN, MD
Professor, Department of Neurology, University of Michigan; Chief, Neuroscience Research, Veterans Affairs Medical Center, Ann Arbor, Michigan

TETSUO ASHIZAWA, MD
Department of Neurology, Center for Movement Disorders and Neurorestoration College of Medicine, McKnight Brain Institute, University of Florida, Gainesville, Florida

KAILASH P. BHATIA, FRCP
Sobell Department of Motor Neuroscience and Movement Disorders, University College London Institute of Neurology, London, United Kingdom

ANNA CZLONKOWSKA, MD, PhD
2nd Department of Neurology, Institute Psychiatry and Neurology; Department of Experimental and Clinical Pharmacology, Medical University, Warsaw, Poland

PRAVEEN DAYALU, MD
Clinical Assistant Professor, Department of Neurology, University of Michigan, Ann Arbor, Michigan

GÜNTHER DEUSCHL, MD
Professor, Department of Neurology, University-Hospital Schleswig-Holstein, Christian-Albrechts-University Kiel, Kiel, Germany

ATBIN DJAMSHIDIAN-TEHRANI, MD
Department of Neurology, Innsbruck Medical University, Innsbruck, Austria

PETR DUSEK, MD, PhD
Department of Neurology and Centre of Clinical Neuroscience, First Faculty of Medicine and General University Hospital in Prague, Charles University in Prague, Prague, Czech Republic; Institute of Neuroradiology, University Medicine Goettingen, Göttingen, Germany

STEWART A. FACTOR, DO
Department of Neurology, Emory University, School of Medicine, Atlanta, Georgia

CHRISTOS GANOS, MD
Sobell Department of Motor Neuroscience and Movement Disorders, University College London Institute of Neurology, London, United Kingdom; Department of Neurology, University Medical Center Hamburg-Eppendorf (UKE), Hamburg, Germany

JOSEPH JANKOVIC, MD
Professor of Neurology, Department of Neurology, Distinguished Chair in Movement Disorders, Director, Parkinson's Disease Center and Movement Disorders Clinic, Baylor College of Medicine, Houston, Texas

H.A. JINNAH, MD, PhD
Professor, Departments of Neurology, Human Genetics and Pediatrics, Emory University School of Medicine, Atlanta, Georgia

TOMASZ LITWIN, MD, PhD
2nd Department of Neurology, Institute Psychiatry and Neurology, Warsaw, Poland

DAVIDE MARTINO, PhD
Neurology Department, King's College Hospital NHS Foundation Trust; Department of Neurology, Queen Elizabeth Hospital, Lewisham and Greenwich NHS Trust, London, United Kingdom

SHYAMAL H. MEHTA, MD, PhD
Assistant Professor of Neurology, Mayo Clinic Arizona, Scottsdale, Arizona

JOHN C. MORGAN, MD, PhD
Associate Professor of Neurology, Georgia Health Sciences University, Augusta, Georgia

STEPHEN MULLIN, BSc, MRCP
Leonard Wolfson Clinical Research Fellow, Department of Clinical Neurosciences, University College London Institute of Neurology, London, United Kingdom

CHRISTIANA OSSIG, MD
Division of Neurodegenerative Diseases, Department of Neurology, Dresden University of Technology Dresden, Germany; Department of Neuropsychiatry and Laboratory of Molecular Psychiatry, Charité-Universitätsmedizin Berlin, Berlin, Germany

WERNER POEWE, MD
Professor of Neurology, Director, Department of Neurology, Innsbruck Medical University, Innsbruck, Austria

HEINZ REICHMANN, MD, PhD, FRCP, FAAN
Professor, Department of Neurology, Dresden University of Technology, Dresden, Germany

ANTHONY H.V. SCHAPIRA, MD, DSc, FRCP, FMedSci
Head, Department of Clinical Neurosciences, University College London Institute of Neurology, London, United Kingdom

SUSANNE A. SCHNEIDER, MD, PhD
Department of Neurology, University-Hospital Schleswig-Holstein, Christian-Albrechts-University Kiel, Kiel, Germany

KAPIL D. SETHI, MD, FRCP (UK), FAAN
Director, Movement Disorders Program, Professor of Neurology, Georgia Health Sciences University, Augusta, Georgia; Senior Medical Expert, Merz Pharmaceuticals, Greensboro, North Carolina

MARIA STAMELOU, MD, PhD
Second Department of Neurology, Attiko Hospital, University of Athens, Athens, Greece; Department of Neurology, Philipps Universität, Marburg, Germany; Sobell Department of Motor Neuroscience and Movement Disorders, University College London Institute of Neurology, London, United Kingdom

MARY ANN THENGANATT, MD
Assistant Professor of Neurology, Department of Neurology, Parkinson's Disease Center and Movement Disorders Clinic, Baylor College of Medicine, Houston, Texas

OLGA WALN, MD
Department of Neurology, Houston Methodist Neurological Institute, Houston, Texas

Contents

VIDEOS: Movement Disorders

Videos demonstrating clinical examples of movement disorders accompany this publication: Jankovic: Movement Disorders. All can be viewed online at www.neurologic.theclinics.com associated with this issue as well as on Science Direct. Videos are listed below in association with the article in which they appear

Stamelous: Atypical Parkinsonism: Diagnosis and Treatment

Video: Progressive Supranuclear Palsy

Jinnah: Diagnosis and Treatment of Dystonia

Video 1: Typical cervical dystonia and response to botulinum toxin
Video 2: Tremor-dominant cervical dystonia
Video 3: Blepharospasm
Video 4: Hand dystonia – "writer's cramp" involving the entire hand
Video 5: Hand dystonia – "writer's cramp" involving one finger
Video 6: Foot dystonia with tremor
Video 7: Oromandibular dystonia
Video 8: Axial dystonia

Waln & Jankovic: Paroxysmal Movement Disorders

Video 1: Paroxysmal kinesigenic dyskinesia (PKD)
Video 2: Paroxysmal kinesigenic dyskinesia (PKD)

Thenganatt & Jankovic: Psychogenic Movement Disorders (PMD)

Video 1: Convergance spasm in PMD
Video 2: Classic clinical features of psychogenic tremor
Video 3: Psychogenic dystonia
Video 4: Psychogenic myoclonus
Video 5: Psychogenic parkinsonism
Video 6: Psychogenic tics
Video 7: Organic movement disorder in PMD
Video 8: Psychogenic gait disorder
Video 9: Psychogenic chorea
Video 10: Psychogenic facial movements

Dusek, Litwin, Czlonkowska: Wilson Disease and other Neurodegenerations with Metal Accumulations

Video 1: Neurologic presentation of Wilson Disease
Video 2: Neurologic presentation of Wilson Disease
Video 3: Pantothenate kinase-associated neurodegeneration (PKAN)
Video 4: Mitochondrial membrane protein-associated neurodegeneration (MPAN)

Jankovic: Gait Disorders

Video 1: Parkinsonian gait
Video 2: Parkinsonian gait
Video 3: Subcortical gait pattern
Video 4: Cautious gait disorder
Video 5: Gait disorder of Non-neurologic, psychogenic origin

Poewe & Djamshidian: Movement Disorders in Systemic Disorders

Video 1: Movement disorder in cerebral toxoplasmosis
Video 2: Movement disorder as part of clinical presentation of Anti-NMDA receptor encephalitis

NEUROLOGIC CLINICS

FORTHCOMING ISSUES

May 2015
Cerebrovascular Disease
William Powers, *Editor*

August 2015
Neuro-otology
David Newman-Toker, Kevin Kerber, Jonathan Edlow, and William Meurer, *Editors*

November 2015
Motor Neuron Disease
Richard Barohn, MD, and Mazen Dimachkie, MD, *Editors*

RECENT ISSUES

November 2014
Cerebellar Diseases
Alireza Minagar, and Alejandro A. Rabinstein, *Editors*

August 2014
Myopathies
Mazen M. Dimachkie, and Richard J. Barohn, *Editors*

May 2014
Secondary Headache
Randolph W. Evans, *Editor*

RELATED INTEREST

Imaging of Movement Disorders, February 2010 (Vol. 20, No. 1)
In Neuroimaging Clinics
Tarek Yousry, MD, and Andrew J. Lees, MD, *Authors*

Preface

Movement Disorders

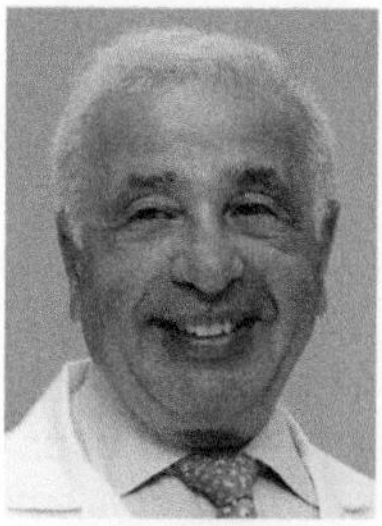

Joseph Jankovic, MD
Editor

Movement disorders is a group of neurologic conditions that can be divided phenomenologically into slow movements (hypokinetic disorders) and abnormal involuntary movements (hyperkinesias). The hypokinetic disorders are characterized not only by slowness of movement but also by paucity of movement. The most characteristic feature of hypokinetic movement disorder is bradykinesia, typically present in Parkinson disease and other parkinsonian disorders. Hyperkinetic movement disorders are subdivided into tremors, dystonia, tics, chorea, athetosis, ballism, stereotypy, and akathisia. Furthermore, ataxia, gait disorders, and spasticity are also often included among movement disorders. While the basal ganglia and their connections have been implicated in the pathophysiology of most of the movement disorders, some are caused by altered peripheral input as exemplified by hemifacial spasm and other peripherally induced movement disorders. A subset of movement disorders with varied phenomenology is caused by psychological factors, hence referred to as "psychogenic movement disorders." Because the diagnosis of a movement disorder is based on recognition of specific phenomenological features, clinicians who encounter patients with movement disorders must use their powers of observation to carefully characterize the disorder. The phenomenological categorization is absolutely critical for formulation of differential etiologic diagnosis and for selection of the most appropriate treatment.

There has been remarkable progress in the field of Movement Disorders since 2009, when I edited the last issue of *Neurologic Clinics* devoted to this topic. In planning this special issue, I carefully considered and eventually selected the most important topics and invited the best experts to provide authoritative reviews. I am pleased that I was able to assemble the most outstanding, internationally renowned, faculty. This comprehensive issue, which includes 14 different topics, should be of interest not only to neurologists who are asked to evaluate and treat patients with Parkinson disease and other movement disorders but also to other clinicians and clinical investigators, as well as basic neuroscientists and other researchers pursuing answers to some

Neurol Clin 33 (2015) xv–xvi
http://dx.doi.org/10.1016/j.ncl.2014.10.001
0733-8619/15/$ – see front matter

of the unanswered questions about the pathogenesis of this challenging group of disorders. The authors were encouraged to provide the most up-to-date reviews and submit as many figures, tables, and videos as possible to enhance the clinical and scientific value of each article. Indeed, this is the first issue in the history of *Neurologic Clinics* that uses patient videos to illustrate the phenomenology and other aspects of the movement disorder. In addition, the authors were instructed to highlight the most important aspects in "key points." One of the many reasons all invited authors accepted the challenge to provide the comprehensive and well-balanced reviews is that *Neurologic Clinics* is a well-established and prestigious brand of scientific and clinical publication. Furthermore, a unique feature of *Neurologic Clinics* is that the issues are not only viewed as books but also as collections of articles, cited in PubMed.

I wish to thank all the authors for their scholarly and timely contributions. I also wish to thank the editorial staff of Elsevier, particularly Joanne Husovski, Senior Editor, *Clinics*, and Donald Mumford, Senior Developmental Editor, for their professionalism and hard work. I also thank my colleague, friend, and tennis partner, Randolph Evans, MD, the Consulting Editor, who inspired this issue. Finally, I wish to express my deep appreciation to my wife, Cathy, for her support throughout this project and over the many decades of our shared lives.

Joseph Jankovic, MD
Professor of Neurology, Distinguished Chair in Movement Disorders
Director, Parkinson's Disease Center and Movement Disorders Clinic
Department of Neurology
Baylor College of Medicine
Houston, TX 77030, USA

E-mail address:
josephj@bcm.edu

Pathogenic Mechanisms of Neurodegeneration in Parkinson Disease

Stephen Mullin, BSc, MRCP,
Anthony H.V. Schapira, MD, DSc, FRCP, FMedSci*

KEYWORDS

- Parkinson disease • α-Synuclein • Lewy bodies • Mitochondrial dysfunction

KEY POINTS

- Sporadic Parkinson disease (PD) represents an accelerated extreme of the normal spectrum of human senescence.
- Recent discoveries have shown that it is likely to result from the effect of many small but quantifiable genetic risk factors, in combination possibly with the effect of certain environmental insults.
- α-Synuclein is the presynaptic protein that constitutes the principal component of Lewy bodies, the pathologic hallmark of PD. Its transformation to fibrillar and oligomeric forms appears to be the key to its neuronal toxicity.
- Although its exact role in the etiology of sporadic PD is unclear, mitochondrial dysfunction appears to play a major role in its pathogenesis.
- The basis for the selective toxicity to dopaminergic cells that characterizes PD remains unclear.

HISTOLOGY, EPIDEMIOLOGY AND GENETICS OF SPORADIC PARKINSON DISEASE

Lewy bodies (LB), discovered in 1912 by Frederic Lewy, remain the pathologic hallmark of Parkinson disease (PD). Their distribution is thought to follow a sequential appearance within the dorsal motor nucleus, olfactory bulbs and nucleus, locus ceruleus, and subsequently, in the substantia nigra pars compacta (SNc).[1] Neuronal cell loss in PD appears first in the dopaminergic cells of the SNc. It has been estimated that dopamine levels in the striatum are reduced to approximately 60% to 70% of normal values at the time of diagnosis. Degeneration of non-dopaminergic neurons

Department of Clinical Neurosciences, UCL Institute of Neurology, Rowland Hill Street, Hampstead, London NW3 2PF, UK
* Corresponding author.
E-mail address: a.schapira@ucl.ac.uk

Neurol Clin 33 (2015) 1–17
http://dx.doi.org/10.1016/j.ncl.2014.09.010 neurologic.theclinics.com

also occurs in PD, but usually later in the course of the disease. The cholinergic nucleus basalis of Meynert, the serotoninergic neurons of the raphe nucleus, and the hypocretin-containing neurons of the hypothalamus suffer neuron loss with advanced disease.[1]

Consistently, age is the greatest risk factor for sporadic PD.[2,3] In the United States, the age-adjusted incidence is 13.5 to 13.9 per 100,000 person-years.[2,4] Age-adjusted prevalence is approximately 115 per 100,000, estimated as 1.3 per 100,000 under age 45 years, and 1192.9 per 100,000 in patients aged 75 to 85 years.[4] Conversely, a prevalence study in Holland found 3100 cases per 100,000 aged 75 to 85 years and 4300 per 100,000 for those older than 85 years.[5] The pathological progression of PD occurs in advance of symptomatic motor PD, with the so-called premotor symptoms, including rapid eye movement sleep disturbance, constipation, subcortical cognitive impairment, and hyposmia potentially preceding it by decades.[6] Imaging with positron emission tomography (PET) suggests the preclinical period of cell loss within the SNc is around 8 years, with the greatest rate of decline in the early stages of the disease.[7] LB have been found within the brains of normal aged subjects,[8,9] perhaps the best indication that PD as a disease entity should be viewed as the accelerated extreme of the "normal" spectrum of senescence. Conversely, in dementia with LB, Lewy pathology with an extremely similar distribution to that in advanced PD[10] leads to a progressive subcortical dementia with or without Parkinsonism,[11] highlighting the variable penetrance of the motor PD phenotype and Lewy pathology's lack of specificity to it.

Although caution must be exercised when correlating the histological stigmata of PD with its clinical and, specifically, its motor signs, the PD phenotype remains remarkably robust. Genome-wide association studies (GWAS) correlate single-nucleotide polymorphisms (SNPs) within the genomes of disease carrying subjects and compare them to controls to calculate (expressed as an odds ratio) the risk associated with those SNPs.[12] The success of GWAS in the context of the PD phenotype attests to its specificity. GWAS studies have confirmed the importance of several gene loci, associated with mendelian forms of PD[13,14] (see later discussion). With the exception of *LRRK2*, truly mendelian pathogenic mutations are comparatively rare. However, haplotypes within the same gene loci confer a smaller PD risk with a much greater frequency. In addition, SNPs in novel loci, not previously associated with PD risk, have been identified and confirmed as risk factors for PD.[14] The most prominent example is the consistent recording of the microtubule associated protein τ (*MAPT*), more commonly associated with the pathogenesis of Alzheimer disease, as a major risk allele locus for PD, the implications of which on the established LB centric model of PD remain unclear.

Age and genetic predispositions aside, other environmental factors have been proposed as risk associations in the pathogenesis of sporadic PD. Consistently, chronic tobacco smoke inhalation and coffee drinking have been shown to reduce the risk for PD. In the case of the former, the relationship appears to be dose-dependent and occurs even when the added burden of mortality from the complications of smoking are taken into account.[15] Pesticide exposure, rural living, and farming seem to confer an increased risk of the development of PD, although it is not clear whether farming represents a confounding association with pesticide exposure.[16] Nonsteroidal anti-inflammatory drug exposure, traumatic brain injury, and several other environmental risk factors[17] have also been identified as contributory; however, the odds ratios (ORs) of any of these risks are not sufficient to cause PD in isolation. Their role in the pathogenesis of PD therefore seems likely to be small, probably in conjunction with a (or a combination of) predisposing genetic risk factor(s).

An as yet underdeveloped field which almost certainty makes a significant contribution to PD risk is that of epigenetics. Epigenetic modifications provide phenotypic plasticity, allowing adaptation to a change in the environment without modifying the genotype. Hence, through processes such as methylation, phosphorylation, acetylation, and generation of micro-RNAs (miRNA), expression of genes can be modulated in response to environmental stimuli.[18] Although the field is in its infancy, there are promising signs that it may yield fruitful insights into potentially modifiable epigenetic processes contributing to PD pathogenesis. There is, for instance, evidence that epigenetic methylation of the α-synuclein (*SNCA*) locus upregulates its translation, with methylation levels being reduced in the substantia nigra of sporadic PD brains.[19,20] Similarly, sporadic PD patients have been shown to have differential expression of various miRNA probes, including miR-34b/c, which has been associated with the development mitochondrial dysfunction.[21,22]

α-SYNUCLEIN

The first indication of the significance of the presynaptic protein SNCA in the pathogenesis of PD came with the discovery of the A53T mutation of the *SNCA* gene, which gives rise to an autosomal-dominant form of familial PD in the fifth to sixth decade.[23] Subsequently, SNCA was discovered to be the principal component of LB.[24] Further autosomal-dominant mutations at E46K and A30P leading to PD in the third to fifth and fifth to seventh decade, respectively,[25,26] were identified along with, more recently, two putative pathogenic substitutions at H50Q and G51D.[27–29] In vitro work subsequently revealed that heterozygous A53T and A30P transgenic mice develop certain aspects of the motor and histological PD phenotype.[30]

The next breakthrough came with the discovery that *SNCA* gene triplications and subsequent duplications led to PD in a dose-dependent manner. A family with an autosomal-dominant form of PD with onset in the fourth decade was found to have a triplication in the *SNCA* gene,[31,32] while subjects with a duplication were found to develop PD from the fifth decade, with relative SNCA expression levels being in proportion to the gene copy number "dosage."[33–35] GWAS have shown that overexpression of *SNCA* mediated by the Rep1 promotor region confers an increased risk of sporadic PD.[36–38] The *SNCA* locus is consistently the most frequent association in GWAS quantifying the risk of PD associated with SNPs.[14]

Despite SNCA's evident significance to the pathogenesis of PD, the pressing question of its physiological function remains unsolved. Pertinently, homozygous *SNCA* knockout mice do not display a Parkinsonian phenotype, although some groups report mild impairment to vesicle trafficking and dopamine release.[39–41] SNCA is predominately a presynaptic terminal protein associated with the distal synaptic reserve. Knockdown or depletion of SNCA in transgenic mice and primary hippocampal neurons deplete synaptic vesicles and impair their mobilization to the presynaptic terminus, although intriguingly it seems to be a viable phenotype.[41,42]

SNCA's conformational properties appear to be a key factor in its pathogenicity. It exists as a monomer in its native state, but has a propensity to defer to a β-sheet-rich amyloid aggregate following, among other factors, oxidative stress, post translational modification, or contact with lipids.[43–45] Oligomeric then protofibrillar intermediaries are precursors to this aggregated form, and it is this transition and these conformations that are thought to confer toxicity.[46,47] This theme is borne out in the finding that familial mutations of *SNCA* have faster (A53T, E46K, H50Q)[48–50] or slower (A30P) aggregation[47,51] compared with wild type and that within LBs SNCA is predominately in its fibrillar and aggregated forms.[52–54]

SNCA's conformational properties have been further brought into focus by the unexpected finding that it may in exhibit "prion-like" properties. Prions are aberrantly folded "infectious" proteins, which, in the absence of nucleic acids, propagate their misfolded β-sheet-rich and aggregated structure to the adjacent native state proteins.[55] The relevance of these proteins to the pathogenesis of PD was sparked by the finding that healthy neurons implanted into PD brains (as part of a therapeutic trial) developed LBs some eleven to sixteen years later pathology which was present 16 months following transplantation.[56–58] Subsequently, it was shown in a variety of models that SNCA can enter the cell via endocytosis, interact directly with and propagate through adjacent cells.[59,60] This aggregated and "transplanted" SNCA from "infected" cells was able to induce aggregation of host SNCA. The same study was able to show in *vivo* transfer of misfolded SNCA to grafted neurons in the striatum of mice overexpressing SNCA,[60] findings that were replicated in the striatum of rats.[57] Similarly preformed fibrils of SNCA injected directly into the striatum of mice have been shown to result in progressive Lewy-derived neuronal toxicity in anatomically adjacent areas. In this study, a progressive reduction of dopamine concentration and impaired motor performance were noted in comparison with mice injected with phosphate-buffered saline, pathology that could be partially rescued with knock-out of the *SNCA* gene.[61] These studies provide some correlation with Braak's clinical and histopathological observation that Lewy pathology spreads consecutively from the first, ninth, and tenth cranial nerves/nuclei through the brainstem, cortex, and on to the neocortex.[1] Accordingly, the "seeding" observed in *vitro* and in *vivo* may be analogous to the progression of LBs in humans, with SNCA aggregation "transmitted" from these selectively vulnerable cranial nerve structures.

There is evidence that SNCA may compromise autophagic cellular degradation mechanisms. Autophagy, which broadly speaking degrades long-lived intracellular proteins, comprises 3 mechanisms: macroautophagy, microautophagy, and chaperone-mediated autophagy (CMA). In macroautophagy, double-membraned autophagosomes fuse with lysosomes to deliver cytoplasmic contents, including misfolded or aggregated proteins for digestion, while microautophagy delivers the same outcome by lysosomal pinocytosis of cytoplasmic contents. CMA depends on the protein chaperone hsc70 and its binding to LAMP-2A, a lysosomal surface receptor.[36] A highly specific subset of cytosolic proteins with a KFREQ motif is recognized by the hsc70 chaperone and internalized for degradation by LAMP-2A lysosomal membrane receptors.[62]

There is abnormal expression of lysosomal proteins in the substantia nigra of PD brains, implying activation of lysosomal pathways common to all 3 autophagial mechanisms.[63] More specifically, SNCA's pentapeptide sequence is consistent with LAMP-2A binding[64] and in lysosomal preparations of SNCA have been shown to be degraded following binding to it. In this system, mutant *SNCA* was bound to this lysosomal receptor with high affinity but was not translocated across the membrane and appeared to block these receptors, thereby inhibiting the CMA pathway, suggesting mutant SNCA may differentially accumulate through CMA inhibition by SNCA mutants.[65] Macroautophagic inhibition with bafilomycin has been shown to cause accumulation of mutant SNCA; conversely, macroautophagial enhancement with rapamycin accelerates clearance of both wild type and mutant SNCA.[66] Overexpression of beclin 1 (another macroautophagial inducer) was able to reduce SNCA levels in mouse brains, providing in *vitro* correlation of macroautophagy's involvement in SNCA clearance SNCA.[67] Moreover, the proteosomal system, which is responsible for the removal of short-lived proteins, has also been implicated in SNCA degradation, although its exact role is controversial. It has been reported that oligomeric SNCA is targeted to the 26S subunit of the proteasome, which, in the process of trying to degrade the protein, is functionally inhibited by it.[68] Conversely, 26S depletion in mice causes early neurodegeneration and striatal accumulation of SNCA.[69] There is at present no consensus as to the significance of these findings, or indeed, what the exact role of the lysosomal and proteosomal degradation of SNCA in PD is. It may be that SNCA's degradation pathway is determined by its conformational state, with monomeric and smaller oligomeric species being degraded by proteosomal and CMA pathways, while larger fibrillar and aggregated forms require bulk disposal with macroautophagy. What is clear is that protein degradation pathways represent a promising area for therapeutic innovation, with upregulation potentially providing an accessible means of removing toxic oligomeric and fibrillar SNCA from the brain.

GLUCOCEREBROSIDASE

The role of glucocerebrosidase (GBA) in the pathogenesis of PD has begun to come to prominence in recent years. GBA is a lysosomal hydrolase, which, through β-cleavage of the β-glucosidic linkage, degrades glucosylceramide to ceramide within the lysosome. Mutations in *GBA* lead to the autosomal-recessive condition Gaucher disease, a lysosomal storage disorder, common among Ashkenazi Jews, resulting in glucosylceramide accumulation in visceral organs and a variety of clinical phenotypes.[70] A decade ago, it was observed that a higher proportion of Gaucher's patients developed motor features of PD[71–73] and subsequently that there was a higher incidence of PD among the pedigree of homozygous mutation carriers, many of whom were obligate heterozygotes.[74] Conversely, it was found that heterozygous carriers of *GBA* mutants had a variable penetrance of the PD phenotype.[75,76] In turn, compared with controls, heterozygous Gaucher's patients were found to have a combined odds ratio (OR) of 5.43 of developing PD,[77] with the N370S mutation having an OR of 3.51 based on a candidate gene approach in a GWAS meta-analysis.[14] Recent data suggest that heterozygote states confer a cumulative risk of developing PD of 5% at age 60 rising to 15% at age 80.[78] Numerically, *GBA* is now the greatest genetic risk factor for PD, with mutation prevalence estimated between 2.3% and 9.4% in non-Ashkenazi PD populations.[79]

Intriguingly, there appears to be evidence of an interaction between GBA and SNCA. Analysis of postmortem brains of sporadic PD patients without *GBA* mutations showed reduced levels of GBA activity,[80] while several studies have demonstrated that inhibition or knockdown of *GBA* causes accumulation of SNCA in cell lines expressing pathogenic PD mutations.[81–83] Conversely, overexpression of SNCA leads to reduced GBA activity.[84] Such an interaction could explain the limited penetrance of parkinsonism in heterozygous Gaucher carriers, with the "priming" effect of a predisposition to SNCA aggregation bringing out the pathogenicity of the GBA mutant.

Evidence for the dysfunctional autophagic disposal of SNCA has already been outlined above; however, an important and developing strand of thinking relating to the pathogenicity of mutant *GBA* is that it acts to impair SNCA autophagy. A recent study found evidence of increased autophagic markers in *GBA* homozygous knockout primary neuronal culture,[85] while another demonstrated that impaired GBA activity contributed to reduced lysosomal activity. The same study also indicated that GBA mutations promote the aggregation to and stabilization of oligomeric SNCA species and, conversely, that SNCA overexpression causes GBA to be sequestered within the endoplasmic reticulum (ER), leading to an increase in reactive oxygen species production and cellular stress.[84] Encouragingly, treatment of disease-carrying fibroblasts and neuroblastoma cells with the ambroxol, a pH-dependent mixed type inhibitor of GBA, appears to restore GBA activity and reduce SNCA expression in GBA cell lines.[86,87] It has been postulated that this occurs by correction of aberrant GBA folding, facilitating trafficking of GBA through the ER.[88]

LEUCINE-RICH REPEAT KINASE 2

An autosomal-dominant form of PD commonly presenting in the sixth decade caused by a mutation in Leucine-rich repeat kinase 2 (*LRRK2*) was first identified in a Japanese family in 2002,[89] with further kindreds identified in the subsequent years,[90,91] including, in 2005, G2019S, the most common mutation.[92] Although there is widespread variation in mutation frequency dependent on ethnicity, it is clear that *LRRK2* is a common mutation that exhibits incomplete penetrance, with the PD phenotype emerging in an age-dependent fashion.[93] In the case of G2019S, for instance, between 0.5% and 12.4% of familial and 0.1% to 4.3% of sporadic Caucasian PD cases carry the mutation, while figures as high as 43% and 33%, respectively, have been recorded in Arabic populations.[94]

LRRK2 is a cytosolic protein of unknown function that has been implicated in a variety of roles, including neurite growth, cytoskeleton maintenance, vesicle trafficking, and autophagy.[46,95–98] It contains a kinase and a GTPase domain; however, at present, its substrate is unknown. As well as the PD phenotype, mutants have been implicated in the pathogenesis of inflammatory bowel disease,[99] a variety of cancers, and leprosy.[100] It can display a more heterogenous pathologic picture than other forms of PD, with tau, neurofibrillary tangles, and anterior horn cell pathology occasionally described with or without LB and nigrostriatal degeneration.[101–104] Apart from its high-allele frequency, of particular interest is its apparent characteristic to exhibit pathogenicity in a gain of function-dependent manner, whereby pharmacological kinase inhibition appears to stabilize neuronal cell death in *LRRK2* cell lines[105,106] and presents a tantalizing therapeutic target, although to date, efforts to produce a viable disease-modifying kinase inhibitor have been disappointing.

MITOCHONDRIA IN PARKINSON DISEASE

Mitochondrial dysfunction is recognized as a pathway in the pathogenesis of PD.[107] The scientific community was first alerted to the potential role of mitochondria in PD by discovery of levodopa-responsive parkinsonism following intravenous injection by drug addicts in California of 1-methyl-4-phenyl-1,2,3,6-tetrahydropyridine (MPTP), a potent inhibitor of complex I of the mitochondrial respiratory chain. Primates who were administered MPTP were found to develop clinical and pathological features of PD,[108,109] and mice were found to develop dopamine depletion in the substantia nigra.[110] Epidemiologic and in vitro work subsequently implicated rotenone, another complex I inhibitor, in the etiology of PD.[110–112] Analysis of platelets in postmortem PD brains has revealed mitochondrial complex I inhibition in the SNc.[113]

Further evidence of the role of mitochondria in PD came with the discovery that disruption of the mechanisms underlying mitochondria quality control cause PD. Mitochondria are controlled and regulated both endogenously (by the genes of mitochondria's own DNA, mtDNA) and exogenously (by those within the nuclear DNA, nDNA) of the host cell. Quality control and exchange of mtDNA within the mitochondrial pool are accomplished by a constant and dynamic process of fission, fusion, and autophagic destruction (mitophagy). The autosomal-recessive nuclear mutations *PINK1* and *PARKIN* lead to PD onset in the fourth[114,115] and third decades, respectively.[116,117] Defective mitochondria are marked for destruction by the externalization to the outer mitochondrial membrane protein by PINK1, which allows recruitment and subsequent ubiquitylation by PARKIN of external mitochondrial proteins, earmarking it for destruction by autophagic machinery.[118,119] These mutations lead to morphologically aberrant and functionally impaired mitochondria.[120–122] In addition to *PINK1* and *PARKIN*, morphological and bioenergetic mitochondrial dysfunction has been described in a significant number of mutations implicated in mendelian and sporadic PD,[85,123–125] implying that mitochondrial damage may be the downstream consequence of these functionally distinct pathogenic mechanisms.

Conversely, parkinsonism has been reported as a component of maternally inherited mitochondrial disease.[126] The pathogenesis of these conditions is a consequence of specific inherited mutations of maternal mtDNA, resulting in clonal expansion and the presence of the mutation within all host mitochondria. These homoplasmic mutations are in contrast to those with a heteroplasmic origin, whereby spontaneous point mutations, which subsequently become clonally expanded, accumulate in a portion of host mitochondria. Specific pathogenic homoplasmic point mutations or the cumulative burden of heteroplasmic mutations past a critical threshold cause disruption of oxidative phosphorylation and hence ATP production, leading to impaired energy supply and ultimately increased susceptibility to cellular death. Heteroplasmic mutations have been recognized as a key component of human senescence, with mtDNA mutation load closely correlates with age,[127] an observation which, given the striking age dependence of sporadic PD, has alerted many researchers to mitochondrial heteroplasmy's possible role in its pathogenesis. An increased mutation burden was found in Parkinsonian brains at postmortem,[127] while variation in mitochondrial haplotype (where evolutionarily conserved homoplasmic mutations in mtDNA are shared in subjects of the same or similar ethinicity) has been found to correlate with increased or decreased risk of sporadic PD.[128] Interestingly, reports have emerged of an unexpectedly high number of HIV patients with prolonged exposure to nucleoside reverse transcriptase inhibitors (which cause a prematurely high level of mtDNA heteroplasmy[129]), developing PD at a comparatively young age, although as yet the association remains unproven.[130,131] Moreover, mutations in the polymerase $\gamma1$ (*Polg1*), a nuclear protein that acts as a "proof reading" mechanism for mitochondrial DNA, leads to Parkinsonism. Some reports have suggested variation in *Polg1* may also be a risk factor for sporadic PD, although results are contradictory. Accordingly, mutation load within mtDNA appears to play a role in PD etiology, although the precise understanding of it remains unclear.

The predominately cytosolic protein SNCA associates with both the inner and the outer mitochondrial membranes.[99,132–135] Overexpressed or A53T SNCA cause morphological and functional disruption of mitochondria and inhibition of complex I,[135,136] while SNCA concentration within the mitochondria appears to directly correlate with the degree of complex I inhibition.[137] Thus, there is evidence of an interaction between SNCA and mitochondria; however, its details and, more pertinently, its bioenergetic consequences remain poorly understood.

SELECTIVE VULNERABILITY OF DOPAMINERGIC NEURONS IN PARKINSON DISEASE

An as yet unresolved question is why the neuronal toxicity is PD is predominately confined to dopaminergic cells of the SNc. Initial attention was focused on whether this selective toxicity was a property of dopamine itself. Dopamine has been found to induce cell toxicity in the presence of SNCA that was not produced with SNCA in isolation[138] and has been shown induce aggregation of SNCA in vitro[139]; this has led to speculation that the oxidation of cytosolic dopamine and the free radical production it generates increases cellular stress and in turn leads to neuronal degeneration. If this were the case, then treatment of PD with L-3,4-dihydroxyphenylalanine (L-dopa) would be expected to accelerate the course of the disease; however, this remains an open question. In one large study, for instance, it was shown that L-dopa may slow the rate of clinical PD progression; however, conversely, single-photon emission CT brain imaging revealed reduced dopamine uptake, implying a decline in dopamine transporter integrity (hence, reduced dopamine levels).[140] This model fails to explain why PD involves a minority of nondopaminergic neurons[141] and equally why many dopaminergic neurons outside the SNc are spared in PD.[142,143]

More recently, attention has focused on the intrinsic physiological pacemaking properties of neurons within the SNc and other parts of the mesencephalon and brainstem. This activity, essential in the case of the dopaminergic cells of the SNc for maintenance of basal dopamine levels (and hence movement), requires rapid spontaneous firing of neurons, which are highly dependent on transmembrane calcium currents. It is suggested that these currents make mitochondria particularly prone to damage, possibly by way of these neurons' characteristic inability to buffer such calcium flux.[144] A promising extension of this line of enquiry is the epidemiologic finding that the use of dihydropyridines, commonly used antihypertensives that antagonize L-type calcium channels, seems to exhibit a protective effect against PD.[145,146] A theoretically attractive hypothesis is that blocking of these channels limits pathologic calcium flux, reducing neuronal toxicity during periods of enhanced energy demand, slowing the progression of PD.

SUMMARY

The principal impediment to progress in the understanding of PD has been the complexity of its etiology. What is certain is that a condition that was once viewed as the prototypical sporadic disease is heavily influenced by the genetic predispositions to it. The presence of toxic oligomeric and fibrillar SNCA species appears to be critical to its the pathogenesis, yet it is still unclear what SNCA's physiological function is. Recent discoveries implicating other such proteins, such as LRRK2 and MAPT, which do not to adhere to the SNCA centric model of PD, have muddied the waters. Equally, the finding through GWAS of multiple novel risk alleles with unknown or unclear modes of action complicate the picture still further. Such findings begin to make sense if, as there is significant evidence to suggest, sporadic PD is viewed as an accelerated variant of normal ageing, with multiple, possibly interacting, genetic predispositions, complemented potentially by epigenetic and environmental insults, resulting in dopaminergic cell death. The putative interaction between GBA and SNCA may serve as a template for such a multifaceted etiological model. Equally, a recurring finding across a spectrum of familial PD cell lines is that mitochondrial dysfunction, delivered by a variety of mechanisms, gives rise to the PD phenotype. These findings imply mitochondrial damage may be the common and irreversible downstream consequence of these mechanisms. Even more critical is why dopaminergic cells of the SNc are selectively vulnerable to PD-induced neuronal damage. Although significant progress has been made to date, this remains an unresolved question. Thus, although remarkable insights into the pathogenesis of PD have emerged in recent years, considerable work and many challenges remain before a coherent and comprehensive model can emerge. Principal among these will be reconciling the diverse and at times contradictory range of pathogenic mechanisms identified to date. It is clear that effective therapeutic interventions to slow the progress of PD will depend on an improved understanding of both its etiology and its pathogenesis.

ACKNOWLEDGMENTS

This work was funded by the Leonard Wolfson Experimental Neurology Center, the Wellcome Trust/MRC Joint Call in Neurodegeneration award (WT089698) to the UK Parkinson's Disease Consortium (UKPDC), Parkinson's UK, the Javon trust, the Kattan Trust and was supported by the National Institute for Health Research University College London Hospitals Biomedical Research Centre.

REFERENCES

1. Braak H, Tredici KD, Rüb U, et al. Staging of brain pathology related to sporadic Parkinson's disease. Neurobiol Aging 2003;24(2):197–211. http://dx.doi.org/10.1016/S0197-4580(02)00065-9.
2. Bower JH, Maraganore DM, McDonnell SK, et al. Incidence and distribution of parkinsonism in Olmsted County, Minnesota, 1976-1990. Neurology 1999;52(6):1214–20.
3. Van Den Eeden SK, Tanner CM, Bernstein AL, et al. Incidence of Parkinson's disease: variation by age, gender, and race/ethnicity. Am J Epidemiol 2003;157(11):1015–22.
4. Mayeux R, Marder K, Cote LJ, et al. The frequency of idiopathic Parkinson's disease by age, ethnic group, and sex in northern Manhattan, 1988-1993. Am J Epidemiol 1995;142(8):820–7.
5. de Rijk MC, Breteler MM, Graveland GA, et al. Prevalence of Parkinson's disease in the elderly: the Rotterdam Study. Neurology 1995;45(12):2143–6.
6. Siderowf A, Jennings D, Eberly S, et al. Impaired olfaction and other prodromal features in the Parkinson At-Risk Syndrome Study. Mov Disord 2012;27(3):406–12. http://dx.doi.org/10.1002/mds.24892.
7. Hilker R, Schweitzer K, Coburger S, et al. Nonlinear progression of Parkinson disease as determined by serial positron emission tomographic imaging of striatal fluorodopa F 18 activity. Arch Neurol 2005;62(3):378–82. http://dx.doi.org/10.1001/archneur.62.3.378.
8. Markesbery WR, Jicha GA, Liu H, et al. Lewy body pathology in normal elderly subjects. J Neuropathol Exp Neurol 2009;68(7):816–22. http://dx.doi.org/10.1097/NEN.0b013e3181ac10a7.
9. Jellinger KA. Age-associated prevalence and risk factors of Lewy body pathology in a general population. Acta Neuropathol 2003;106(4):383–4. http://dx.doi.org/10.1007/s00401-003-0751-9.
10. Tsuboi Y, Uchikado H, Dickson DW. Neuropathology of Parkinson's disease dementia and dementia with Lewy bodies with reference to striatal pathology. Parkinsonism Relat Disord 2007;13(Suppl 3):S221–4. http://dx.doi.org/10.1016/S1353-8020(08)70005-1.
11. Del Ser T, McKeith I, Anand R, et al. Dementia with lewy bodies: findings from an international multicentre study. Int J Geriatr Psychiatry 2000;15(11):1034–45.
12. Manolio TA. Genomewide association studies and assessment of the risk of disease. N Engl J Med 2010;363(2):166–76. http://dx.doi.org/10.1056/NEJMra0905980.
13. International Parkinson Disease Genomics Consortium, Nalls MA, Plagnol V, et al. Imputation of sequence variants for identification of genetic risks for Parkinson's disease: a meta-analysis of genome-wide association studies. Lancet 2011;377(9766):641–9. http://dx.doi.org/10.1016/S0140-6736(10)62345-8.
14. Lill CM, Roehr JT, McQueen MB, et al. Comprehensive research synopsis and systematic meta-analyses in Parkinson's disease genetics: the PDGene

database. PLoS Genet 2012;8(3):e1002548. http://dx.doi.org/10.1371/journal.pgen.1002548.
15. Hernán MA, Takkouche B, Caamaño-Isorna F, et al. A meta-analysis of coffee drinking, cigarette smoking, and the risk of Parkinson's disease. Ann Neurol 2002;52(3):276–84. http://dx.doi.org/10.1002/ana.10277.
16. Tanner CM, Ross GW, Jewell SA, et al. Occupation and risk of parkinsonism: a multicenter case-control study. Arch Neurol 2009;66(9):1106–13. http://dx.doi.org/10.1001/archneurol.2009.195.
17. Kieburtz K, Wunderle KB. Parkinson's disease: evidence for environmental risk factors. Mov Disord 2013;28(1):8–13. http://dx.doi.org/10.1002/mds.25150.
18. Ammal Kaidery N, Tarannum S, Thomas B. Epigenetic landscape of Parkinson's disease: emerging role in disease mechanisms and therapeutic modalities. Neurotherapeutics 2013;10(4):698–708. http://dx.doi.org/10.1007/s13311-013-0211-8.
19. Jowaed A, Schmitt I, Kaut O, et al. Methylation regulates alpha-synuclein expression and is decreased in Parkinson's disease patients' brains. J Neurosci 2010;30(18):6355–9. http://dx.doi.org/10.1523/JNEUROSCI.6119-09.2010.
20. Matsumoto L, Takuma H, Tamaoka A, et al. CpG demethylation enhances alpha-synuclein expression and affects the pathogenesis of Parkinson's disease. PLoS One 2010;5(11):e15522. http://dx.doi.org/10.1371/journal.pone.0015522.
21. Margis R, Margis R, Rieder CR. Identification of blood microRNAs associated to Parkinson's disease. J Biotechnol 2011;152(3):96–101. http://dx.doi.org/10.1016/j.jbiotec.2011.01.023.
22. Miñones-Moyano E, Porta S, Escaramís G, et al. MicroRNA profiling of Parkinson's disease brains identifies early downregulation of miR-34b/c which modulate mitochondrial function. Hum Mol Genet 2011;20(15):3067–78. http://dx.doi.org/10.1093/hmg/ddr210.
23. Polymeropoulos MH, Lavedan C, Leroy E, et al. Mutation in the α-synuclein gene identified in families with Parkinson's disease. Science 1997;276:2045–7.
24. Spillantini MG, Schmidt ML, Lee VM, et al. Alpha-synuclein in Lewy bodies. Nature 1997;388(6645):839–40. http://dx.doi.org/10.1038/42166.
25. Krüger R, Kuhn W, Müller T, et al. Ala30Pro mutation in the gene encoding alpha-synuclein in Parkinson's disease. Nat Genet 1998;18(2):106–8. http://dx.doi.org/10.1038/ng0298-106.
26. Zarranz JJ, Alegre J, Esteban JG. The new mutation, E46K, of α-synuclein causes parkinson and Lewy body dementia. Ann Neurol 2004;55:164–73.
27. Kiely AP, Asi YT, Kara E, et al. α-Synucleinopathy associated with G51D SNCA mutation: a link between Parkinson's disease and multiple system atrophy? Acta Neuropathol 2013;125(5):753–69. http://dx.doi.org/10.1007/s00401-013-1096-7.
28. Appel-Cresswell S, Vilarino-Guell C, Encarnacion M, et al. Alpha-synuclein p.H50Q, a novel pathogenic mutation for Parkinson's disease. Mov Disord 2013;28(6):811–3. http://dx.doi.org/10.1002/mds.25421.
29. Proukakis C, Dudzik CG, Brier T, et al. A novel α-synuclein missense mutation in Parkinson disease. Neurology 2013;80(11):1062–4. http://dx.doi.org/10.1212/WNL.0b013e31828727ba.
30. Magen I, Chesselet MF. Genetic mouse models of Parkinson's disease the state of the art. Prog Brain Res 2010;184:53–87. http://dx.doi.org/10.1016/S0079-6123(10)84004-X.
31. Singleton AB, Farrer M, Johnson J, et al. Alpha-synuclein locus triplication causes Parkinson's disease. Science 2003;302(5646):841. http://dx.doi.org/10.1126/science.1090278.

32. Muenter MD, Forno LS, Hornykiewicz O. Hereditary form of parkinsonism—dementia. Ann Neurol 1998;43:768–81.
33. Miller DW, Hague SM, Clarimon J, et al. Alpha-synuclein in blood and brain from familial Parkinson disease with SNCA locus triplication. Neurology 2004;62(10):1835–8.
34. Ibáñez P, Bonnet AM, Débarges B, et al. Causal relation between alpha-synuclein gene duplication and familial Parkinson's disease. Lancet 2004;364(9440):1169–71. http://dx.doi.org/10.1016/S0140-6736(04)17104-3.
35. Chartier-Harlin MC, Kachergus J, Roumier C, et al. Alpha-synuclein locus duplication as a cause of familial Parkinson's disease. Lancet 2004;364(9440):1167–9. http://dx.doi.org/10.1016/S0140-6736(04)17103-1.
36. Tan CC, Yu JT, Tan MS, et al. Autophagy in aging and neurodegenerative diseases: implications for pathogenesis and therapy. Neurobiol Aging 2014;35(5):941–57. http://dx.doi.org/10.1016/j.neurobiolaging.2013.11.019.
37. Pals P, Lincoln S, Manning J, et al. Alpha-Synuclein promoter confers susceptibility to Parkinson's disease. Ann Neurol 2004;56(4):591–5. http://dx.doi.org/10.1002/ana.20268.
38. Krüger R, Vieira-Saecker AM, Kuhn W, et al. Increased susceptibility to sporadic Parkinson's disease by a certain combined alpha-synuclein/apolipoprotein E genotype. Ann Neurol 2001;45(5):611–7. http://dx.doi.org/10.1002/1531-8249(199905)45:5<611::AID-ANA9>3.0.CO;2-X.
39. Cabin DE, Shimazu K, Murphy D, et al. Synaptic vesicle depletion correlates with attenuated synaptic responses to prolonged repetitive stimulation in mice lacking alpha-synuclein. J Neurosci 2002;22(20):8797–807.
40. Chandra S, Fornai F, Kwon HB, et al. Double-knockout mice for alpha- and beta-synucleins: effect on synaptic functions. Proc Natl Acad Sci U S A 2004;101(41):14966–71. http://dx.doi.org/10.1073/pnas.0406283101.
41. Abeliovich A, Schmitz Y, Fariñas I, et al. Mice lacking alpha-synuclein display functional deficits in the nigrostriatal dopamine system. Neuron 2000;25(1):239–52.
42. Murphy DD, Rueter SM, Trojanowski JQ, et al. Synucleins are developmentally expressed, and alpha-synuclein regulates the size of the presynaptic vesicular pool in primary hippocampal neurons. J Neurosci 2000;20(9):3214–20.
43. Hashimoto M, Hsu LJ, Xia Y, et al. Oxidative stress induces amyloid-like aggregate formation of NACP/α-synuclein in vitro. Neuroreport 1999;10(4):717.
44. Oueslati A, Fournier M, Lashuel HA. Role of post-translational modifications in modulating the structure, function and toxicity of alpha-synuclein: implications for Parkinson's disease pathogenesis and therapies. Prog Brain Res 2010;183:115–45. http://dx.doi.org/10.1016/S0079-6123(10)83007-9.
45. Cole NB, Murphy DD, Grider T, et al. Lipid droplet binding and oligomerization properties of the Parkinson's disease protein α-Synuclein. J Biol Chem 2002;277(8):6344–52.
46. Winner B, Melrose HL, Zhao C, et al. Adult neurogenesis and neurite outgrowth are impaired in LRRK2 G2019S mice. Neurobiol Dis 2011;41(3):706–16. http://dx.doi.org/10.1016/j.nbd.2010.12.008.
47. Conway KA, Lee SJ, Rochet JC, et al. Acceleration of oligomerization, not fibrillization, is a shared property of both α-synuclein mutations linked to early-onset Parkinson's disease: implications for pathogenesis and therapy. Proc Natl Acad Sci U S A 2000;97(2):571–6.
48. Ghosh D, Mondal M, Mohite GM, et al. The Parkinson's disease-associated H50Q mutation accelerates α-synuclein aggregation in vitro. Biochemistry 2013;52(40):6925–7. http://dx.doi.org/10.1021/bi400999d.

49. Pandey JP. Genomewide association studies and assessment of risk of disease. N Engl J Med 2010;363(21):2076–7. http://dx.doi.org/10.1056/NEJMc1010310#SA1 [author reply: 2077].
50. Narhi L. Both familial Parkinson's disease mutations accelerate alpha-synuclein aggregation. J Biol Chem 1999;274(14):9843–6. http://dx.doi.org/10.1074/jbc.274.14.9843.
51. Li J, Uversky VN, Fink AL. Effect of familial Parkinson's disease point mutations A30P and A53T on the structural properties, aggregation, and fibrillation of human alpha-synuclein. Biochemistry 2001;40(38):11604–13.
52. Kosaka K. Diffuse lewy body disease in Japan. J Neurol 1990;237(3):197–204. http://dx.doi.org/10.1007/BF00314594.
53. Dickson DW, Crystal H, Mattiace LA, et al. Diffuse Lewy body disease: light and electron microscopic immunocytochemistry of senile plaques. Acta Neuropathol 1989;78(6):572–84.
54. Baba M, Nakajo S, Tu PH, et al. Aggregation of alpha-synuclein in Lewy bodies of sporadic Parkinson's disease and dementia with Lewy bodies. Am J Pathol 1998;152(4):879–84.
55. Prusiner SB. Nobel lecture: prions. Proc Natl Acad Sci U S A 1998;95(23):13363–83. http://dx.doi.org/10.1073/pnas.95.23.13363.
56. Li Y, Sekine T, Funayama M, et al. Clinicogenetic study of GBA mutations in patients with familial Parkinson's disease. Neurobiol Aging 2014;35(4):935.e3–8. http://dx.doi.org/10.1016/j.neurobiolaging.2013.09.019.
57. Kordower JH, Chu Y, Hauser RA, et al. Lewy body-like pathology in long-term embryonic nigral transplants in Parkinson's disease. Nat Med 2008;14(5):504–6. http://dx.doi.org/10.1038/nm1747.
58. Kordower JH, Freeman TB, Snow BJ, et al. Neuropathological evidence of graft survival and striatal reinnervation after the transplantation of fetal mesencephalic tissue in a patient with Parkinson's disease. N Engl J Med 1995;332(17):1118–24. http://dx.doi.org/10.1056/NEJM199504273321702.
59. Desplats P, Lee HJ, Bae EJ, et al. Inclusion formation and neuronal cell death through neuron-to-neuron transmission of alpha-synuclein. Proc Natl Acad Sci U S A 2009;106(31):13010–5. http://dx.doi.org/10.1073/pnas.0903691106.
60. Hansen C, Angot E, Bergström AL, et al. α-Synuclein propagates from mouse brain to grafted dopaminergic neurons and seeds aggregation in cultured human cells. J Clin Invest 2011;121(2):715–25. http://dx.doi.org/10.1172/JCI43366.
61. Luk KC, Kehm V, Carroll J, et al. Pathological α-synuclein transmission initiates Parkinson-like neurodegeneration in nontransgenic mice. Science 2012;338(6109):949–53. http://dx.doi.org/10.1126/science.1227157.
62. Majeski AE, Dice JF. Mechanisms of chaperone-mediated autophagy. Int J Biochem Cell Biol 2004;36(12):2435–44. http://dx.doi.org/10.1016/j.biocel.2004.02.013.
63. Anglade P, Vyas S, Hirsch EC, et al. Apoptosis in dopaminergic neurons of the human substantia nigra during normal aging. Histol Histopathol 1997;12(3):603–10.
64. Dice JF. Peptide sequences that target cytosolic proteins for lysosomal proteolysis. Trends Biochem Sci 1990;15(8):305–9.
65. Cuervo AM, Stefanis L, Fredenburg R, et al. Impaired degradation of mutant alpha-synuclein by chaperone-mediated autophagy. Science 2004;305(5688):1292–5. http://dx.doi.org/10.1126/science.1101738.
66. Webb JL, Ravikumar B, Atkins J, et al. Alpha-Synuclein is degraded by both autophagy and the proteasome. J Biol Chem 2003;278(27):25009–13. http://dx.doi.org/10.1074/jbc.M300227200.

67. Spencer B, Potkar R, Trejo M, et al. Beclin 1 gene transfer activates autophagy and ameliorates the neurodegenerative pathology in alpha-synuclein models of Parkinson's and Lewy body diseases. J Neurosci 2009;29(43):13578–88. http://dx.doi.org/10.1523/JNEUROSCI.4390-09.2009.
68. Emmanouilidou E, Stefanis L, Vekrellis K. Cell-produced alpha-synuclein oligomers are targeted to, and impair, the 26S proteasome. Neurobiol Aging 2010; 31(6):953–68. http://dx.doi.org/10.1016/j.neurobiolaging.2008.07.008.
69. Bedford L, Hay D, Devoy A, et al. Depletion of 26S proteasomes in mouse brain neurons causes neurodegeneration and Lewy-like inclusions resembling human pale bodies. J Neurosci 2008;28(33):8189–98. http://dx.doi.org/10.1523/JNEUROSCI.2218-08.2008.
70. Grabowski GA. Phenotype, diagnosis, and treatment of Gaucher's disease. Lancet 2008;372(9645):1263–71. http://dx.doi.org/10.1016/S0140-6736(08)61522-6.
71. Tayebi N, Callahan M, Madike V, et al. Gaucher disease and parkinsonism: a phenotypic and genotypic characterization. Mol Genet Metab 2001;73(4): 313–21. http://dx.doi.org/10.1006/mgme.2001.3201.
72. Várkonyi J, Simon Z, Soós K, et al. Gaucher disease type I complicated with Parkinson's syndrome. Haematologia (Budap) 2002;32(3):271–5.
73. Neudorfer O, Giladi N, Elstein D, et al. Occurrence of Parkinson's syndrome in type I Gaucher disease. QJM 1996;89(9):691–4.
74. Halperin A, Elstein D, Zimran A. Increased incidence of Parkinson disease among relatives of patients with Gaucher disease. Blood Cells Mol Dis 2006; 36(3):426–8. http://dx.doi.org/10.1016/j.bcmd.2006.02.004.
75. Anheim M, Elbaz A, Lesage S, et al. Penetrance of Parkinson disease in glucocerebrosidase gene mutation carriers. Neurology 2012;78(6):417–20. http://dx.doi.org/10.1212/WNL.0b013e318245f476.
76. Rosenbloom B, Balwani M, Bronstein JM, et al. The incidence of Parkinsonism in patients with type 1 Gaucher disease: data from the ICGG Gaucher Registry. Blood Cells Mol Dis 2011;46(1):95–102. http://dx.doi.org/10.1016/j.bcmd.2010.10.006.
77. Sidransky E, Nalls MA, Aasly JO, et al. Multicenter analysis of glucocerebrosidase mutations in Parkinson's disease. N Engl J Med 2009;361(17):1651–61. http://dx.doi.org/10.1056/NEJMoa0901281.
78. McNeill A, Duran R, Hughes DA, et al. A clinical and family history study of Parkinson's disease in heterozygous glucocerebrosidase mutation carriers. J Neurol Neurosurg Psychiatry 2012;83(8):853–4. http://dx.doi.org/10.1136/jnnp-2012-302402.
79. Sidransky E, Lopez G. The link between the GBA gene and parkinsonism. Lancet Neurol 2012;11(11):986–98. http://dx.doi.org/10.1016/S1474-4422(12)70190-4.
80. Gegg ME, Burke D, Heales SJ, et al. Glucocerebrosidase deficiency in substantia nigra of Parkinson disease brains. Ann Neurol 2012;72(3):455–63. http://dx.doi.org/10.1002/ana.23614.
81. Cullen V, Sardi SP, Ng J, et al. Acid β-glucosidase mutants linked to Gaucher disease, Parkinson disease, and Lewy body dementia alter α-synuclein processing. Ann Neurol 2011;69(6):940–53. http://dx.doi.org/10.1002/ana.22400.
82. Cleeter MW, Chau KY, Gluck C, et al. Glucocerebrosidase inhibition causes mitochondrial dysfunction and free radical damage. Neurochem Int 2013; 62(1):1–7. http://dx.doi.org/10.1016/j.neuint.2012.10.010.
83. Manning-Boğ AB, Schüle B, Langston JW. Alpha-synuclein-glucocerebrosidase interactions in pharmacological Gaucher models: a biological link between

Gaucher disease and parkinsonism. Neurotoxicology 2009;30(6):1127–32. http://dx.doi.org/10.1016/j.neuro.2009.06.009.
84. Mazzulli JR, Xu YH, Sun Y, et al. Gaucher disease glucocerebrosidase and α-synuclein form a bidirectional pathogenic loop in synucleinopathies. Cell 2011;146(1):37–52. http://dx.doi.org/10.1016/j.cell.2011.06.001.
85. Osellame LD, Rahim AA, Hargreaves IP, et al. Mitochondria and quality control defects in a mouse model of Gaucher disease–links to Parkinson's disease. Cell Metab 2013;17(6):941–53. http://dx.doi.org/10.1016/j.cmet.2013.04.014.
86. McNeill A, Magalhaes J, Shen C, et al. Ambroxol improves lysosomal biochemistry in glucocerebrosidase mutation-linked Parkinson disease cells. Brain 2014; 137(Pt 5):1481–95. http://dx.doi.org/10.1093/brain/awu020.
87. Maegawa GH, Tropak MB, Buttner JD, et al. Identification and characterization of ambroxol as an enzyme enhancement agent for Gaucher disease. J Biol Chem 2009;284(35):23502–16. http://dx.doi.org/10.1074/jbc.M109.012393.
88. Bendikov-Bar I, Maor G, Filocamo M, et al. Ambroxol as a pharmacological chaperone for mutant glucocerebrosidase. Blood Cells Mol Dis 2013;50(2): 141–5. http://dx.doi.org/10.1016/j.bcmd.2012.10.007.
89. Funayama M, Hasegawa K, Kowa H, et al. A new locus for Parkinson's disease (PARK8) maps to chromosome 12p11.2-q13.1. Ann Neurol 2002;51(3): 296–301.
90. Paisán-Ruíz C, Jain S, Evans EW, et al. Cloning of the gene containing mutations that cause PARK8-linked Parkinson's disease. Neuron 2004;44(4):595–600. http://dx.doi.org/10.1016/j.neuron.2004.10.023.
91. Zimprich A, Biskup S, Leitner P, et al. Mutations in LRRK2 cause autosomal-dominant parkinsonism with pleomorphic pathology. Neuron 2004;44(4): 601–7. http://dx.doi.org/10.1016/j.neuron.2004.11.005.
92. Kachergus J, Mata IF, Hulihan M, et al. Identification of a novel LRRK2 mutation linked to autosomal dominant parkinsonism: evidence of a common founder across European populations. Am J Hum Genet 2005;76(4):672–80. http://dx.doi.org/10.1086/429256.
93. Sierra M, González-Aramburu I, Sánchez-Juan P, et al. High frequency and reduced penetrance of LRRK2 G2019S mutation among Parkinson's disease patients in Cantabria (Spain). Mov Disord 2011;26(13):2343–6. http://dx.doi.org/10.1002/mds.23965.
94. Correia Guedes L, Ferreira JJ, Rosa MM, et al. Worldwide frequency of G2019S LRRK2 mutation in Parkinson's disease: a systematic review. Parkinsonism Relat Disord 2010;16(4):237–42. http://dx.doi.org/10.1016/j.parkreldis.2009.11.004.
95. Dächsel JC, Behrouz B, Yue M, et al. A comparative study of Lrrk2 function in primary neuronal cultures. Parkinsonism Relat Disord 2010;16(10):650–5. http://dx.doi.org/10.1016/j.parkreldis.2010.08.018.
96. Tong Y, Giaime E, Yamaguchi H, et al. Loss of leucine-rich repeat kinase 2 causes age-dependent bi-phasic alterations of the autophagy pathway. Mol Neurodegener 2012;7:2. http://dx.doi.org/10.1186/1750-1326-7-2.
97. Ren Y, Liu W, Jiang H, et al. Selective vulnerability of dopaminergic neurons to microtubule depolymerization. J Biol Chem 2005;280(40):34105–12. http://dx.doi.org/10.1074/jbc.M503483200.
98. Piccoli G, Condliffe SB, Bauer M, et al. LRRK2 controls synaptic vesicle storage and mobilization within the recycling pool. J Neurosci 2011;31(6):2225–37. http://dx.doi.org/10.1523/JNEUROSCI.3730-10.2011.
99. Liu G, Zhang C, Yin J, et al. alpha-Synuclein is differentially expressed in mitochondria from different rat brain regions and dose-dependently down-regulates

complex I activity. Neurosci Lett 2009;454(3):187–92. http://dx.doi.org/10.1016/j.neulet.2009.02.056.
100. Lewis PA, Manzoni C. LRRK2 and human disease: a complicated question or a question of complexes? Sci Signal 2012;5(207):pe2. http://dx.doi.org/10.1126/scisignal.2002680.
101. Ujiie S, Hatano T, Kubo SI, et al. LRRK2 I2020T mutation is associated with tau pathology. Parkinsonism Relat Disord 2012;18(7):819–23. http://dx.doi.org/10.1016/j.parkreldis.2012.03.024.
102. Khan NL, Jain S, Lynch JM, et al. Mutations in the gene LRRK2 encoding dardarin (PARK8) cause familial Parkinson's disease: clinical, pathological, olfactory and functional imaging and genetic data. Brain 2005;128(Pt 12):2786–96. http://dx.doi.org/10.1093/brain/awh667.
103. Gaig C, Martí MJ, Ezquerra M, et al. G2019S LRRK2 mutation causing Parkinson's disease without Lewy bodies. J Neurol Neurosurg Psychiatry 2007;78(6):626–8. http://dx.doi.org/10.1136/jnnp.2006.107904.
104. Rajput A, Dickson DW, Robinson CA, et al. Parkinsonism, Lrrk2 G2019S, and tau neuropathology. Neurology 2006;67(8):1506–8. http://dx.doi.org/10.1212/01.wnl.0000240220.33950.0c.
105. Greggio E, Jain S, Kingsbury A, et al. Kinase activity is required for the toxic effects of mutant LRRK2/dardarin. Neurobiol Dis 2006;23(2):329–41. http://dx.doi.org/10.1016/j.nbd.2006.04.001.
106. Smith WW, Pei Z, Jiang H, et al. Kinase activity of mutant LRRK2 mediates neuronal toxicity. Nat Neurosci 2006;9(10):1231–3. http://dx.doi.org/10.1038/nn1776.
107. Schapira AH. Mitochondria in the aetiology and pathogenesis of Parkinson's disease. Lancet Neurol 2008;7(1):97–109. http://dx.doi.org/10.1016/S1474-4422(07)70327-7.
108. Chiueh CC, Markey SP, Burns RS, et al. Neurochemical and behavioral effects of 1-methyl-4-phenyl-1,2,3,6- tetrahydropyridine (MPTP) in rat, guinea pig, and monkey. Psychopharmacol Bull 1984;20(3):548–53.
109. Langston JW, Quik M, Petzinger G, et al. Investigating levodopa-induced dyskinesias in the parkinsonian primate. Ann Neurol 2000;47(4 Suppl 1):S79–89.
110. Sherer TB, Richardson JR, Testa CM, et al. Mechanism of toxicity of pesticides acting at complex I: relevance to environmental etiologies of Parkinson's disease. J Neurochem 2007;100(6):1469–79. http://dx.doi.org/10.1111/j.1471-4159.2006.04333.x.
111. Betarbet R, Sherer TB, MacKenzie G, et al. Chronic systemic pesticide exposure reproduces features of Parkinson's disease. Nat Neurosci 2000;3(12):1301–6. http://dx.doi.org/10.1038/81834.
112. Gorell JM, Johnson CC, Rybicki BA, et al. The risk of Parkinson's disease with exposure to pesticides, farming, well water, and rural living. Neurology 1998;50(5):1346–50.
113. Schapira AH, Cooper JM, Dexter D, et al. Mitochondrial complex I deficiency in Parkinson's disease. Lancet 1989;1(8649):1269.
114. Hatano Y, Li Y, Sato K, et al. Novel PINK1 mutations in early-onset parkinsonism. Ann Neurol 2004;56(3):424–7. http://dx.doi.org/10.1002/ana.20251.
115. Valente EM, Abou-Sleiman PM, Caputo V, et al. Hereditary early-onset Parkinson's disease caused by mutations in PINK1. Science 2004;304(5674):1158–60. http://dx.doi.org/10.1126/science.1096284.
116. Ishikawa A, Tsuji S. Clinical analysis of 17 patients in 12 Japanese families with autosomal-recessive type juvenile parkinsonism. Neurology 1996;47(1):160–6.

117. Kitada T, Asakawa S, Hattori N, et al. Mutations in the parkin gene cause autosomal recessive juvenile parkinsonism. Nature 1998;392(6676):605–8. http://dx.doi.org/10.1038/33416.
118. Dupuis L. Mitochondrial quality control in neurodegenerative diseases. Biochimie 2014;100:177–83. http://dx.doi.org/10.1016/j.biochi.2013.07.033.
119. McLelland GL, Soubannier V, Chen CX, et al. Parkin and PINK1 function in a vesicular trafficking pathway regulating mitochondrial quality control. EMBO J 2014;33(4):282–95. http://dx.doi.org/10.1002/embj.201385902.
120. Wood-Kaczmar A, Gandhi S, Yao Z, et al. PINK1 is necessary for long term survival and mitochondrial function in human dopaminergic neurons. PLoS One 2008;3(6):e2455. http://dx.doi.org/10.1371/journal.pone.0002455.
121. Cui M, Tang X, Christian WV, et al. Perturbations in mitochondrial dynamics induced by human mutant PINK1 can be rescued by the mitochondrial division inhibitor mdivi-1. J Biol Chem 2010;285(15):11740–52. http://dx.doi.org/10.1074/jbc.M109.066662.
122. Lutz AK, Exner N, Fett ME, et al. Loss of parkin or PINK1 function increases Drp1-dependent mitochondrial fragmentation. J Biol Chem 2009;284(34):22938–51. http://dx.doi.org/10.1074/jbc.M109.035774.
123. Papkovskaia TD, Chau KY, Inesta-Vaquera F, et al. G2019S leucine-rich repeat kinase 2 causes uncoupling protein-mediated mitochondrial depolarization. Hum Mol Genet 2012;21(19):4201–13. http://dx.doi.org/10.1093/hmg/dds244.
124. Mortiboys H, Johansen KK, Aasly JO, et al. Mitochondrial impairment in patients with Parkinson disease with the G2019S mutation in LRRK2. Neurology 2010;75(22):2017–20. http://dx.doi.org/10.1212/WNL.0b013e3181ff9685.
125. Choubey V, Safiulina D, Vaarmann A, et al. Mutant A53T alpha-synuclein induces neuronal death by increasing mitochondrial autophagy. J Biol Chem 2011;286(12):10814–24. http://dx.doi.org/10.1074/jbc.M110.132514.
126. Orsucci D, Ienco EC, Mancuso M. POLG1-related and other "mitochondrial Parkinsonisms": an overview. J Mol Neurosci 2011;44:17–24.
127. Bender A, Krishnan KJ, Morris CM, et al. High levels of mitochondrial DNA deletions in substantia nigra neurons in aging and Parkinson disease. Nat Genet 2006;38(5):515–7. http://dx.doi.org/10.1038/ng1769.
128. Hudson G, Nalls M, Evans JR, et al. Two-stage association study and meta-analysis of mitochondrial DNA variants in Parkinson disease. Neurology 2013;80:2042–58.
129. Payne BA, Wilson IJ, Hateley CA, et al. Mitochondrial aging is accelerated by anti-retroviral therapy through the clonal expansion of mtDNA mutations. Nat Genet 2011;43(8):806–10. http://dx.doi.org/10.1038/ng.863.
130. Tisch S, Brew BJ. HIV, HAART, and Parkinson's disease: co-incidence or pathogenetic link? Mov Disord 2010;25:2257–8.
131. Tisch S, Brew B. Parkinsonism in hiv-infected patients on highly active antiretroviral therapy. Neurology 2009;73(5):401–3. http://dx.doi.org/10.1212/WNL.0b013e3181b04b0d.
132. Cole NB, Dieuliis D, Leo P, et al. Mitochondrial translocation of alpha-synuclein is promoted by intracellular acidification. Exp Cell Res 2008;314(10):2076–89. http://dx.doi.org/10.1016/j.yexcr.2008.03.012.
133. Shavali S, Brown-Borg HM, Ebadi M, et al. Mitochondrial localization of alpha-synuclein protein in alpha-synuclein overexpressing cells. Neurosci Lett 2008;439(2):125–8. http://dx.doi.org/10.1016/j.neulet.2008.05.005.
134. Nakamura K, Nemani VM, Wallender EK, et al. Optical reporters for the conformation of alpha-synuclein reveal a specific interaction with mitochondria. J Neurosci 2008;28(47):12305–17. http://dx.doi.org/10.1523/JNEUROSCI.3088-08.2008.

135. Hsu LJ, Sagara Y, Arroyo A, et al. Alpha-synuclein promotes mitochondrial deficit and oxidative stress. Am J Pathol 2000;157(2):401–10.
136. Martin LJ. Biology of mitochondria in neurodegenerative diseases. Prog Mol Biol Transl Sci 2012;107:355–415. http://dx.doi.org/10.1016/B978-0-12-385883-2.00005-9.
137. Devi L, Raghavendran V, Prabhu BM, et al. Mitochondrial import and accumulation of alpha-synuclein impair complex I in human dopaminergic neuronal cultures and Parkinson disease brain. J Biol Chem 2008;283(14):9089–100. http://dx.doi.org/10.1074/jbc.M710012200.
138. Xu J, Kao SY, Lee FJ, et al. Dopamine-dependent neurotoxicity of alpha-synuclein: a mechanism for selective neurodegeneration in Parkinson disease. Nat Med 2002;8(6):600–6. http://dx.doi.org/10.1038/nm0602-600.
139. Moussa CE, Mahmoodian F, Tomita Y, et al. Dopamine differentially induces aggregation of A53T mutant and wild type alpha-synuclein: insights into the protein chemistry of Parkinson's disease. Biochem Biophys Res Commun 2008;365(4):833–9. http://dx.doi.org/10.1016/j.bbrc.2007.11.075.
140. Fahn S, Parkinson Study Group. Does levodopa slow or hasten the rate of progression of Parkinson's disease? J Neurol 2005;252(Suppl 4):IV37–42. http://dx.doi.org/10.1007/s00415-005-4008-5.
141. McCarthy A, McKinley J, Lynch T. The inherent susceptibility of dorsal motor nucleus cholinergic neurons to the neurodegenerative process in Parkinson's Disease. Front Neurol 2012;3:189. http://dx.doi.org/10.3389/fneur.2012.00189.
142. Matzuk MM, Saper CB. Preservation of hypothalamic dopaminergic neurons in Parkinson's disease. Ann Neurol 1985;18(5):552–5. http://dx.doi.org/10.1002/ana.410180507.
143. Damier P, Hirsch EC, Agid Y, et al. The substantia nigra of the human brain. II. Patterns of loss of dopamine-containing neurons in Parkinson's disease. Brain 1999;122(Pt 8):1437–48.
144. Surmeier DJ, Schumacker PT. Calcium, bioenergetics, and neuronal vulnerability in Parkinson's disease. J Biol Chem 2013;288(15):10736–41. http://dx.doi.org/10.1074/jbc.R112.410530.
145. Ascherio A, Tanner CM. Use of antihypertensives and the risk of Parkinson disease. Neurology 2009;72(6):578–9. http://dx.doi.org/10.1212/01.wnl.0000344171.22760.24.
146. Ritz B, Rhodes SL, Qian L, et al. L-type calcium channel blockers and Parkinson disease in Denmark. Ann Neurol 2010;67(5):600–6. http://dx.doi.org/10.1002/ana.21937.

Treatment Strategies in Early and Advanced Parkinson Disease

Christiana Ossig, MD[a,b,c,*], Heinz Reichmann, MD, PhD, FRCP[b]

KEYWORDS

- Parkinson's disease • Levodopa • Dyskinesia • Hypokinesia • Dopamine agonists
- Continuous dopaminergic stimulation

KEY POINTS

- Parkinson disease (PD) is a progressive neurodegenerative disease.
- Patients diagnosed with PD have to be treated individually with respect to their predominant symptom and clinical presentation.
- A broad knowledge of medical treatment options as well as invasive therapeutic approaches is necessary to support patients and improve their quality of life.

PATHOPHYSIOLOGY AND PRECLINICAL STAGES OF PARKINSON DISEASE

Parkinson's disease (PD) is a progressive disorder and the second most common neurodegenerative disease in the elderly. The diagnosis of PD is made on clinical grounds. The presence of bradykinesia together with rigidity, resting tremor, or postural instability is required. When symptoms appear, the dopamine levels in the striatum are already reduced by 60% to 80%. At this point, more than half of the dopaminergic neurons within the substantia nigra (SN) are already destroyed, and the progression of PD proceeds inexorably. In the prodromal phase, nonmotor symptoms such as hyposmia, rapid eye movement (REM) sleep behavior disorder

Disclosures: C. Ossig has received speaker honorary from UCB. H. Reichmann was acting on advisory boards and gave lectures and received research grants from Abbott, AbbVie, Bayer Healthcare, Boehringer Ingelheim, Brittania, Cephalon, Desitin, GSK, Lundbeck, Nedtronic, Merck-Serono, Novartis, Orion, TEVA, UCB Pharma and Valeant received a research grant from Pfizer (CABAS-067-051).

[a] Division of Neurodegenerative Diseases, Department of Neurology, Dresden University of Technology, Fetscherstraße 74, Dresden 01307, Germany; [b] Department of Neurology, Dresden University of Technology, Fetscherstraße 74, Dresden 01307, Germany; [c] Department of Neuropsychiatry and Laboratory of Molecular Psychiatry, Charité-Universitätsmedizin Berlin, Berlin 10117, Germany

* Corresponding author. Department of Neuropsychiatry and Laboratory of Molecular Psychiatry, Charité-Universitätsmedizin Berlin, Berlin 10117, Germany.
E-mail address: christiana.ossig@charite.de

Neurol Clin 33 (2015) 19–37
http://dx.doi.org/10.1016/j.ncl.2014.09.009 neurologic.theclinics.com
0733-8619/15/$ – see front matter

(RBD), depression, and constipation may already be apparent. This progression implies that PD does not start in the SN; a theory further supported by the findings of Braak and colleagues,[1,2] who neuropathologically investigated patients with PD over several years. They observed that defectively folded aggregates of alpha-synuclein, the so-called Lewy bodies and Lewy neurites, are initially found in the olfactory bulb and the medulla oblongata (stage 1 and 2). As the disease progresses, these characteristic pathologic findings appear in the SN, in the nuclei of the midbrain, and in the frontobasal parts of the brain (stage 3 and 4). In stage 5 and 6, Lewy body disorder is found in the cortex, and therefore emotional and cognitive symptoms, such as hallucinations and dementia, may occur. However, the clinical presentation of patients with PD is heterogeneous and does not necessarily follow the classic progression. Alpha-synuclein deposition is not synonymous with neurodegeneration, and moreover alpha-synucleinopathies can occur without clinical symptoms of PD or dementia (eg, in incidental Lewy body disease). Because PD does not originate in the SN, it may be possible to identify at-risk individuals in the preclinical stage, and initiate any neuroprotective treatments that may be available in the future.

Nonmotor symptoms like hyposmia, constipation, depression, and RBD are prodromal markers of PD. Hyposmia is the most sensitive marker (80%–90%), followed by autonomic dysfunction (50%–80%) and RBD (40%); however, with the exception of RBD, the specificity is low.

More than 80% of patients with PD have hyposmia, and patients are unaware of this in half of the cases.[3] Testing for hyposmia (eg, using the University of Pennsylvania Smell Identification Test or the Sniffin' Sticks test) is often necessary. The hyposmia is bilateral, even though the motor symptoms are generally unilateral in the beginning of the disease. Smelling deficits correlate with the disease duration, the disease severity, and striatal innervation, as measured by dopamine transporter (DaT) single-photon emission computed tomography (SPECT).[4] The sensitivity of hyposmia in PD is more than 80%, but hyposmia is not specific for PD. Prospective studies have shown that hyposmia increases the relative risk for developing PD, but the prodromal phase may range from as little as 2 years to as long as 50 years.

Many patients complain of constipation long before the manifestation of motor symptoms in PD. Another autonomic disturbance is the postganglionic sympathetic denervation of the heart, which can be measured by iodine-123-metaiodobenzylguanidine SPECT.[5] Patients with idiopathic RBD may also show a significant reduction of heart rate variability. RBD is characterized by a loss of atony during REM sleep,[6] and patients with RBD physically and verbally act out their dreams. Studies show that RBD is a risk factor for neurodegenerative diseases,[7] with a conversion rate of up to 45% within 5 years, up to 73% within 10 years, and up to 81% within a period of 16 years.[8–10] The specificity for PD in patients with RBD is high, but only half of patients with PD have RBD, and moreover RBD may also occur in atypical Parkinson syndromes such as multisystem atrophy and dementia with Lewy bodies.[11] Patients with PD with RBD more often have additional autonomic dysfunction, and develop a hypokinetic rigid Parkinson syndrome. The presence of RBD seems to have a worse impact if conversion to PD evolves.[12]

Therapeutic strategies for these prodromal symptoms are scarce. Clonazepam is the first-line therapy for RBD. Melatonin may be prescribed if patients do not tolerate clonazepam or have relative contraindications to the medication.[13] Laxatives may be used for treating constipation. Depression should be treated with a selective serotonin reuptake inhibitor or a serotonin-norepinephrine reuptake inhibitor, although there is a lack of evidence regarding the recent study results.[14,15]

CLINICAL PRESENTATION OF IDIOPATHIC PARKINSON DISEASE

Idiopathic Parkinson syndrome is one of the most frequent neurologic disorders, with a prevalence of 200 per 100,000 and an incidence of 4 to 20 per 100,000 per year. The mean age at disease onset is 55 to 60 years, with an increased incidence in older age. The incidence of PD varies by ethnicity, with white people more frequently affected than Asians or Africans.[16]

PD is characterized by bradykinesia, tremor, and rigidity, as well as postural instability. In addition to motor symptoms, various nonmotor features may occur at different stages throughout the disease. Besides treating motor symptoms these nonmotor features have to be addressed, but are generally more difficult to treat.

According to the criteria of the UK Brain Bank, bradykinesia and either rigidity or resting tremor and postural instability have to be present to make the diagnosis. Atypical Parkinson syndromes and secondary Parkinson syndromes have to be ruled out. PD is classically an asymmetric disease. It is expected that, throughout the course of the progression of the disease, a good levodopa response and eventually levodopa-induced dyskinesia evolve; if not, the patient has to be reevaluated retrospectively.

PD is subdivided into 3 subtypes according to the clinical presentation: hypokinetic/akinetic-rigid Parkinson syndrome; tremor-dominant Parkinson syndrome, and a combination of the two: the equivalent Parkinsonian syndrome. This classification seems to be important because, in patients with tremor-dominant PD, for example, the disease course is often slow. The most frequently used and preferred clinical classification is the Hoehn and Yahr[17] scale. For rating the severity of motor symptoms, the Unified Parkinson Disease Rating Scale (UPDRS), consisting of 5 subcategories, is used. Also the Schwab and England ADL (activity of daily life) scale is important in clinical practice.

In addition, there are various rating scales that help the examiner to assess levodopa-induced side effects; the impact of symptoms on the quality of life in patients with PD; and nonmotor symptoms like psychiatric, cognitive, and autonomic features.

Later in this article, treatment options commonly used in PD, their pathophysiology, and frequent side effects are presented (**Table 1**), followed by a practical approach to how therapy in a patient with PD can be managed.

LEVODOPA: MIRACLE DRUG WITH SIDE EFFECTS

In the 1980s, levodopa was, apart from anticholinergics and amantadine, the only medication available for PD. Dyskinesia and motor fluctuations were the downside of this so-called miracle drug, and neurologists began to hold back this treatment option in order not to endanger their patients with these side effects.

The results of studies performed in cell cultures in the 1990s suggested that levodopa may even harm dopaminergic cells.[18] Animal studies showed that, under levodopa treatment, the production of hydroxyl radicals in the SN was increased.[19] Neurologists feared that these hydroxyl radicals might harm the SN and lead to further worsening of the disease. However, the ELLDOPA study provided both relief and hope for the therapists.[20] This double-blind study showed that levodopa leads to a dose-dependent improvement of motor symptoms in patients with PD at an early stage of treatment. After a treatment period of 38 weeks, motor symptoms of patients treated with levodopa improved significantly compared with the control group. Even at week 40, after a 2-week washout period, in which no levodopa was administered, patients who had previously received levodopa did not show any deterioration in their motor symptoms compared with the control group.

Table 1
Treatment in PD

Medication Class	Dosage	Adverse Effects
Levodopa + decarboxylase inhibitor (Carbidopa/ Benserazide)	Initial dose: 3 × 100/25 mg thrice daily, maximum 1500/375 mg/d based on symptoms	Nausea, orthostatic hypotension, dyskinesia, hallucinations
MAO-B Inhibitor		
Rasagiline	1 mg/d	Headache, arthralgia, conjunctivitis, rhinitis, dermatitis, dyspepsia, depression, dyskinesia in combination with levodopa
Selegiline	Initial dose: 2.5 mg/d, maximum 10 mg/d	Stimulant effect, nausea, headache, dizziness, dyskinesia in combination with levodopa
COMT Inhibitor		
Entacapone	200 mg with each dose of levodopa, maximum 8 × 200 mg/d	Brownish orange discoloration of urine, diarrhea, dyskinesia in combination with levodopa
Tolcapone	3 × 200 mg/d	Hepatotoxicity, brownish orange discoloration of urine, diarrhea, dyskinesia in combination with levodopa
Dopamine Agonist		
Piribedil	Initial dose: 3 × 50 mg/d, maximum 250 mg/d	Nausea, hallucinations, confusion, orthostatic hypotension, ICDs, ankle edema
Pramipexole	Initial dose: 3 × 0.125 mg, maximum 24 mg/d. Prolonged release: initial dose 0.52 mg, maximum 3.15 mg/d	Nausea, hallucinations, confusion, orthostatic hypotension, ICDs, ankle edema, increased sleepiness, sleep attacks
Ropinirole	Initial dose: 3 × 0.25 mg, maximum 24 mg/d. Prolonged release: initial dose: 6 mg, maximum 24 mg/d	Nausea, hallucinations, confusion, orthostatic hypotension, ICDs, ankle edema, increased sleepiness, sleep attacks
Rotigotine	Initial dose: 2 mg/24 h, maximum 16 mg/24 h	Nausea, hallucinations, confusion, orthostatic hypotension, ICDs, ankle edema, increased sleepiness, sleep attacks
Others		
Amantadine	Initial dose: 1 × 100 mg, maximum 4 × 100 mg/d	Livedo reticularis, nausea, dry mouth, hallucinations, confusion, ankle edema, constipation, sleep disorder, dizziness, cardiac arrhythmia
Budipine	Initial dose: 3 × 10 mg/d, maximum 60 mg/d	Hallucinations, confusion, cardiac arrhythmia, nausea, diarrhea, ICDs

(*continued on next page*)

Table 1
(*continued*)

Medication Class	Dosage	Adverse Effects
Anticholinergics		
Trihexyphenidyl	Initial dose: 1 mg/d, maximum 3 × 2 mg/d	Cognitive impairment, hallucinations, confusion, dry mouth, urinary retention, constipation
Neuroleptics		
Clozapine	Initial dose: 6.25–12.5 mg at night, maximum 150 mg/d	Agranulocytosis, orthostatic hypotension, myocarditis, seizures
β-Blocker		
Propranolol	Initial dose: 2 × 40 mg/d, maximum 320 mg/d	Dizziness, fatigue

Abbreviations: COMT, catechol-O-methyl transferase; ICD, impulse control disorder; MAO-B inhibitor, monoamine oxidase B inhibitor.

Levodopa is always administered with a decarboxylase inhibitor (carbidopa or benserazide). This inhibitor is needed to reduce peripheral dopaminergic side effects like nausea and hypotension and to increase the amount of medication that crosses the blood-brain barrier. Individual patients may respond better to one or the other decarboxylase inhibitor, therefore, if treatment is unsatisfactory, it may be necessary to switch the inhibitor used. It is important to know that, in order to completely inhibit the peripheral decarboxylase, at least 75 mg of carbidopa or benserazide per day are required along with levodopa.

Besides the standard formula, soluble and prolonged forms of levodopa are available. These formulas show differences in time of onset and uptake of levodopa, although the half-life (1.5 hours) is the same for each formulation. Soluble levodopa begins to act 30 minutes after it is administered, compared with standard levodopa, which acts after 45 to 90 minutes, and prolonged levodopa, which begins to act after 60 to 150 minutes. Prolonged levodopa should be used at nighttime to treat nocturnal hypokinesia and if patients report that sleep no longer has its recuperative powers. Soluble levodopa may be prescribed to overcome early morning akinesia or sudden akinesia appearing during the day. However, administering extra doses of levodopa is disadvantageous, because it may lead to levodopa-induced side effects. If the daily dose of levodopa exceeds more than 600 mg/d, the onset of motor fluctuations and dyskinesia may occur after between 5 to 6 months and 2 years of treatment time. The underlying pathophysiology of levodopa-induced fluctuations and dyskinesia is unknown, but the discontinuous phasic stimulation of the striatal dopamine receptors as opposed to the continuous supply of dopamine in the healthy individual might play an important role.[21] Patients, with a PD onset before the age of 50 years of age and patients with high intake of levodopa are especially at risk of developing motor fluctuations and dyskinesia.[22] Motor fluctuations can present as end-of-dose or wearing-off phenomena, sometimes even with unpredictable "off" episodes. The efficacy of a single levodopa dose is reduced by the progressive loss in the ability to store dopamine in presynaptic nigrostriatal neurons. A delayed "on" or "no-on" response after medication intake may also occur.

Dyskinesia may appear at the highest level of levodopa effectiveness, known as peak-dose dyskinesia, but may also present as biphasic dyskinesia, before and after levodopa intake or as end-of-dose dystonia. The cause for peak-dose dyskinesia is still unclear, but an imbalance in the stimulation of dopaminergic D1 and D2 receptors, as well as long-term pulsatile stimulation of the receptors through high-dose levodopa medication periodically applied throughout the day, may be the reason. Biphasic dyskinesia is rare and occurs only when good and poor motility alternate. As yet there is no pathophysiologic explanation of these alternating periods. End-of-dose dystonia is associated with low plasma levodopa levels and often presents as painful dystonic cramps.

Further side effects of levodopa treatment are nausea, hypotension, hallucinations, and the dopa-dysregulation syndrome (DDS); a form of addictive behavior with compulsive overuse of short-acting soluble levodopa.

MONOAMINE OXIDASE B INHIBITOR: A NEURONAL PROTECTOR?

Selegiline and rasagiline are the main irreversible monoamine oxidase B (MAO-B) inhibitors used. Both inhibitors lead to a delayed central degradation of dopamine and therefore prolong the stimulation of dopamine receptors in the striatum. In cell culture and in animal experiments both inhibitors have been shown to be neuroprotective, raising the hope that MAO-B inhibitors might also be neuroprotective in humans and possibly delay disease progression. Selegiline was the first MAO-B inhibitor approved by the US Food and Drug Administration (in 1996). Daily treatment with 10 mg of selegiline leads to an improvement of 3 points on the total UPDRS and 1.7 points on the motor subscale of the UPDRS after 3 months of treatment.[23] Because the metabolites of selegiline, methamphetamine, and amphetamine inhibit the peripheral monoamine oxidase A (MAO-A), and may therefore pose a risk of causing dietary tyramine–provoked hypertensive crisis, dosages of more than 10 mg/d of selegiline should be avoided.

Early initiation of rasagiline provides long-term clinical benefit, as shown by the TEMPO study.[24,25] The ADAGIO study was also designed to investigate the disease-modifying effect of rasagiline in PD.[26] Again, a control group with delayed administration of rasagiline was compared with 2 groups that either received 1 mg or 2 mg of rasagiline. Early treatment with 1 mg of rasagiline provides clinical benefits, consistent with a possible disease-modifying effect; however, this effect was not replicated with 2 mg of the drug. Because of the proven clinical benefit of early-start rasagiline compared with delayed-start rasagiline, these two important studies may lead to the conclusion that rasagiline might play a role in neuronal protection and may therefore be of particular benefit in early PD.[27] Nonetheless, rasagiline also serves as an add-on medication to levodopa therapy, because a significant reduction in "off" time and an increase in "on" time have been shown in the PRESTO[28] and LARGO studies.[29,30] Rasagiline may also be beneficial when addressing early morning akinesia, freezing, or dopamine agonist–induced fatigue. Besides common side effects like dizziness, headache, and constipation, MAO-B inhibitors may exacerbate levodopa adverse effects and, when used in combination with another serotonergic medication, there is a theoretic risk of developing serotonin syndrome.

CATECHOL-O-METHYL TRANSFERASE INHIBITORS: THE WEARING-OFF MEDICATION

Levodopa is partly metabolized by catechol O-methyl transferase (COMT). Inhibitors of COMT increase the elimination half-life of levodopa and boost the effect of each tablet by approximately 30%. Two selective inhibitors are commonly used: entacapone, a peripheral COMT inhibitor, and tolcapone, a peripheral and central-acting COMT inhibitor. Tolcapone has the potential of causing greater COMT inhibition because of a longer half-life[31] and has to be administered 3 times per day. Entacapone needs to be taken with every levodopa dose. Sporadic cases of fatal hepatotoxicity under treatment with tolcapone have been reported and therefore monitoring of liver function is mandatory.

COMT inhibitors are ideally prescribed together with levodopa when patients report wearing-off symptoms (eg, before taking the next levodopa tablet). This approach might also be effective in treating nonmotor symptoms like excessive sweating, sialorrhea, and pain.

Addition of a COMT inhibitor to levodopa treatment leads to an increase in "on" time, a reduction in "off" time, and an improvement of motor scores in fluctuating patients with PD[32]; however, it does not delay the time of onset or reduce the frequency of dyskinesia, as shown in the STRIDE-PD study.[33] A combination of MAO-B inhibitors and COMT inhibitors may have beneficial effects on mobility in patients with PD without increasing the frequency of side effects. Levodopa and entacapone treatment may result in dyskinesia, particularly when the patient is younger than 65 years of age, male, has a body weight of more than 75 kg, a disease duration of less than 2 years, and is receiving a MAO-B inhibitor or dopamine agonist.

Nausea, orthostatic hypotension, and harmless brownish orange discoloration of urine are known side effects of COMT inhibitors. Diarrhea may potentially develop under treatment, in which case a COMT inhibitor intake break for 3 weeks, followed by a slow uptitration, may reduce the risk of recurrence of this side effect.

AMANTADINE: MULTIPLE APPLICATION POSSIBILITIES

The mode of action of amantadine is presumably its inhibition of dopamine reuptake, the promotion of dopamine distribution, and its peripheral anticholinergic effect. In addition, amantadine possesses an antiglutamatergic effect, which is used in the treatment of influenza A virus infection. In PD, amantadine is used as an add-on drug when dyskinesia develops under levodopa treatment, as an infusion in akinetic crisis, and to treat fatigue, which is a nonmotor symptom often reported by patients with PD.[34] Amantadine is also used in patients with traumatic brain injury to treat fatigue. Side effects include nausea, dry mouth, ankle edema, and livedo reticularis, and hallucinations and confusion may also develop.

BUDIPINE AND ANTICHOLINERGICS

Budipine has its primary effect in successfully treating tremor in PD, but is rarely used because ventricular tachycardia has been noted in patients under treatment. Like amantadine, budipine acts mainly via an antiglutamatergic mode.[35]

Anticholinergics such as trihexyphenidyl have been used since the nineteenth century to treat PD symptoms, in particular tremor, but may also be effective in treating sialorrhea and excessive sweating.[36] In common with budipine, anticholinergics are not commonly used because of their side effects. Anticholinergics may lead to hallucinations and cognitive impairment, mainly in older patients.

DOPAMINE AGONISTS: TREATMENT OF PATIENTS WITH EARLY PARKINSON DISEASE

Dopamine agonists directly stimulate the postsynaptic receptor in the striatum without the requirement for further metabolism within the dopaminergic neurons. Stimulation of presynaptic dopaminergic receptors also takes place, leading to a reduced distribution of endogenous dopamine and a reduced dopamine turnover within the dopaminergic neuron. This effect, along with studies of dopamine agonists in animal models and cell culture, has contributed to the debate as to whether dopamine agonists have neuroprotective or disease-modifying abilities.[37,38]

The older dopamine agonists are the ergot derivatives (bromocriptine, cabergoline, lisuride, and pergolide), which may cause valvular heart disease and are therefore only rarely administered or have even been taken off the market. The commonly used nonergot derivatives are apomorphine, piribedil (unavailable in North America), pramipexole, ropinirole, and rotigotine. Piribedil, pramipexole, and ropinirole are orally administered, and rotigotine is administered via a transdermal patch. Apomorphine is applied via subcutaneous injections using a pen or pump. The RECOVER study showed that addition of a 24-hour transdermal rotigotine patch is associated with significant benefits in the management of early morning motor impairment, nocturnal sleep disturbances, and nonmotor daytime symptoms such as fatigue and mood changes.[39] Dopamine agonists possess a significantly longer half-life compared with levodopa, thus leading to a continuous stimulation of dopamine receptors. Because of their equal effectiveness but lower dyskinesia rate compared with levodopa, dopamine agonists are preferred in early PD stages. However, in the later stages of the disease, additional treatment with levodopa has to be added. In contrast, studies show that fluctuations can be significantly reduced when a dopamine agonist is added to a levodopa regimen. This finding has been shown for pramipexole[40] and ropinirole.[41]

Side effects reported by patients under dopamine agonist treatment are skin irritations when rotigotine patch is applied, orthostatic hypotension, nausea, ankle edema, dizziness, and excessive daytime sleepiness or even sleep attacks. A slow uptitration may reduce these side effects. Another important side effect under dopamine agonist therapy is impulse control disorder (ICD), which can present as hypersexuality, compulsive shopping or gambling, punding, and binge eating. In general, patients with PD tend to develop ICD for various reasons and a history of obsessive-compulsive disorder, impulsive personality, or addictive behaviors increases the likelihood of developing an ICD.[42] The risk of developing ICDs is increased under therapy with dopamine agonists, as shown in a multivariate analysis in which 3000 patients with PD were examined. Seventeen percent of patients treated with dopamine agonists, compared with 7% of patients treated with levodopa, developed ICDs.[43] It is important to educate patients and their relatives about the risk of this potential side effect. ICDs should be monitored regularly in patients with PD.

CONTINUOUS DOPAMINERGIC DRUG DELIVERY: ALTERNATIVE STRATEGY IN PATIENTS WITH ADVANCED PARKINSON DISEASE

Apomorphine is a liquid D1/D2 receptor dopamine agonist that is equally effective as levodopa in patients with symptomatic PD. The onset of the subcutaneously applied apomorphine is 5 to 15 minutes, with a short half-life of 30 to 90 minutes. Subcutaneous apomorphine injections via pen provide rapid delivery to reduce "off" periods and to conquer end-of-dose biphasic dyskinesia, and can easily be added to any medical regimen.[44]

Continuous infusion of apomorphine via pump is considered as an alternative therapeutic strategy in patients with severe motor fluctuations, mainly hypokinesia under oral treatment. A programmed infusion rate can be installed when the apomorphine pump is used. In general, apomorphine is dispensed within a 12-hour to 16-hour regimen, but does not have to be discontinued overnight and can be given within a 24-hour cycle, which may result in reduced nocturnal "off" time. Furthermore, a specifically defined bolus application can be given whenever needed, as with the pen application. Treatment should be started under medical supervision and a premedication with domperidone (not available in the United States) should be used to reduce side effects.[45] A Coombs test should be performed beforehand to exclude circulating antibodies against erythrocytes. One of the main side effects is skin reactions, located at the injection side, resulting in the formation of small nodules.[46] Other side effects include increased daytime sleepiness, nausea, dizziness, renal impairment, and orthostatic hypotension, comparable with the known side effects under dopamine agonist treatment.[47,48] Neuropsychiatric changes like hallucinations and psychosis are rare but can be observed with high doses of apomorphine. Similar to levodopa treatment, DDS may be noted under apomorphine treatment.

Levodopa-carbidopa intestinal gel (LCIG), a combination of levodopa (20 mg/mL) and carbidopa (5 mg/mL), is another method of continuous dopaminergic drug delivery (CDDD). LCIG is efficient in improving mobility, showing a significant reduction of "off" time and a significant increase of "on" time in patients with advanced PD as well as reducing levodopa-associated motor fluctuations and dyskinesia in patients under oral medication,[49,50] and it also improves nonmotor symptoms such as sleep and pain, gastrointestinal and urologic disturbances, and cognition.[51] A test application period of LCIG via a nasoduodenal catheter system is mandatory before proceeding with permanent therapy. If this is well tolerated by the patient and motor symptoms improve, a percutaneous endoscopic gastrostomy (PEG) is performed and LCIG is dispensed via a gastrostomy catheter. LCIG can be applied as a monotherapy. If the pump is taken off at night, prolonged-release levodopa has to be administered before bedtime. Adverse effects are mainly caused by technical problems such as dislocation, obstruction, and breakage of the gastrostomy catheter. PEG-related side effects might occur, including peritonitis and local stoma inflammation. Other side effects are the same as those associated with levodopa therapy.

DEEP BRAIN STIMULATION

Deep brain stimulation (DBS) involves the implantation of electrodes connected to a pulse generator and the modulation of neuronal activity via high-frequency stimulation of the targeted brain area. The implanted electrodes can be adjusted by changing the voltage, the pulse width, and the frequency in order to improve symptoms and reduce potential side effects. In PD, the stimulation of either the subthalamic nuclei (STN) or the internal global pallidum (GPi) is performed. In tremor-dominant Parkinson syndrome, the stimulation of the ventral intermediate nucleus, which is traditionally targeted for DBS in essential tremor, can be considered. All targeted areas are located within the basal ganglia–thalamocortical loop. The mode of action of DBS in patients with PD is not fully understood; however, the stimulation of STN or GPi via DBS may lead to an inhibition and partial normalization of the disordered basal ganglia–thalamocortical loop caused by PD.

DBS is an alternative therapy for patients with PD in advanced stages with severe motor complications and fluctuations uncontrollable by oral medications. The best predictor for a favorable result is a good levodopa response[52] and the best medical "on" state is the best possible condition achievable by DBS. An exception to this rule is tremor in PD, which can be greatly improved with DBS even if oral medications have failed.

Careful testing of patients with PD before surgery is mandatory. The most important contraindications are dementia, brain atrophy in MRI scan, an increased susceptibility to bleeding or infection, or a concomitant life-limiting disease. Age is not an exclusion criterion per se, but reduced benefit and increased incidence of cognitive decline is noted in patients with PD who are more than 70 years of age.[53,54]

The bilateral implantation of electrodes into the STN is mainly performed in patients with PD. Studies show that STN stimulation leads to significant reduction in "off" phase (50%) and dyskinesia (70%).[55] On/off fluctuations decrease and oral medication can be reduced by 50% to 60 %. These effects seem to last for a considerable number of years, as shown by long-term follow-up studies[56,57]; however, the underlying disease progresses and a further deterioration has to be expected.

The stimulation of GPi also results in significant improvement of motor complications in advanced PD. Motor symptoms improve by 35% measured by the UPDRS, dyskinesia rate is reduced by 65%, as well as "off" motor fluctuations by 35%.[58] Compared with STN stimulation, oral medication can rarely be diminished. Long-term effects regarding the clinical outcome after GPi DBS seem to vary and are not as stable as in STN DBS.[59] In contrast, side effects seem to be more common after STN stimulation than after GPi stimulation. Psychiatric symptoms like depression and anhedonia and a 13-fold increased risk of suicide within the first year after STN DBS are causes for concern.[60] Stimulation-induced side effects include dysarthria, paresthesia, and apraxia of eyelid opening but are generally controlled by adjustment of stimulation parameters or oral medication. Mortality is low in DBS, but neurosurgical complications such as intracranial hemorrhage, infection of the implanted system, or technical problems (eg, lead breakage, extension wire failure, and impulse generator malfunctions) can occur.

TREATMENT MANAGEMENT IN PARKINSON DISEASE

Patients less than the age of 40 years presenting with a hypokinetic-rigid syndrome, tremor, or dystonic features should always be screened for Wilson disease. MRI of the brain should be normal in patients with PD and is routinely done. DaT SPECT or, if possible, ^{18}F-dihydroxyphenylalanine PET can be useful if the clinical presentation is atypical, but is unnecessary and too expensive in a typical PD case.

A distinction is made between patients with PD according to the age of onset: onset before the age of 70 years is referred to as early-onset PD and after the age of 70 years is referred to as late-onset PD. As described earlier, PD can be subdivided into 3 subtypes based on the predominant symptom: the hypokinetic/akinetic-rigid Parkinson syndrome, the tremor-dominant Parkinson syndrome, and a combination of the two, the equivalent Parkinson syndrome (compare **Fig. 1**).

WHEN TO START TREATMENT

The transition of a healthy individual into a patient with PD is fluxionary. Different studies have provided different estimates as to the rate at which motor disability progresses in patients with de-novo PD. The rate of progression measured by the total UPDRS score was 6.5 points per year in the ADAGIO study, compared with 14 points in the DATATOP study.[27,61]

No drug has yet proved to be neuroprotective in PD; however, some studies have suggested that MAO-B inhibitors might have a disease-modifying effect.[27] After diagnosis, patients may not think it necessary to start treatment; however, we think that treatment with an MAO-B inhibitor should be considered, especially in patients less than the age of 70 years, because of the potential disease-modifying effect. There have been suggestions that the early initiation of any treatment in PD might improve subsequent response, but this is still unproved. Nowadays, most neurologists initiate treatment when patients with PD report motor impairment or are

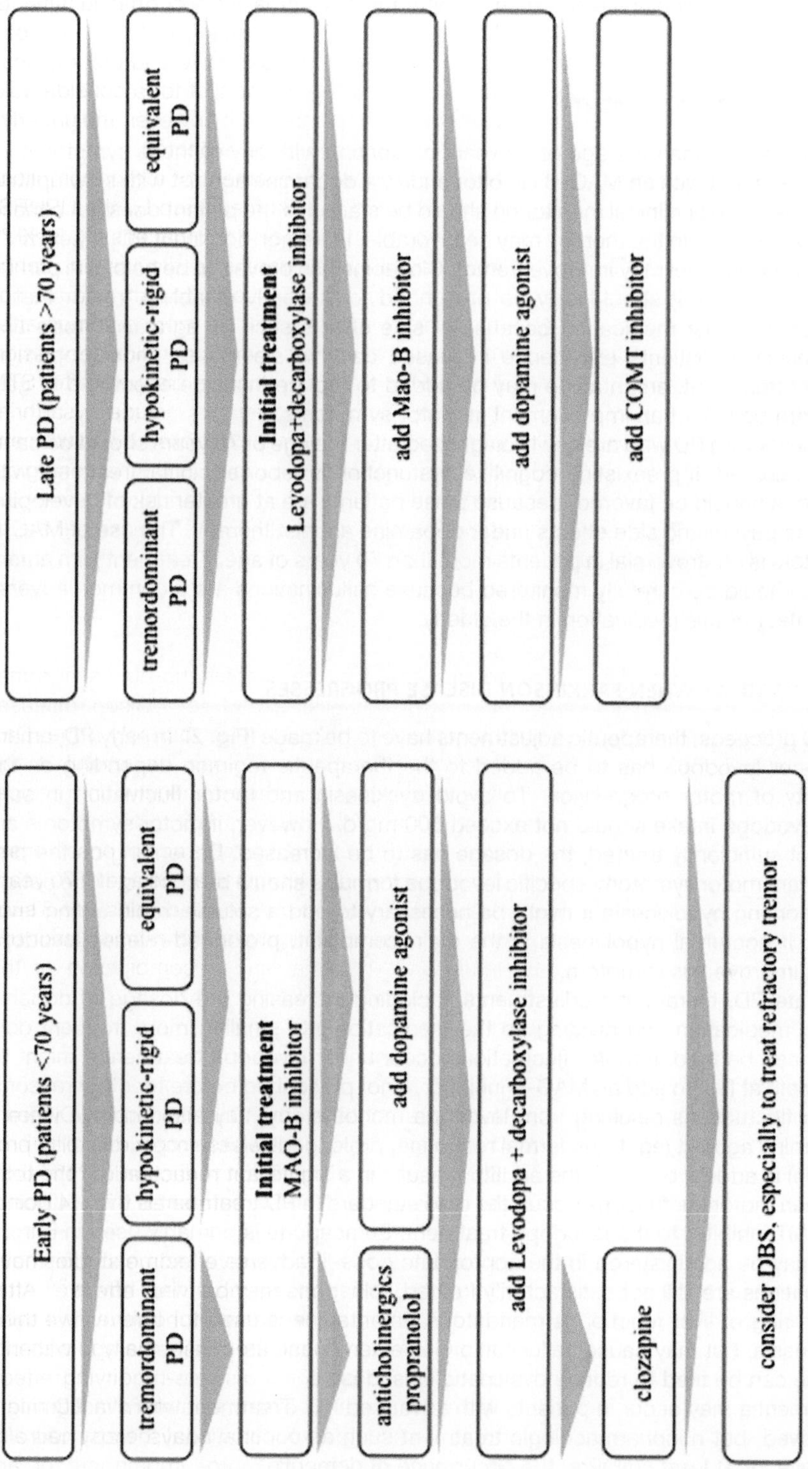

Fig. 1. Algorithm for the treatment of PD.

embarrassed in social life because of symptoms such as tremor, bradykinesia, or rigidity.

HOW TO START TREATMENT

In patients less than the age of 70 years presenting with any of these symptoms an initial treatment with an MAO-B inhibitor and/or a dopamine agonist with slow uptitration under regular clinical monitoring should be started. If the patient does not benefit, adding levodopa to the therapy may be favorable. In tremor-dominant PD, trihexyphenidyl or propranolol may improve tremor. Clozapine has proved to be helpful in parkinsonian tremor, but should only be prescribed for severely disabling tremor that is resistant to other medication because of side effects such as agranulocytosis and leukopenia. If patients experience increased daytime sleepiness under dopamine agonist treatment, amantadine may be added to reduce this side effect and to gain the extra benefit of an improvement in motor symptoms.

Patients with PD who are newly diagnosed after the age of 70 years should be carefully evaluated. If preexisting cognitive dysfunction is reported, initial treatment with levodopa should be favored, because these patients are at greater risk of developing adverse psychiatric side effects under dopamine agonist therapy. The use of MAO-B inhibitors is controversial in patients more than 70 years of age. Treatment with amantadine should be carefully monitored because hallucinations are a common adverse side effect of this medication in the elderly.

HOW TO TREAT WHEN PARKINSON DISEASE PROGRESSES

As PD proceeds, therapeutic adjustments have to be made (**Fig. 2**). In early PD, amantadine or levodopa has to be added to the therapeutic regimen depending on the severity of motor progression. To avoid dyskinesia and motor fluctuation in early PD, levodopa intake should not exceed 600 mg/d. However, if motor symptoms are still not sufficiently treated, the dosage has to be increased. Depending on the predominant motor symptom, specific levodopa formulas should be applied. If the patient has morning hypokinesia it might be necessary to add a soluble, rapid-acting levodopa. If nocturnal hypokinesia is the main complaint, prolonged-release levodopa might improve this symptom.

In late PD, therapeutic adjustments, including increasing the dosage of dopaminergic medication and dividing up the medication into smaller, more frequent dosages, can be tried. If motor fluctuations occur under levodopa treatment it might be of benefit at first to add an MAO-B inhibitor, if not prescribed before for other reasons. Motor fluctuations resulting from levodopa monotherapy may also improve when a dopamine agonist (eg, transdermal rotigotine, prolonged-release ropinirole, or pramipexole) is added, because the addition results in a significant reduction of “off” time.

When motor fluctuations occur, the gold standard in PD treatment is the addition of a COMT inhibitor to the levodopa treatment. Entacapone is primarily used in Europe and may be administered in the appropriate dose. If adverse effects occur or motor fluctuations are still not satisfactorily treated, tolcapone may be tried; however, strict monitoring of liver function is mandatory. Amantadine is used for improving severe dyskinesia, but may cause hallucinations in elderly patients. Again, therapy with clozapine can be tried to reduce dyskinetic episodes.

Dementia may occur in patients with advanced PD. Treatment with rivastigmine is approved, but nonpharmacologic treatment such as occupational therapy can also improve, or at least stabilize, the occurrence of dementia.

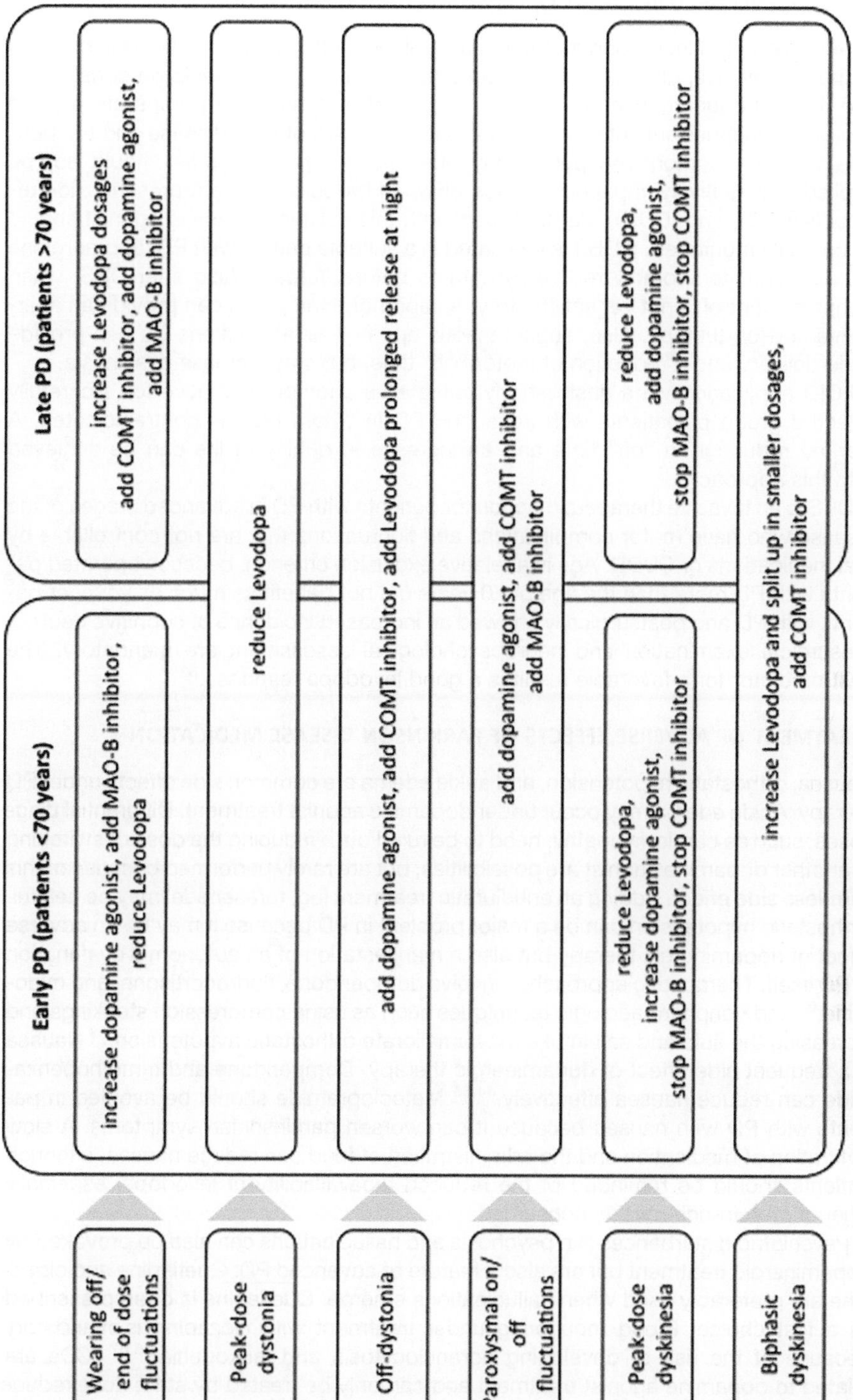

Fig. 2. Algorithm for treatment options in advanced PD.

INVASIVE THERAPEUTIC OPTIONS

When severe dyskinesia and motor fluctuations occur that disable patients in their activities of daily life, alternative therapeutic options like CDDD should be considered, and this is frequently used in Europe. In general, apomorphine pumps are a good choice for younger patients with a good understanding of their disease and the benefits that an apomorphine pump may offer. Apomorphine pumps should not be applied in cognitively impaired patients or when hallucinations are present. Side effects like DDS and ICDs under treatment with this soluble dopamine agonist should be carefully monitored. If DBS is evaluated in a suitable patient with PD, apomorphine pumps might temporarily relieve symptoms before surgery. Also after DBS, when symptom control is not yet satisfactory, an apomorphine pump can provide an alternative add-on therapy. Also, subcutaneous apomorphine injections via pen provide rapid delivery and a reduction of motor "off" time, but may increase dyskinesia.

LCID application via a gastrostomy catheter is another alternative for a carefully selected group of patients with advanced PD in whom DBS is contraindicated. A marked reduction in "off" time and an increase in quality of life can be achieved with this approach.

DBS is an invasive therapeutic option for patients with PD in advanced stages of the disease who have motor complications and fluctuations that are not controllable by oral medications or CDDD. Age is a relative exclusion criterion, because operated patients with PD more than the age of 70 years did not benefit as much as younger patients with PD and postsurgically showed an increased incidence of cognitive decline. Presurgical examination and neuropsychological assessment are mandatory. The best predictor for a favorable result is a good levodopa response.[52]

TREATMENT OF ADVERSE EFFECTS OF PARKINSON DISEASE MEDICATION

Nausea, orthostatic hypotension, and ankle edema are common side effects under PD therapy. Ankle edema may occur under dopamine agonist treatment. Differential diagnoses, such as cardiomyopathy, need to be ruled out. Reducing the dose or switching to another dopamine agonist are possibilities, but are rarely performed because of this harmless side effect. Adding an antidiuretic treatment (eg, torasemide) may be helpful. Orthostatic hypotension can be a major problem in PD because it may be an adverse effect of dopaminergic therapy but also a manifestation of an autonomic dysfunction of PD itself. Therapeutic approaches involve domperidone, fludrocortisone, and midodrine,[62] and nonpharmacologic techniques such as using compression stockings and increasing the fluid and salt intake may ameliorate orthostatic hypotension.[63] Nausea is a frequent side effect of dopaminergic therapy. Domperidone and trimethobenzamide can reduce nausea effectively.[64,65] Metoclopramide should be avoided in patients with PD with nausea because it can worsen parkinsonian symptoms. A slow uptitration of medication and the administration of food can reduce nausea, although patients should be reminded of the reduced bioavailability of levodopa, especially when a protein-rich meal is consumed.

Psychiatric disturbances like psychosis and hallucinations can also be provoked by dopaminergic treatment but are also a feature of advanced PD. Quetiapine and clozapine are preferably used when hallucinations emerge. Quetiapine is often prescribed as a first choice. Blood monitoring under treatment with clozapine is mandatory because of the risk of developing agranulocytosis and leukopenia.[66,67] ICDs are related to dopamine agonist treatment and can only be treated by strict dose reduction or even discontinuation of dopamine agonist treatment. Medical approaches with zonisamide,[68] valproate,[69] topiramate,[70] and amantadine[71] have been effective in case series. Reduction of levodopa or apomorphine is necessary in the management of DDS. In a small case series, 4 patients with DDS responded to valproate.[72]

TREATMENT OF NONMOTOR SYMPTOMS IN PARKINSON DISEASE

Nonmotor symptoms like hyposmia, constipation, depression, and RBD may be present before motor symptoms occur and are therefore regarded as prodromal markers. However, throughout the course of the disease, nonmotor symptoms may manifest and are generally difficult to treat. Fatigue is a major nonmotor symptom in PD. Adding amantadine to the therapeutic regimen may be helpful.[67] Anticholinergics with low central activity are effective for treatment of sialorrhea but may cause systemic adverse effects including delirium and hallucinations, especially in older patients. Injections of botulinum toxin into the parotid and submandibular gland can significantly improve drooling frequency and saliva quantity.[73] Pain and paresthesia might be caused by insufficient dopaminergic treatment, but internal and orthopedic diseases have to be ruled out. In some cases, analgesic treatment with ibuprofen, gabapentin, or pregabalin, or even administration of morphine derivatives, may be needed for relief of neuropathic pain.[74] Fear and panic attacks can be related to "off" symptoms and increasing dopaminergic therapy may be necessary; however, in some cases benzodiazepines are administered and additional psychotherapy has to be performed. Dysphagia is regarded as both a motor and nonmotor symptom and therefore may be treated with an increase of dopaminergic therapy as well as with nonpharmacologic approaches. In general, all of the nonmotor symptoms mentioned earlier can ameliorate when additional physical therapy, speech therapy, and occupational therapy are implemented.

SUMMARY

Managing the multifaceted symptoms of PD remains challenging and requires individual treatment. Adverse effects of the medication should particularly be evaluated and addressed. In newly diagnosed patients the different therapeutic approaches in early and late PD should be considered. In advanced stages of the disease similar treatment options are available. In patients with PD who are less than the age of 70 years DBS or CDDD should be evaluated to increase the patients' quality of life.

Nonmotor symptoms are difficult to treat satisfactory. In most studies, the outcome measures for most nonmotor features have been inconsistent and the observation period has been too short to establish treatment guidelines. The greatest unaccomplished therapeutic need is the identification of an effective disease-modifying and neuroprotective treatment option in order to slow the disease progression.

REFERENCES

1. Braak H, Del Tredici K, Rub U, et al. Staging of brain pathology related to sporadic Parkinson's disease. Neurobiol Aging 2003;24(2):197–211.
2. Braak H, Del Tredici K, Bratzke H, et al. Staging of the intracerebral inclusion body pathology associated with idiopathic Parkinson's disease (preclinical and clinical stages). J Neurol 2002;249(Suppl 3):III/1–5.
3. Haehner A, Boesveldt S, Berendse HW, et al. Prevalence of smell loss in Parkinson's disease–a multicenter study. Parkinsonism Relat Disord 2009;15(7):490–4.
4. Deeb J, Shah M, Muhammed N, et al. A basic smell test is as sensitive as a dopamine transporter scan: comparison of olfaction, taste and DaTSCAN in the diagnosis of Parkinson's disease. QJM 2010;103(12):941–52.

5. Oka H, Toyoda C, Yogo M, et al. Cardiovascular dysautonomia in de novo Parkinson's disease without orthostatic hypotension. Eur J Neurol 2011;18(2):286–92.
6. Schenck CH, Mahowald MW. REM sleep behavior disorder: clinical, developmental, and neuroscience perspectives 16 years after its formal identification in SLEEP. Sleep 2002;25(2):120–38.
7. Schenck CH, Montplaisir JY, Frauscher B, et al. Rapid eye movement sleep behavior disorder: devising controlled active treatment studies for symptomatic and neuroprotective therapy–a consensus statement from the International Rapid Eye Movement Sleep Behavior Disorder Study Group. Sleep Med 2013;14(8): 795–806.
8. Iranzo A, Molinuevo JL, Santamaria J, et al. Rapid-eye-movement sleep behaviour disorder as an early marker for a neurodegenerative disorder: a descriptive study. Lancet Neurol 2006;5(7):572–7.
9. Postuma RB, Gagnon JF, Vendette M, et al. Quantifying the risk of neurodegenerative disease in idiopathic REM sleep behavior disorder. Neurology 2009; 72(15):1296–300.
10. Iranzo A, Tolosa E, Gelpi E, et al. Neurodegenerative disease status and postmortem pathology in idiopathic rapid-eye-movement sleep behaviour disorder: an observational cohort study. Lancet Neurol 2013;12(5):443–53.
11. Olichney JM, Murphy C, Hofstetter CR, et al. Anosmia is very common in the Lewy body variant of Alzheimer's disease. J Neurol Neurosurg Psychiatr 2005; 76(10):1342–7.
12. Jennum P, Mayer G, Ju YE, Postuma R. Morbidities in rapid eye movement sleep behavior disorder. Sleep Med 2013;14(8):782–7.
13. Aurora RN, Zak RS, Maganti RK, et al. Best practice guide for the treatment of REM sleep behavior disorder (RBD). J Clin Sleep Med 2010;6(1):85–95.
14. Troeung L, Egan SJ, Gasson N. A meta-analysis of randomised placebo-controlled treatment trials for depression and anxiety in Parkinson's disease. PLoS One 2013;8(11):e79510.
15. Liu J, Dong J, Wang L, et al. Comparative efficacy and acceptability of antidepressants in Parkinson's disease: a network meta-analysis. PLoS One 2013; 8(10):e76651.
16. Morens DM, Davis JW, Grandinetti A, et al. Epidemiologic observations on Parkinson's disease: incidence and mortality in a prospective study of middle-aged men. Neurology 1996;46(4):1044–50.
17. Hoehn MM, Yahr MD. Parkinsonism: onset, progression and mortality. Neurology 1967;17(5):427–42.
18. Gille G, Hung ST, Reichmann H, et al. Oxidative stress to dopaminergic neurons as models of Parkinson's disease. Ann N Y Acad Sci 2004;1018:533–40.
19. Michel PP, Hefti F. Toxicity of 6-hydroxydopamine and dopamine for dopaminergic neurons in culture. J Neurosci Res 1990;26(4):428–35.
20. Fahn S, Oakes D, Shoulson I, et al. Levodopa and the progression of Parkinson's disease. N Engl J Med 2004;351(24):2498–508.
21. Olanow CW, Obeso JA, Stocchi F. Continuous dopamine-receptor treatment of Parkinson's disease: scientific rationale and clinical implications. Lancet Neurol 2006;5(8):677–87.
22. Kostic V, Przedborski S, Flaster E, et al. Early development of levodopa-induced dyskinesias and response fluctuations in young-onset Parkinson's disease. Neurology 1991;41(2 (Pt 1)):202–5.
23. Palhagen S, Heinonen E, Hagglund J, et al. Selegiline slows the progression of the symptoms of Parkinson disease. Neurology 2006;66(8):1200–6.

24. Parkinson Study Group. A controlled trial of rasagiline in early Parkinson disease: the TEMPO Study. Arch Neurol 2002;59(12):1937–43.
25. Hauser RA, Lew MF, Hurtig HI, et al. Long-term outcome of early versus delayed rasagiline treatment in early Parkinson's disease. Mov Disord 2009;24(4):564–73.
26. Rascol O, Fitzer-Attas CJ, Hauser R, et al. A double-blind, delayed-start trial of rasagiline in Parkinson's disease (the ADAGIO study): prespecified and post-hoc analyses of the need for additional therapies, changes in UPDRS scores, and non-motor outcomes. Lancet Neurol 2011;10(5):415–23.
27. Olanow CW, Rascol O, Hauser R, et al. A double-blind, delayed-start trial of rasagiline in Parkinson's disease. N Engl J Med 2009;361(13):1268–78.
28. Parkinson Study Group. A randomized placebo-controlled trial of rasagiline in levodopa-treated patients with Parkinson disease and motor fluctuations: the PRESTO study. Arch Neurol 2005;62(2):241–8.
29. Stocchi F, Rabey JM. Effect of rasagiline as adjunct therapy to levodopa on severity of OFF in Parkinson's disease. Eur J Neurol 2011;18(12):1373–8.
30. Rascol O, Brooks DJ, Melamed E, et al. Rasagiline as an adjunct to levodopa in patients with Parkinson's disease and motor fluctuations (LARGO, Lasting effect in Adjunct therapy with Rasagiline Given Once daily, study): a randomised, double-blind, parallel-group trial. Lancet 2005;365(9463):947–54.
31. Deane KH, Spieker S, Clarke CE. Catechol-O-methyltransferase inhibitors for levodopa-induced complications in Parkinson's disease. Cochrane Database Syst Rev 2004;(4):CD004554.
32. Entacapone improves motor fluctuations in levodopa-treated Parkinson's disease patients. Parkinson Study Group. Ann Neurol 1997;42(5):747–55.
33. Stocchi F, Rascol O, Kieburtz K, et al. Initiating levodopa/carbidopa therapy with and without entacapone in early Parkinson disease: the STRIDE-PD study. Ann Neurol 2010;68(1):18–27.
34. Ferreira JJ, Katzenschlager R, Bloem BR, et al. Summary of the recommendations of the EFNS/MDS-ES review on therapeutic management of Parkinson's disease. Eur J Neurol 2013;20(1):5–15.
35. Reichmann H. Budipine in Parkinson's tremor. J Neurol Sci 2006;248(1–2):53–5.
36. Katzenschlager R, Sampaio C, Costa J, et al. Anticholinergics for symptomatic management of Parkinson's disease. Cochrane Database Syst Rev 2003;(2):CD003735.
37. Zou L, Jankovic J, Rowe DB, et al. Neuroprotection by pramipexole against dopamine- and levodopa-induced cytotoxicity. Life Sci 1999;64(15):1275–85.
38. Iida M, Miyazaki I, Tanaka K, et al. Dopamine D2 receptor-mediated antioxidant and neuroprotective effects of ropinirole, a dopamine agonist. Brain Res 1999; 838(1–2):51–9.
39. Trenkwalder C, Kies B, Rudzinska M, et al. Rotigotine effects on early morning motor function and sleep in Parkinson's disease: a double-blind, randomized, placebo-controlled study (RECOVER). Mov Disord 2011;26(1):90–9.
40. Parkinson Study Group. Pramipexole vs levodopa as initial treatment for Parkinson disease: a randomized controlled trial. Parkinson Study Group. JAMA 2000;284(15):1931–8.
41. Rascol O, Brooks DJ, Korczyn AD, et al. A five-year study of the incidence of dyskinesia in patients with early Parkinson's disease who were treated with ropinirole or levodopa. 056 Study Group. N Engl J Med 2000;342(20):1484–91.
42. Weiss HD, Marsh L. Impulse control disorders and compulsive behaviors associated with dopaminergic therapies in Parkinson disease. Neurol Clin Pract 2012; 2(4):267–74.

43. Barone P, Poewe W, Albrecht S, et al. Pramipexole for the treatment of depressive symptoms in patients with Parkinson's disease: a randomised, double-blind, placebo-controlled trial. Lancet Neurol 2010;9(6):573–80.
44. Frankel JP, Lees AJ, Kempster PA, et al. Subcutaneous apomorphine in the treatment of Parkinson's disease. J Neurol Neurosurg Psychiatr 1990;53(2):96–101.
45. Bowron A. Practical considerations in the use of apomorphine injectable. Neurology 2004;62(6 Suppl 4):S32–6.
46. Deleu D, Hanssens Y, Northway MG. Subcutaneous apomorphine: an evidence-based review of its use in Parkinson's disease. Drugs Aging 2004;21(11): 687–709.
47. Manson AJ, Hanagasi H, Turner K, et al. Intravenous apomorphine therapy in Parkinson's disease: clinical and pharmacokinetic observations. Brain 2001;124(Pt 2): 331–40.
48. Stocchi F, Vacca L, De Pandis MF, et al. Subcutaneous continuous apomorphine infusion in fluctuating patients with Parkinson's disease: long-term results. Neurol Sci 2001;22(1):93–4.
49. Antonini A, Mancini F, Canesi M, et al. Duodenal levodopa infusion improves quality of life in advanced Parkinson's disease. Neurodegener Dis 2008;5(3–4):244–6.
50. Eggert K, Schrader C, Hahn M, et al. Continuous jejunal levodopa infusion in patients with advanced Parkinson disease: practical aspects and outcome of motor and non-motor complications. Clin Neuropharmacol 2008;31(3):151–66.
51. Honig H, Antonini A, Martinez-Martin P, et al. Intrajejunal levodopa infusion in Parkinson's disease: a pilot multicenter study of effects on nonmotor symptoms and quality of life. Mov Disord 2009;24(10):1468–74.
52. Charles PD, Van Blercom N, Krack P, et al. Predictors of effective bilateral subthalamic nucleus stimulation for PD. Neurology 2002;59(6):932–4.
53. Russmann H, Ghika J, Villemure JG, et al. Subthalamic nucleus deep brain stimulation in Parkinson disease patients over age 70 years. Neurology 2004;63(10): 1952–4.
54. Saint-Cyr JA, Trepanier LL, Kumar R, et al. Neuropsychological consequences of chronic bilateral stimulation of the subthalamic nucleus in Parkinson's disease. Brain 2000;123(Pt 10):2091–108.
55. Kleiner-Fisman G, Herzog J, Fisman DN, et al. Subthalamic nucleus deep brain stimulation: summary and meta-analysis of outcomes. Mov Disord 2006; 21(Suppl 14):S290–304.
56. Krack P, Batir A, Van Blercom N, et al. Five-year follow-up of bilateral stimulation of the subthalamic nucleus in advanced Parkinson's disease. N Engl J Med 2003; 349(20):1925–34.
57. Schupbach WM, Chastan N, Welter ML, et al. Stimulation of the subthalamic nucleus in Parkinson's disease: a 5 year follow up. J Neurol Neurosurg Psychiatr 2005;76(12):1640–4.
58. Deep-Brain Stimulation for Parkinson's Disease Study Group. Deep-brain stimulation of the subthalamic nucleus or the pars interna of the globus pallidus in Parkinson's disease. N Engl J Med 2001;345(13):956–63.
59. Ghika J, Villemure JG, Fankhauser H, et al. Efficiency and safety of bilateral contemporaneous pallidal stimulation (deep brain stimulation) in levodopa-responsive patients with Parkinson's disease with severe motor fluctuations: a 2-year follow-up review. J Neurosurg 1998;89(5):713–8.
60. Voon V, Krack P, Lang AE, et al. A multicentre study on suicide outcomes following subthalamic stimulation for Parkinson's disease. Brain 2008;131(Pt 10): 2720–8.

61. DATATOP: a multicenter controlled clinical trial in early Parkinson's disease. Parkinson Study Group. Arch Neurol 1989;46(10):1052–60.
62. Jankovic J, Gilden JL, Hiner BC, et al. Neurogenic orthostatic hypotension: a double-blind, placebo-controlled study with midodrine. Am J Med 1993;95(1): 38–48.
63. Schoffer KL, Henderson RD, O'Maley K, et al. Nonpharmacological treatment, fludrocortisone, and domperidone for orthostatic hypotension in Parkinson's disease. Mov Disord 2007;22(11):1543–9.
64. Parkes JD. Domperidone and Parkinson's disease. Clin Neuropharmacol 1986; 9(6):517–32.
65. Gunzler SA. Apomorphine in the treatment of Parkinson disease and other movement disorders. Expert Opin Pharmacother 2009;10(6):1027–38.
66. Shotbolt P, Samuel M, David A. Quetiapine in the treatment of psychosis in Parkinson's disease. Ther Adv Neurol Disord 2010;3(6):339–50.
67. Seppi K, Weintraub D, Coelho M, et al. The Movement Disorder Society evidence-based medicine review update: treatments for the non-motor symptoms of Parkinson's disease. Mov Disord 2011;26(Suppl 3):S42–80.
68. Bermejo PE, Ruiz-Huete C, Anciones B. Zonisamide in managing impulse control disorders in Parkinson's disease. J Neurol 2010;257(10):1682–5.
69. Hicks CW, Pandya MM, Itin I, et al. Valproate for the treatment of medication-induced impulse-control disorders in three patients with Parkinson's disease. Parkinsonism Relat Disord 2011;17(5):379–81.
70. Bermejo PE. Topiramate in managing impulse control disorders in Parkinson's disease. Parkinsonism Relat Disord 2008;14(5):448–9.
71. Thomas A, Bonanni L, Gambi F, et al. Pathological gambling in Parkinson disease is reduced by amantadine. Ann Neurol 2010;68(3):400–4.
72. Sriram A, Ward HE, Hassan A, et al. Valproate as a treatment for dopamine dysregulation syndrome (DDS) in Parkinson's disease. J Neurol 2013;260(2):521–7.
73. Lagalla G, Millevolte M, Capecci M, et al. Botulinum toxin type A for drooling in Parkinson's disease: a double-blind, randomized, placebo-controlled study. Mov Disord 2006;21(5):704–7.
74. Ha AD, Jankovic J. Pain in Parkinson's disease. Mov Disord 2012;27(4):485–91.

Atypical Parkinsonism

Diagnosis and Treatment

Maria Stamelou, MD, PhD[a,b,c,*], Kailash P. Bhatia, FRCP[c]

KEYWORDS

- Progressive supranuclear palsy • Corticobasal degeneration
- Multiple system atrophy • Atypical parkinsonism • Diagnosis

KEY POINTS

- Careful clinical examination is important for the differential diagnosis of atypical parkinsonism from Parkinson disease.
- The expanding phenotypic spectrum of atypical parkinsonism and the expanding pathologic spectrum of classic atypical parkinsonian phenotypes make the early differential diagnosis challenging.
- Investigations may be supportive, but their sensitivity and specificity are low.
- There are currently no biomarkers available.
- There are currently no neuroprotective treatments available, although there are some symptomatic and supportive treatments with usually no sustained effect.

Video of progressive supranuclear palsy accompanies this article at http://www.neurologic.theclinics.com/

INTRODUCTION

Parkinsonism is defined according to the UK Brain Bank Criteria as the presence of bradykinesia and at least one of the following: rest tremor, rigidity, or postural instability.[1] Once the presence of parkinsonism has been established, the main question for the clinician is whether the patient has the most common cause of parkinsonism (eg, Parkinson disease [PD]) or an atypical parkinsonian condition [AP]. Although the term "atypical" implies the presence of features "atypical" for PD, and there are numerous disorders causing parkinsonism,[2] typically this term is used to describe 3 particular sporadic parkinsonian conditions, namely progressive supranuclear palsy

Financial disclosure: See last page of the article.

[a] Second Department of Neurology, Attiko Hospital, University of Athens, Rimini 1, Athens 12462, Greece; [b] Department of Neurology, Philipps Universität, Baldingerstrasse, Marburg 35039, Germany; [c] Sobell Department of Motor Neuroscience and Movement Disorders, UCL Institute of Neurology, Queen Square, London WC1N 3BG, UK

* Corresponding author. Second Department of Neurology, Attiko Hospital, University of Athens, Rimini 1, Athens 12462, Greece.

E-mail address: mariastamelou@gmail.com

Neurol Clin 33 (2015) 39–56
http://dx.doi.org/10.1016/j.ncl.2014.09.012 neurologic.theclinics.com
0733-8619/15/$ – see front matter

(PSP), corticobasal degeneration (CBD), and multiple system atrophy (MSA), which are the conditions that are further discussed here.

PSP, CBD, and MSA are distinct pathologic entities. Despite ongoing research, their cause and pathophysiology are still unknown, and there are no biomarkers or effective treatments available. One important reason that may account for that is that their early differential diagnosis is still challenging. Clinicopathologic studies have shown that the most common misdiagnoses occur between these 3 disorders and also PD, Lewy-body dementia, frontotemporal lobar degeneration, and Alzheimer disease (AD).[3–8] Moreover, the early differential diagnosis is complicated by patients with pathologically proven PSP, CBD, or MSA that may present clinically with phenotypes other than the classic ones.[9–12] Conversely, patients with the classic AP phenotypes may turn out to have other pathologic abnormalities.[9–12] Here, a guide on how to diagnose these conditions is provided and the limited available treatment options are discussed.

PROGRESSIVE SUPRANUCLEAR PALSY

PSP is a neurodegenerative disease characterized by symmetric parkinsonism, supranuclear palsy of vertical gaze, early postural instability with falls backwards, subcortical dementia, dysarthria, and dysphagia.[7] The prevalence of PSP is approximately 5 per 100,000, and men and women are equally affected. Average age at onset is 63, and mean time from symptom onset to death is 7 years. No pathologic proven cases have begun before the age of 40.[7]

PSP is a tauopathy with an unknown cause. PSP is almost always sporadic, and only a few familial cases have been reported, mostly carrying mutations in the *MAPT* (microtubuli associated protein τ) gene.[13,14] A genome-wide association study has confirmed that the most common risk allele for PSP is the H1 haplotype of the *MAPT* gene, and further risk loci have been identified.[15] Mitochondrial dysfunction and oxidative stress have been implicated in the pathophysiology of PSP.[16]

Diagnostic Approach to Progressive Supranuclear Palsy

Clinical features

PSP is typically characterized by symmetric and axial parkinsonism, postural instability with early falls particularly usually backwards, vertical supranuclear gaze palsy, and a frontal-subcortical dementia. This classic PSP phenotype is now termed Richardson syndrome (RS; see Phenotypic spectrum of PSP section). Postural instability and falls occur also in PD, however usually later in the disease course. In PSP, the prevailing axial rigidity causes head and trunk hyperextension sometimes with retrocollis (although rarely), unlike the posture in flexion in PD. The typical pill-rolling asymmetric rest-tremor typically seen in PD is usually absent (**Table 1**).[3,7,17,18] Gait may be slightly broad-based and typically not the short-stepped gait seen in PD. Freezing of gait is common and may lead to diagnostic confusion with MSA.

The characteristic sign of PSP is the supranuclear palsy of vertical gaze followed by abnormalities of horizontal gaze (Video 1). The ocular motor dysfunction begins with a slowing of vertical saccadic movements, downward in particular. Markedly reduced blink rate and closure of eyelids due to eyelid dystonia or levator inhibition (also known as apraxia of eyelid opening) results in overactivity of the frontalis muscle, in an attempt to keep eyelids open, leading to a characteristic surprised look. Horizontal saccade intrusions named square wave-jerks, occurring while staring at an object, are frequently present in PSP patients, while ocular-vestibular reflexes are preserved. Thus, on doll's eye maneuver, there is improved range, as vestibulo-ocular reflex is preserved, confirming the supranuclear nature of the gaze palsy.[7,18–25]

Table 1
Clinical features helpful to distinguish Parkinson disease, multiple system atrophy, progressive supranuclear palsy, and corticobasal degeneration

	PD	MSA	PSP	CBD
Mean age at onset	60	55	63	63
Youngest reported age of onset	Childhood	31	40	45
Family history	Possible, particularly if onset <50 y	Rarely If present, consider genetic MSA look alikes **(Table 2)**	Rarely If present, consider genetic PSP look alikes **(Table 2)**	Rarely If present, consider genetic CBD look alikes **(Table 2)**
Parkinsonism	Asymmetric	Symmetric or asymmetric	Symmetric Axial	Asymmetric Axial
Eye movement abnormalities	Usually normal at initial stages	Square wave jerks, jerky pursuit, nystagmus	Square wave jerks, slowed vertical saccades, supranuclear gaze palsy	Delayed initiation of saccades
Dementia	Usually later in the disease course	Not an early prominent feature	Frontal, subcortical prominent feature	Frontal, subcortical prominent feature
Tremor	Often present	Often present, rarely pill-rolling	Uncommon in RS May be present in PSP-P	Jerky
Falls	May occur after some years of symptoms	Common early in course of disease	Very common early in course of disease, mostly backwards	Common early in course of disease
Freezing	Can be present	Can be present	Can be present, in particular in PAGF	Can be present
Levodopa response	Good, prolonged, may develop dyskinesia	May cause facial dystonia, no prolonged response	Occasional response, not usually prolonged	Very occasional, short-lived response
Cardiovascular autonomic failure	May develop, but often late in disease	Usually a prominent early feature	Very rare	Very rare
Bladder disturbance	Urgency, frequency, incontinence secondary to immobility	Urgency, frequency, incontinence, incomplete bladder emptying	Urgency, frequency, incontinence, incomplete bladder emptying	Urgency, frequency, incontinence secondary to immobility
Other features	RBD	Myoclonus, stridor, RBD	Levator inhibition	Apraxia, cortical sensory loss, myoclonus, alien limb

Table 2
Other disorders that may present as progressive supranuclear palsy, corticobasal degeneration, or multiple system atrophy look alikes

	PSP	CBD	MSA
Sporadic neurodegenerative disorders	CBD[7,8,90] FTD[7,8,90] PD[7,8,90] DLB[7,8,90] MSA[7,8,90] Cerebral amyloid angiopathy and motor neurone disease[91] MM2 sCJD[92] Caribbean parkinsonism[93] Motor neuron disease[94] AD[95]	PSP[7,8,90] FTD[7,8,90] AD PD[7,8,90] DLB[7,8,90] MSA[7,8,90] sCJD Motor neurone disease-inclusion body dementia[94] Caribbean parkinsonism[93] Neurofilament inclusion body disease[96,97] Basophilic inclusion body disease	PD[7,8,90] DLB[7,8,90] Neurofilament inclusion body disease Primary lateral sclerosis[98]
Vascular	Cerebrovascular disease[99–102] Intracranial dural arteriovenous fistula Thoracic aneurysm surgery[103]	Small vessel disease[104] Carotid artery occlusion[105]	Vascular parkinsonism[106]
Infectious	Whipple disease[107,108] Neurosyphilis[109,110] HIV[111]	Neurosyphilis[112] PML[113]	—
Auto-immune	Paraneoplastic (Ma2 encephalitis)[114–117] Antiphospholipid syndrome PERM (anti-glycine antibodies)[118] Neurosarcoidosis[119]	Antiphospholipid syndrome[120,121]	Primary progressive multiple sclerosis
Genetic conditions	Genetic FTDs (*MAPT, PGRN, C9ORF72*) Perry syndrome (*DCTN1*) Kufor-Rakeb (*ATP13A2*) Gaucher disease Mitochondrial disorders CADASIL (*NOTCH3*) Leucoencephalopathy with axonal spheroids (*CSF1R*)	Genetic FTDs (*MAPT, PGRN, C9ORF72*) Perry syndrome (*DCTN1*) Gaucher disease Cerebrotendinous xanthomatosis	Perry syndrome (*DCTN1*) Spinocerebellar ataxias Fragile-X-tremor ataxia syndrome (*FMR1*)

Abbreviations: AD, Alzheimer disease; C9ORF72, chromosome 9 open reading frame 72; CSF1R, colony stimulating factor 1; DCTN1, dynactin; DLB, dementia with Lewy bodies; FMR1, fragile-X mental retardation 1; HIV, human immunodeficiency virus; MAPT, microtubule-associated τ; PERM, progressive encephalomyelitis with rigidity and myoclonus; PGRN, progranulin; PML, progressive multifocal encephalopathy; sCJD, sporadic Creutzfeld-Jakob disease.

Pseudobulbar palsy with dysarthria and dysphagia is very common and appears earlier in the disease course compared with PD. Subcortical-type dementia is present in PSP patients having a dramatically slowed information processing and motor execution as well as difficulty in planning and shifting conceptual sets. Apathy and withdrawal are very common and may initially be confused with depression. Reduced verbal fluency, motor perseveration, which can be detected with the "applause sign," echopraxia, echolalia, and frontal release signs are often present.[20,26] Patients often display motor recklessness where, despite frequent falls, they display no caution in the way they walk, throwing themselves into and out of chairs, taking no account of their lack of balance ("the rocket sign").[21,22]

There are several sets of criteria proposed to diagnose PSP, but the most widely used are the National Institute of Neurological Disorders and Stroke and Society for Progressive Supranuclear Palsy.[7] These criteria have shown high specificity but low sensitivity to diagnose PSP.[7,23] Pathology remains the gold standard for definite diagnosis (see Pathology of PSP section).

The phenotypic spectrum of progressive supranuclear palsy

The typical PSP phenotype described above is now termed Richardson syndrome.[9] The second most common phenotype seems to be PSP-parkinsonism, which may resemble PD at least at the initial stages, with asymmetric parkinsonism, rest-tremor, better levodopa response, and a longer mean survival of 9 years compared with RS.[9] Further phenotypes include pure akinesia with gait freezing (PSP-PAGF), corticobasal syndrome (PSP-CBS), frontotemporal dementia (PSP-FTD), progressive nonfluent aphasia.[10] In particular, the PAGF phenotype is characterized by severe freezing of gait and speech, and only later in the disease course the characteristic eye abnormalities may occur.[10] The relative frequency and natural distribution of these phenotypes are not known, and there is currently no clinical sign to predict PSP pathologic abnormality accurately in the non-RS phenotypes.

Investigations

PSP remains largely a clinical diagnosis. However, several abnormalities in MRI have been proposed as possible candidates to differentiate between AP syndromes.[24] However, their sensitivity and specificity, assessed retrospectively in pathologically proven cases, were found almost equal to that of clinical diagnosis.[24,25,27] The most clinically useful MRI abnormalities seen in PSP are signs of midbrain atrophy, superior cerebellar peduncle atrophy.[24,25,27] The "morning glory flower sign" and the "humming bird sign" are quite specific but show low sensitivity (50% and 68.4%, respectively) in one retrospective study.[27]

With regard to functional imaging, dopamine transporters imaging (DATscan) is abnormal in PD and all AP syndromes and, therefore, not useful in their differential diagnosis. To differentiate with PD, [123]meta-iodobenzylguanidine (MIBG) and 123I-iodobenzamide (IBZM) SPECT may be useful. MIBG is abnormal in PD because of postganglionic sympathetic denervation, but is typically normal in PSP. IBZM SPECT assessing the postsynaptic receptors is abnormal in PSP and normal in PD. However, IBZM SPECT is abnormal in all APs and therefore cannot differentiate between PSP and other AP conditions such as MSA or CBD.[28,29] Novel diagnostic approaches and biomarkers such as proteins in cerebrospinal fluid (a-synuclein, τ, and so forth) are still being researched.[30,31] In this regard, neurofilament light chain may be proven useful as a biomarker in the future.[32]

Pathology

PSP is a tauopathy, a disorder associated with abnormal aggregates of τ protein (4-repeat τ, 4R tauopathy). PSP is characterized pathologically by degeneration of several subcortical structures, including the substantia nigra, the subthalamic nucleus, and the midbrain. Neurofibrillary tangles are present in these areas. Tufted astrocytes (Gallyas-positive) are the hallmark feature of PSP that differentiates it in pathology from other 4R tauopathies such as CBD (astrocytic plaques).[33]

Treatment

Currently, there are no effective symptomatic or neuroprotective treatments for PSP.[34] Proposed treatments are based largely on small, uncontrolled studies with no pathologic or retrospective confirmation. Supportive treatment, particularly regarding swallowing and prevention of falls, may prolong survival and improve quality of life.

- A trial of levodopa (up to 1 g/d) and amantadine (up to 450 mg/d) is worthwhile.
- Botulinum toxin injections can be used to treat levator inhibition.
- Serotonin reuptake inhibitors (SSRIs) may be used for apathy with no clear benefit.
- A small study with Coenzyme Q10 has shown a statistically significant improvement in clinical scales and magnetic resonance spectroscopy, but warrants further confirmation.[35]
- Recent large, double-blind studies with GSK-3b inhibitors (Tideglusib, Davunetide) have failed to show any clinical effect.[36,37] However, Tideglusib reduced the rate of brain atrophy in one study.[36]
- Supportive measures such as physiotherapy, walking aids, speech therapy and percutaneous endoscopic gastrostomy (PEG) for advanced dysphagia, may be helpful.

CORTICOBASAL DEGENERATION

CBD is a rare neurodegenerative disorder typically characterized by progressive asymmetric levodopa-resistant parkinsonism, dystonia, myoclonus, and further cortical signs (eg, apraxia, alien limb phenomena, cortical sensory loss).[11,12] The exact prevalence of CBD is unknown, but it is thought to be considerably lower than that of PSP or MSA, and men and women are equally affected. Average time from symptom onset to death is 8 years. CBD is a 4R tauopathy and almost always a sporadic condition.

Diagnostic Approach to Corticobasal Degeneration

Clinical features

Patients typically present with strikingly asymmetric rigidity and bradykinesia affecting one limb, which may be also affected by dystonia and distal, stimulus-sensitive myoclonus.[11] The limb is often described by the patient as "dead" or "useless" and is frequently held postured across the body. "Alien-limb phenomena" may occur, the patients describing this as the affected limb "having a mind of its own," and this may occur in up to 50% of patients. Clinically, the limb may move about, often grabbing objects or interfering with the actions of the unaffected hand (intermanual conflict). Patients with CBD may have difficulty in initiating saccades rather than slow saccades as seen in PSP (see **Table 1**).

Cortical features include apraxia, which can be difficult to demonstrate in the more affected arm because of severe bradykinesia, rigidity, and dystonia, but it is usually also present in the unaffected arm, particularly later in the disease course. Patients will also often have cortical sensory loss (impaired 2-point discrimination, dysgraphesthesia, astereognosis).[3,12,38–40] Dementia is an important part of the phenotype and may be the presenting or predominant clinical feature in CBD. Neuropsychometry typically reveals frontal executive defects together with parietal lobe dysfunction. In contrast with AD, episodic memory is usually well preserved.[41–43]

There are several sets of criteria for the diagnosis of CBD with low sensitivity and specificity. Recently, new clinical criteria are proposed that attempt to take into account the different phenotypes, as described in later discussion, which, however, have not been independently validated yet.[12] Definite CBD requires pathologic confirmation (see Pathology discussion later).

The phenotypic spectrum of corticobasal degeneration

The classic CBD phenotype (that is the combination of an asymmetric parkinsonian syndrome with cortical signs) is now called corticobasal syndrome (CBS). However, patients with pathologically confirmed CBD may present with a FTD, RS, primary progressive aphasia, or a posterior cortical atrophy syndrome.[12] Conversely, patients with other underlying pathologies such as AD, PSP, and FTD may present with CBS.[4,39,44] The prevalence and natural distribution of these phenotypes are not known.

There are some suggestions that certain clinical features may be helpful to suspect the underlying pathology in a patient with CBS. For example, a symmetric bilateral CBS could imply AD pathology,[4] or a patient with RS and earlier age of onset than expected in PSP may have CBD pathology[8]; however, these suggestions need further confirmation. Moreover, the different phenotypes likely represent the distribution (eg, the brain areas affected) of the underlying pathology in each of these disorders, and thus, reflect more likely a spectrum rather than well-defined phenotypes, for which strictly defined clinical criteria can be applied.[10,39,45]

Investigations

MRI in CBD may show asymmetric frontoparietal atrophy.[46] DATscans are abnormal in CBD, as they are in PD, PSP, and MSA. Glucose metabolism measured by fluorodeoxyglucose PET (FDG-PET), and blood flow measured by SPECT scanning, may show asymmetric reduction in frontoparietal regions in CBD, which is not a feature typically seen in PSP, MSA, or PD.[47–49] However, patients that participated in the FDG-PET studies have not been pathologically confirmed; therefore, it is unknown whether the pattern of hypometabolism reflects only the phenotype (eg, CBS) or can be helpful to predict the underlying pathology.

Pathology

CBD is characterized by widespread deposition of hyperphosphorylated τ protein (specifically, 4-R) in the brain. There is marked neuronal degeneration in the substantia nigra and the frontoparietal cortex. The hallmark feature of CBD pathology is the characteristic astrocytic plaques that differentiate CBD from other 4R tauopathies such as PSP (tufted astrocytes).[8]

Treatment

As in PSP, most published data regarding treatment in CBD are anecdotal, with a small number of patients and uncontrolled trials. In clinical practice, treatment options are limited to a levodopa trial (up to 1 g/d) and amantadine for parkinsonism and gait disturbance as well as valproate or levetiracetam for myoclonus.[31] Although not sufficiently studied,[11] Botulinum toxin injections can be helpful to relieve dystonic spasms of the hand ("the dystonic clenched fist"). These injections do not usually restore function, but can help with hand hygiene and pain. No trials of cholinesterase inhibitors for dementia in CBD currently exist. Early management of dysphagia is important, and prompt provision of walking aids or a wheelchair may help preventing falls.

MULTIPLE SYSTEM ATROPHY

MSA is a neurodegenerative disorder characterized by autonomic failure and parkinsonism and/or cerebellar signs. MSA-parkinsonism (MSA-P) is characterized predominantly by parkinsonism and autonomic failure at presentation, whereas in MSA-cerebellar type (MSA-C), cerebellar signs occur with autonomic failure. However, during disease progression, cerebellar signs often develop in patients with MSA-P and parkinsonism in MSA-C.

The prevalence is about 4 per 100,000. Typical age at onset is 53 to 55 and onset before age 30 has never been reported.[50] Men and women are equally affected, and mean survival time is 9 years from symptom onset.[50] MSA is an a-synucleinopathy and usually a sporadic disease; however, rarely, familial cases have been described in which several mutations in *COQ2* gene (essential for biosynthesis of Coenzyme Q10) have been described.[51,52]

Diagnostic Approach to Multiple System Atrophy

Clinical features

Motor symptoms Parkinsonism in MSA is usually symmetric, although asymmetric cases have been described.[53] Classic asymmetric pill-rolling tremor is not often seen in MSA, although it can occur. Usually MSA patients have a jerky poly-mini-myoclonus, which has been suggested to be cortical in origin.[53,54] Focal dystonia of the neck muscles also occurs in MSA, but usually in the form of a mixed antecollis/laterocollis, which can be fixed and painful. MSA can also present with focal dystonia of the vocal cords or a segmental dystonia of trunk muscles, causing lateroflexion (Pisa sign) or anteroflexion (camptocormia) of the trunk. Pyramidal involvement with hyperreflexia and Babinski sign may occur in up to 50% of the patients. However, prominent and severe spasticity should raise suspicion for an alternative diagnosis. Cerebellar signs include jerky pursuit, nystagmus, dysarthria, dysmetria, and gait ataxia.

Autonomic dysfunction Autonomic failure is a prominent clinical feature and essential for a diagnosis of MSA.[55] Both central and peripheral autonomic networks controlling cardiovascular, respiratory, urogenital, gastrointestinal, and sudomotor functions are disrupted. Importantly, autonomic dysfunction can precede the onset of motor symptoms in up to 50% of the patients.[56,57] Urogenital dysfunction precedes orthostatic hypotension in most patients.[56,58,59] Erectile dysfunction, which may precede the onset of urinary symptoms, occurs in up to 97% of men with definite MSA and is reported as the first symptom in up to 48% of patients.[56,58] For female patients, sexual dysfunction is more difficult to assess; therefore, data are missing.

Orthostatic hypotension occurs less frequently than urogenital dysfunction. Symptoms of orthostatic hypotension, such as syncope, postural dizziness, or pain centered in the neck and shoulders (so-called coat-hanger ache), result from cerebral and muscular hypoperfusion. The clinical diagnosis of probable MSA requires a reduction in systolic blood pressure by at least 30 mm Hg or in diastolic blood pressure by at least 15 mm Hg after 3 min of standing compared with a previous 3-minute interval in the recumbent position.[55]

Respiratory symptoms, such as stridor, sleep-related breathing disorders, and respiratory insufficiency, are part of the clinical spectrum of MSA. Deep inspiratory sighs and involuntary gasps are seen commonly in clinical practice and also may be noted by the carers; however, there are insufficient published data regarding those symptoms. Inspiratory stridor, especially at night, is commonly attributed to laryngeal abductor paralysis but might instead result from dystonia of the vocal cords.[60–62] Inspiratory stridor has been documented in 9% to 69% of MSA patients. The frequency of obstructive sleep apnea ranges from 15% to 37% and carries a far worse prognosis than common idiopathic sleep apnea. Central sleep apnea is less common and tends to occur at later stages.[58,63–66]

Other clinical features and "red flags"

- REM sleep behavior disorder (RBD) is very common in MSA and, together with autonomic dysfunction, represents a premotor stage in MSA in many patients and should alert for diagnosis. RBD is also seen, but less frequently, in PD and quite rarely in PSP.[56,58,67–71]
- Early falls and postural instability, also seen in PSP, may also be a feature of MSA and can cause diagnostic difficulties with PSP. Careful examination of eye movement abnormalities and early frontal-subcortical dysfunction which is common in PSP but not in MSA, will aid the diagnosis.
- Dystonia affecting the orofacial muscles occurring spontaneously, or when levodopa treatment is initiated, is rarely the case in PSP or CBD and is a "red flag" for MSA diagnosis.
- Raynaud phenomenon is a common in MSA.
- Freezing of gait may be prominent, early, and severe, causing diagnostic difficulties with PSP and in particular the PAGF phenotype.
- Clinical features that do not support the diagnosis of MSA include early dementia, hallucinations, early slowness of saccades, clinically significant neuropathy, age of onset greater than 75 years, and extensive white matter changes in brain imaging.[72] Especially with regard to dementia, it is considered a nonsupporting feature for the diagnosis of MSA. However, accumulating evidence suggests that there may be cognitive impairment in MSA mainly of frontal-executive dysfunction. However, frank, prominent, early dementia should lead the clinician to other diagnoses.

Investigations

Cardiovascular autonomic function tests may detect early autonomic dysfunction and may also be abnormal in PD, but severe abnormalities within the first 2 to 3 years of symptoms are frequent in MSA and infrequent in PD.[59,73–76]

In MRI, degeneration of the middle cerebellar peduncles (MCP) and pons can cause a cruciform appearance in the pons on axial MRI slices called the "hot cross bun sign,"[27] which is, however, not pathognomonic of MSA.[77] There may be putaminal atrophy with hypointensity and a hyperintense lateral slit-like rim to the putamen.[53,78,79] There may be cerebellar atrophy and hyperintensity of the MCP. In a retrospective study on 13 definite MSA patients, only 50% had putaminal atrophy and 25% had the hyperintense putaminal rim. MCP hyperintensity was found in 50% of the MSA patients, and the hot cross bun sign was found in 58.3%.[27] These findings suggest that better and novel MRI techniques are needed to improve sensitivity and to be able to serve as specific biomarkers for monitoring disease progression.

With regard to functional imaging, DATscans are abnormal in all MSA, PSP, and PD. MIBG scintigraphy is abnormal in PD because of postganglionic sympathetic denervation, but is typically normal in MSA.[28] IBZM SPECT is normal in PD, and abnormal in MSA (but also in PSP and CBD).[29] FDG-PET shows hypometabolism in putamen, pons, and cerebellum and is also considered an additional feature in the criteria for possible MSA.[48,55]

Specific proteins in the cerebrospinal fluid (CSF) may be proven valuable biomarkers in the future. Mollenhauer and colleagues[30] found that a CSF mean α-synuclein levels and not total τ, or Ab42 levels differentiated PD and MSA from neurologic controls (70% sensitivity, 53% specificity). Moreover, a combination of α-synuclein and phosphorylated τ/total τ could differentiate PD from MSA with a sensitivity of 90% and a specificity of 71% in another study.[80] The Flt3 ligand, a cytokine that acts as a neurotrophic and antiapoptotic factor in CNS, could alone differentiate between PD and MSA with a sensitivity of 99% and a specificity of 95%.[80] However, this was not confirmed in a recent study.[81] Confirmation studies on large prospective cohorts are warranted.

Pathology

MSA is a member of a diverse group of neurodegenerative disorders termed α-synucleinopathies, due to the presence of abnormal α-synuclein-positive cytoplasmic inclusions in oligodendrocytes, termed glial cytoplasmic inclusions, mainly found in the basal ganglia, cerebellar structures, and motor cortex. Neuropathologic examination often reveals gross abnormalities of the striatonigral and/or olivopontocerebellar systems, which on microscopic examination are associated with severe neuronal loss, gliosis, myelin pallor, and axonal degeneration.[82,83]

Treatment

Treatment of MSA is currently only symptomatic.

- Parkinsonism: Many patients with MSA show some levodopa or dopamine-agonists response, but this is usually not sustained, may cause craniocervical dystonia, and may worsen postural hypotension. Amantadine may be helpful for gait disturbance.
- Orthostatic hypotension: Conservative measures, such as head-up tilt to the bed at night, high-salt diet, and elastic compression stockings, may be helpful. Pharmacologic measures include fludrocortisone, midodrine (α1-receptor agonist), pyridostigmine, and droxidopa,[84] for postprandial hypotension.
- Urinary dysfunction: Assessment with urodynamics is essential to characterize the nature of bladder dysfunction. Oxybutynin or tolderidone can be helpful for neurogenic bladder, and clean intermittent self-catheterization is helpful for those with a large residual volume. Desmopressin can be helpful for nocturnal polyuria.
- Erectile dysfunction: Sildenafil may be efficacious, but can dramatically worsen postural hypotension. Intracavernosal injections (alprostadil, papaverine) or penile implants may be effective without worsening hypotension.
- Emotional incontinence: May be helped by selective SSRIs or tricyclic antidepressants.
- Recent large controlled studies with rasagiline and rifampicin have shown no effect.[85,86] Neuroprotective or disease-modifying approaches such as with intravenous immunoglobulin and intra-arterial or intravenous injections of autologous mesenchymal stem cells have shown promising results in pilot studies, but need further confirmation.[87,88] Future studies such as α-syn targeting antibodies are currently planned.[89]

"Atypical" Atypical Parkinsonism

Clinicopathologic studies have shown that misdiagnosis occurs mainly between PD and AP as well as further conditions, such as FTD, Alzheimer disease, and others. As summarized above, clinical features and "red flags" will mainly help to distinguish between these disorders, in the absence of reliable biomarkers. However, there are several further conditions that may mimic the classic phenotypes of PSP, CBD, and MSA. With the advent in genetics, the list of these conditions is growing. For example, *PGRN*, *C9ORF72*, and *MAPT* mutation carriers may present with RS or CBS phenotypes, while spinocerebellar ataxias and fragile-X-tremor ataxia syndrome may cause confusion with MSA. Sporadic and genetic prion disorders may present with AP phenotypes, as well as mitochondrial and some neurometabolic disorders (Gaucher disease, Niemann-Pick C, cerebrotendinous xanthomatosis) (**Table 2**).[2] The age of onset, the tempo of progression, a detailed family history, and careful examination for associated clinical features will point the diagnosis toward particular conditions.

Case Study

Case 1 (Video 1): This 70-year-old woman developed a rest-tremor on her right hand at the age of 62. On examination at this age, there was right-sided bradykinesia and reduced arm-swing on the right. She had mild upward gaze restriction but saccade velocity was normal. She was diagnosed with PD and treated with levodopa, with only mild improvement of her tremor. At the age of 68, she started falling backwards. On examination at this age, she presented with supranuclear gaze palsy, axial rigidity, postural instability, and frontal signs. The asymmetric tremor was still present (although not the typical pill-rolling tremor), and the diagnosis was revised to PSP-P. This case highlights the problems in diagnosing some patients with AP early, and the importance of regular follow-up to pick up signs unusual for PD.

FINANCIAL DISCLOSURE

M. Stamelou serves on the editorial board for *Movement Disorders Journal* and *Frontiers in Movement Disorders*, received speaker honoraria from Actelion Pharmaceuticals, K.P. Bhatia serves on the editorial boards of Movement Disorders and Therapeutic Advances in Neurological Disorders; receives royalties from the publication of Oxford Specialist Handbook of Parkinson's Disease and Other Movement Disorders (Oxford University Press, 2008); received speaker honoraria and travel from GlaxoSmithKline, Ipsen, Merz Pharmaceuticals LLC, Novartis, Sun Pharmaceutical Industries Ltd; personal compensation for scientific advisory board for GSK and Boehringer Ingelheim; received research support from Ipsen and from the Halley Stewart Trust through Dystonia Society UK, and the Wellcome Trust MRC strategic neurodegenerative disease initiative award (Ref. number WT089698), a grant from the Dystonia Coalition, and a grant from Parkinson's UK (Ref. number G-1009).

SUPPLEMENTARY DATA

Supplementary data related to this article can be found online at http://dx.doi.org/10.1016/j.ncl.2014.09.012.

REFERENCES

1. Gibb WR, Lees AJ. The significance of the Lewy body in the diagnosis of idiopathic Parkinson's disease. Neuropathol Appl Neurobiol 1989;15:27–44.

2. Stamelou M, Quinn NP, Bhatia KP. "Atypical" atypical parkinsonism: new genetic conditions presenting with features of progressive supranuclear palsy, corticobasal degeneration, or multiple system atrophy-a diagnostic guide. Mov Disord 2013;28:1184–99.
3. Josephs KA, Petersen RC, Knopman DS, et al. Clinicopathologic analysis of frontotemporal and corticobasal degenerations and PSP. Neurology 2006;66:41–8.
4. Josephs KA, Whitwell JL, Boeve BF, et al. Anatomical differences between CBS-corticobasal degeneration and CBS-Alzheimer's disease. Mov Disord 2010;25:1246–52.
5. Nath U, Ben-Shlomo Y, Thomson RG, et al. Clinical features and natural history of progressive supranuclear palsy: a clinical cohort study. Neurology 2003;60:910–6.
6. Kertesz A, McMonagle P. Behavior and cognition in corticobasal degeneration and progressive supranuclear palsy. J Neurol Sci 2010;289:138–43.
7. Litvan I, Mangone CA, McKee A, et al. Natural history of progressive supranuclear palsy (Steele-Richardson-Olszewski syndrome) and clinical predictors of survival: a clinicopathological study. J Neurol Neurosurg Psychiatr 1996;60:615–20.
8. Ling H, O'Sullivan SS, Holton JL, et al. Does corticobasal degeneration exist? A clinicopathological re-evaluation. Brain 2010;133:2045–57.
9. Williams DR, de Silva R, Paviour DC, et al. Characteristics of two distinct clinical phenotypes in pathologically proven progressive supranuclear palsy: Richardson's syndrome and PSP-parkinsonism. Brain 2005;128:1247–58.
10. Williams DR, Lees AJ. Progressive supranuclear palsy: clinicopathological concepts and diagnostic challenges. Lancet Neurol 2009;8:270–9.
11. Stamelou M, Alonso-Canovas A, Bhatia KP. Dystonia in corticobasal degeneration: a review of the literature on 404 pathologically proven cases. Mov Disord 2012;27:696–702.
12. Armstrong MJ, Litvan I, Lang AE, et al. Criteria for the diagnosis of corticobasal degeneration. Neurology 2013;80:496–503.
13. Morris HR, Osaki Y, Holton J, et al. Tau exon 10 +16 mutation FTDP-17 presenting clinically as sporadic young onset PSP. Neurology 2003;61:102–4.
14. Boeve BF, Hutton M. Refining frontotemporal dementia with parkinsonism linked to chromosome 17: introducing FTDP-17 (MAPT) and FTDP-17 (PGRN). Arch Neurol 2008;65:460–4.
15. Hoglinger GU, Melhem NM, Dickson DW, et al. Identification of common variants influencing risk of the tauopathy progressive supranuclear palsy. Nat Genet 2011;43:699–705.
16. Stamelou M, Pilatus U, Reuss A, et al. In vivo evidence for cerebral depletion in high-energy phosphates in progressive supranuclear palsy. J Cereb Blood Flow Metab 2009;29:861–70.
17. Litvan I, Campbell G, Mangone CA, et al. Which clinical features differentiate progressive supranuclear palsy (Steele-Richardson-Olszewski syndrome) from related disorders? A clinicopathological study. Brain 1997;120(Pt 1):65–74.
18. Osaki Y, Ben-Shlomo Y, Lees AJ, et al. Accuracy of clinical diagnosis of progressive supranuclear palsy. Mov Disord 2004;19:181–9.
19. Marx S, Respondek G, Stamelou M, et al. Validation of mobile eye-tracking as novel and efficient means for differentiating progressive supranuclear palsy from Parkinson's disease. Front Behav Neurosci 2012;6:88.
20. Dubois B, Slachevsky A, Litvan I, et al. The FAB: a Frontal Assessment Battery at bedside. Neurology 2000;55:1621–6.

21. Litvan I. Cognitive disturbances in progressive supranuclear palsy. J Neural Transm Suppl 1994;42:69–78.
22. Paviour DC, Winterburn D, Simmonds S, et al. Can the frontal assessment battery (FAB) differentiate bradykinetic rigid syndromes? Relation of the FAB to formal neuropsychological testing. Neurocase 2005;11:274–82.
23. Respondek G, Roeber S, Kretzschmar H, et al. Accuracy of the National Institute for Neurological Disorders and Stroke/Society for Progressive Supranuclear Palsy and Neuroprotection and Natural History in Parkinson Plus Syndromes Criteria for the Diagnosis of Progressive Supranuclear Palsy. Mov Disord 2013;28(4):504–9.
24. Stamelou M, Knake S, Oertel WH, et al. Magnetic resonance imaging in progressive supranuclear palsy. J Neurol 2011;258:549–58.
25. Longoni G, Agosta F, Kostic VS, et al. MRI measurements of brainstem structures in patients with Richardson's syndrome, progressive supranuclear palsy-parkinsonism, and Parkinson's disease. Mov Disord 2011;26:247–55.
26. Wu LJ, Sitburana O, Davidson A, et al. Applause sign in parkinsonian disorders and Huntington's disease. Mov Disord 2008;23:2307–11.
27. Massey LA, Micallef C, Paviour DC, et al. Conventional magnetic resonance imaging in confirmed progressive supranuclear palsy and multiple system atrophy. Mov Disord 2012;27:1754–62.
28. Orimo S, Suzuki M, Inaba A, et al. 123I-MIBG myocardial scintigraphy for differentiating Parkinson's disease from other neurodegenerative parkinsonism: a systematic review and meta-analysis. Parkinsonism Relat Disord 2012;18:494–500.
29. Vlaar AM, de Nijs T, Kessels AG, et al. Diagnostic value of 123I-ioflupane and 123I-iodobenzamide SPECT scans in 248 patients with parkinsonian syndromes. Eur Neurol 2008;59:258–66.
30. Mollenhauer B, Locascio JJ, Schulz-Schaeffer W, et al. Alpha-Synuclein and tau concentrations in cerebrospinal fluid of patients presenting with parkinsonism: a cohort study. Lancet Neurol 2011;10:230–40.
31. Stamelou M, Hoeglinger GU. Atypical parkinsonism: an update. Curr Opin Neurol 2013;26:401–5.
32. Boxer AL, Lang AE, Grossman M, et al. Davunetide in patients with progressive supranuclear palsy: a randomised, double-blind, placebo-controlled phase 2/3 trial. Lancet Neurol 2014;13:676–85.
33. Dickson DW, Ahmed Z, Algom AA, et al. Neuropathology of variants of progressive supranuclear palsy. Curr Opin Neurol 2010;23:394–400.
34. Stamelou M, de Silva R, Arias-Carrion O, et al. Rational therapeutic approaches to progressive supranuclear palsy. Brain 2010;133:1578–90.
35. Stamelou M, Reuss A, Pilatus U, et al. Short-term effects of coenzyme Q10 in progressive supranuclear palsy: a randomized, placebo-controlled trial. Mov Disord 2008;23:942–9.
36. Hoglinger GU, Huppertz HJ, Wagenpfeil S, et al. Tideglusib reduces progression of brain atrophy in progressive supranuclear palsy in a randomized trial. Mov Disord 2014;29:479–87.
37. Tolosa E, Litvan I, Hoglinger GU, et al. A phase 2 trial of the GSK-3 inhibitor tideglusib in progressive supranuclear palsy. Mov Disord 2014;29:470–8.
38. Colosimo C, Morgante L, Antonini A, et al. Non-motor symptoms in atypical and secondary parkinsonism: the PRIAMO study. J Neurol 2010;257:5–14.
39. Kouri N, Murray ME, Hassan A, et al. Neuropathological features of corticobasal degeneration presenting as corticobasal syndrome or Richardson syndrome. Brain 2011;134:3264–75.

40. Lee SE, Rabinovici GD, Mayo MC, et al. Clinicopathological correlations in corticobasal degeneration. Ann Neurol 2011;70:327–40.
41. Borroni B, Alberici A, Agosti C, et al. Pattern of behavioral disturbances in corticobasal degeneration syndrome and progressive supranuclear palsy. Int Psychogeriatr 2009;21:463–8.
42. Lee W, Williams DR, Storey E. Cognitive testing in the diagnosis of parkinsonian disorders: a critical appraisal of the literature. Mov Disord 2012;27:1243–54.
43. Rittman T, Ghosh BC, McColgan P, et al. The Addenbrooke's Cognitive Examination for the differential diagnosis and longitudinal assessment of patients with parkinsonian disorders. J Neurol Neurosurg Psychiatr 2013;84(5):544–51.
44. Chand P, Grafman J, Dickson D, et al. Alzheimer's disease presenting as corticobasal syndrome. Mov Disord 2006;21:2018–22.
45. Hassan A, Whitwell JL, Josephs KA. The corticobasal syndrome-Alzheimer's disease conundrum. Expert Rev Neurother 2011;11:1569–78.
46. Schrag A, Good CD, Miszkiel K, et al. Differentiation of atypical parkinsonian syndromes with routine MRI. Neurology 2000;54:697–702.
47. Hellwig S, Amtage F, Kreft A, et al. [^{18}F]FDG-PET is superior to [^{123}I]IBZM-SPECT for the differential diagnosis of parkinsonism. Neurology 2012;79:1314–22.
48. Tripathi M, Dhawan V, Peng S, et al. Differential diagnosis of parkinsonian syndromes using F-18 fluorodeoxyglucose positron emission tomography. Neuroradiology 2013;55(4):483–92.
49. Zhao P, Zhang B, Gao S. 18F-FDG PET study on the idiopathic Parkinson's disease from several parkinsonian-plus syndromes. Parkinsonism Relat Disord 2012;18(Suppl 1):S60–2.
50. Wenning GK, Geser F, Krismer F, et al. The natural history of multiple system atrophy: a prospective European cohort study. Lancet Neurol 2013;12:264–74.
51. Ozawa T. The COQ2 mutations in Japanese multiple system atrophy: impact on the pathogenesis and phenotypic variation. Mov Disord 2014;29:184.
52. Multiple-System Atrophy Research Collaboration. Mutations in COQ2 in familial and sporadic multiple-system atrophy. N Engl J Med 2013;369:233–44.
53. Batla A, Stamelou M, Mensikova K, et al. Markedly asymmetric presentation in multiple system atrophy. Parkinsonism Relat Disord 2013;19:901–5.
54. Wenning GK, Ben Shlomo Y, Magalhaes M, et al. Clinical features and natural history of multiple system atrophy. An analysis of 100 cases. Brain 1994;117(Pt 4):835–45.
55. Gilman S, Wenning GK, Low PA, et al. Second consensus statement on the diagnosis of multiple system atrophy. Neurology 2008;71:670–6.
56. Iodice V, Lipp A, Ahlskog JE, et al. Autopsy confirmed multiple system atrophy cases: Mayo experience and role of autonomic function tests. J Neurol Neurosurg Psychiatr 2012;83:453–9.
57. Schmidt C, Herting B, Prieur S, et al. Autonomic dysfunction in different subtypes of multiple system atrophy. Mov Disord 2008;23:1766–72.
58. Jecmenica-Lukic M, Poewe W, Tolosa E, et al. Premotor signs and symptoms of multiple system atrophy. Lancet Neurol 2012;11:361–8.
59. Kimpinski K, Iodice V, Burton DD, et al. The role of autonomic testing in the differentiation of Parkinson's disease from multiple system atrophy. J Neurol Sci 2012;317:92–6.
60. Benarroch EE, Schmeichel AM, Sandroni P, et al. Involvement of vagal autonomic nuclei in multiple system atrophy and Lewy body disease. Neurology 2006;66:378–83.

61. Magalhaes M, Wenning GK, Daniel SE, et al. Autonomic dysfunction in pathologically confirmed multiple system atrophy and idiopathic Parkinson's disease–a retrospective comparison. Acta Neurol Scand 1995;91:98–102.
62. Wenning GK, Tison F, Ben Shlomo Y, et al. Multiple system atrophy: a review of 203 pathologically proven cases. Mov Disord 1997;12:133–47.
63. Munschauer FE, Loh L, Bannister R, et al. Abnormal respiration and sudden death during sleep in multiple system atrophy with autonomic failure. Neurology 1990;40:677–9.
64. Kitae S, Murata Y, Tachiki N, et al. Assessment of cardiovascular autonomic dysfunction in multiple system atrophy. Clin Auton Res 2001;11:39–44.
65. Plazzi G, Cortelli P, Montagna P, et al. REM sleep behaviour disorder differentiates pure autonomic failure from multiple system atrophy with autonomic failure. J Neurol Neurosurg Psychiatr 1998;64:683–5.
66. Vetrugno R, D'Angelo R, Cortelli P, et al. Impaired cortical and autonomic arousal during sleep in multiple system atrophy. Clin Neurophysiol 2007;118:2512–8.
67. Ahmed Z, Asi YT, Lees AJ, et al. Identification and quantification of oligodendrocyte precursor cells in multiple system atrophy, progressive supranuclear palsy and Parkinson's disease. Brain Pathol 2013;23(3):263–73.
68. Gilman S, Koeppe RA, Chervin RD, et al. REM sleep behavior disorder is related to striatal monoaminergic deficit in MSA. Neurology 2003;61:29–34.
69. Iranzo A, Santamaria J, Rye DB, et al. Characteristics of idiopathic REM sleep behavior disorder and that associated with MSA and PD. Neurology 2005;65: 247–52.
70. Plazzi G, Corsini R, Provini F, et al. REM sleep behavior disorders in multiple system atrophy. Neurology 1997;48:1094–7.
71. Tison F, Wenning GK, Quinn NP, et al. REM sleep behaviour disorder as the presenting symptom of multiple system atrophy. J Neurol Neurosurg Psychiatr 1995;58:379–80.
72. Gilman S, Low P, Quinn N, et al. Consensus statement on the diagnosis of multiple system atrophy. American Autonomic Society and American Academy of Neurology. Clin Auton Res 1998;8:359–62.
73. Asahina M, Akaogi Y, Yamanaka Y, et al. Differences in skin sympathetic involvements between two chronic autonomic disorders: multiple system atrophy and pure autonomic failure. Parkinsonism Relat Disord 2009;15:347–50.
74. Asahina M, Young TM, Bleasdale-Barr K, et al. Differences in overshoot of blood pressure after head-up tilt in two groups with chronic autonomic failure: pure autonomic failure and multiple system atrophy. J Neurol 2005;252:72–7.
75. Brisinda D, Sorbo AR, Di Giacopo R, et al. Cardiovascular autonomic nervous system evaluation in Parkinson disease and multiple system atrophy. J Neurol Sci 2014;336:197–202.
76. Deguchi K, Ikeda K, Shimamura M, et al. Assessment of autonomic dysfunction of multiple system atrophy with laryngeal abductor paralysis as an early manifestation. Clin Neurol Neurosurg 2007;109:892–5.
77. Marrannes J, Mulleners E. Hot cross bun sign in a patient with SCA-2. JBR-BTR 2009;92:263.
78. Han YH, Lee JH, Kang BM, et al. Topographical differences of brain iron deposition between progressive supranuclear palsy and parkinsonian variant multiple system atrophy. J Neurol Sci 2013;325:29–35.
79. Tha KK, Terae S, Tsukahara A, et al. Hyperintense putaminal rim at 1.5 T: prevalence in normal subjects and distinguishing features from multiple system atrophy. BMC Neurol 2012;12:39.

80. Shi M, Bradner J, Hancock AM, et al. Cerebrospinal fluid biomarkers for Parkinson disease diagnosis and progression. Ann Neurol 2011;69:570–80.
81. Silajdzic E, Constantinescu R, Holmberg B, et al. Flt3 ligand does not differentiate between Parkinsonian disorders. Mov Disord 2014;29(10):1319–22.
82. Ahmed Z, Asi YT, Sailer A, et al. The neuropathology, pathophysiology and genetics of multiple system atrophy. Neuropathol Appl Neurobiol 2012;38:4–24.
83. Dickson DW, Lin W, Liu WK, et al. Multiple system atrophy: a sporadic synucleinopathy. Brain Pathol 1999;9:721–32.
84. Kaufmann H, Freeman R, Biaggioni I, et al, On behalf of the NOH301 Investigators. Droxidopa for neurogenic orthostatic hypotension: a randomized, placebo-controlled, phase 3 trial. Neurology 2014;83(4):328–35.
85. Poewe W, Barone P, Gliadi N, et al. A randomized, placebo-controlled clinical trial to assess the effects of rasagiline in patients with multiple system atrophy of the parkinsonian subtype. Mov Disord 2012;27:1182.
86. Low PA, Robertson D, Gilman S, et al. Efficacy and safety of rifampicin for multiple system atrophy: a randomised, double-blind, placebo-controlled trial. Lancet Neurol 2014;13:268–75.
87. Novak P, Williams A, Ravin P, et al. Treatment of multiple system atrophy using intravenous immunoglobulin. BMC Neurol 2012;12:131.
88. Lee PH, Lee JE, Kim HS, et al. A randomized trial of mesenchymal stem cells in multiple system atrophy. Ann Neurol 2012;72:32–40.
89. Palma JA, Kaufmann H. Novel therapeutic approaches in multiple system atrophy. Clin Auton Res 2014. [Epub ahead of print].
90. Papapetropoulos S, Gonzalez J, Mash DC. Natural history of progressive supranuclear palsy: a clinicopathologic study from a population of brain donors. Eur Neurol 2005;54:1–9.
91. Weeks RA, Scaravilli F, Lees AJ, et al. Cerebral amyloid angiopathy and motor neurone disease presenting with a progressive supranuclear palsy-like syndrome. Mov Disord 2003;18:331–6.
92. Petrovic IN, Martin-Bastida A, Massey L, et al. MM2 subtype of sporadic Creutzfeldt-Jakob disease may underlie the clinical presentation of progressive supranuclear palsy. J Neurol 2013;260(4):1031–6.
93. Lannuzel A, Hoglinger GU, Verhaeghe S, et al. Atypical parkinsonism in Guadeloupe: a common risk factor for two closely related phenotypes? Brain 2007;130:816–27.
94. Gilbert RM, Fahn S, Mitsumoto H, et al. Parkinsonism and motor neuron diseases: twenty-seven patients with diverse overlap syndromes. Mov Disord 2010;25:1868–75.
95. Kasahata N, Uchihara T, Orimo S, et al. Limbic and nigral Lewy bodies and Alzheimer's disease pathology mimicking progressive supranuclear palsy in a 75-year-old man with preserved cardiac uptake of MIBG. J Alzheimers Dis 2012;32(4):889–94.
96. Josephs KA, Holton JL, Rossor MN, et al. Neurofilament inclusion body disease: a new proteinopathy? Brain 2003;126:2291–303.
97. Yokota O, Tsuchiya K, Terada S, et al. Basophilic inclusion body disease and neuronal intermediate filament inclusion disease: a comparative clinicopathological study. Acta Neuropathol 2008;115:561–75.
98. Norlinah IM, Bhatia KP, Ostergaard K, et al. Primary lateral sclerosis mimicking atypical parkinsonism. Mov Disord 2007;22:2057–62.

99. Bonelli RM, Cummings JL. Frontal-subcortical dementias. Neurologist 2008;14: 100–7.
100. Choi SM, Kim BC, Nam TS, et al. Midbrain atrophy in vascular Parkinsonism. Eur Neurol 2011;65:296–301.
101. Daniel SE, de Bruin VM, Lees AJ. The clinical and pathological spectrum of Steele-Richardson-Olszewski syndrome (progressive supranuclear palsy): a re-appraisal. Brain 1995;118(Pt 3):759–70.
102. Favaretto S, Ferrari S, Battistin L, et al. Apraxia of eyelid closure in autopsy-confirmed vascular progressive supranuclear palsy. Parkinsonism Relat Disord 2011;17:708–9.
103. Mokri B, Ahlskog JE, Fulgham JR, et al. Syndrome resembling PSP after surgical repair of ascending aorta dissection or aneurysm. Neurology 2004;62: 971–3.
104. Bhatia KP, Lee MS, Rinne JO, et al. Corticobasal degeneration look-alikes. Adv Neurol 2000;82:169–82.
105. Engelen M, Westhoff D, de Gans J, et al. A 64-year old man presenting with carotid artery occlusion and corticobasal syndrome: a case report. J Med Case Rep 2011;5:357.
106. Horvath J, Burkhard PR, Bouras C, et al. Etiologies of parkinsonism in a century-long autopsy-based cohort. Brain Pathol 2013;23(1):28–33.
107. Lagier JC, Lepidi H, Raoult D, et al. Systemic Tropheryma whipplei: clinical presentation of 142 patients with infections diagnosed or confirmed in a reference center. Medicine (Baltimore) 2010;89:337–45.
108. Mohamed W, Neil E, Kupsky WJ, et al. Isolated intracranial Whipple's disease–report of a rare case and review of the literature. J Neurol Sci 2011;308:1–8.
109. Murialdo A, Marchese R, Abbruzzese G, et al. Neurosyphilis presenting as progressive supranuclear palsy. Mov Disord 2000;15:730–1.
110. Page NG, Lean JS, Sanders MD. Vertical supranuclear gaze palsy with secondary syphilis. J Neurol Neurosurg Psychiatr 1982;45:86–8.
111. Jang W, Kim JS, Ahn JY, et al. Reversible progressive supranuclear palsy-like phenotype as an initial manifestation of HIV infection. Neurol Sci 2011;33(5): 1169–71.
112. Benito-Leon J, Alvarez-Linera J, Louis ED. Neurosyphilis masquerading as corticobasal degeneration. Mov Disord 2004;19:1367–70.
113. Van Zandycke M, Dehaene I. A "cortico-basal degeneration"-like syndrome as first sign of progressive multifocal leukoencephalopathy. Acta Neurol Belg 2000; 100:242–5.
114. Adams C, McKeon A, Silber MH, et al. Narcolepsy, REM sleep behavior disorder, and supranuclear gaze palsy associated with Ma1 and Ma2 antibodies and tonsillar carcinoma. Arch Neurol 2011;68:521–4.
115. Castle J, Sakonju A, Dalmau J, et al. Anti-Ma2-associated encephalitis with normal FDG-PET: a case of pseudo-Whipple's disease. Nat Clin Pract Neurol 2006;2:566–72 [quiz: 573].
116. Jankovic J. Progressive supranuclear palsy: paraneoplastic effect of bronchial carcinoma. Neurology 1985;35:446–7.
117. Tan JH, Goh BC, Tambyah PA, et al. Paraneoplastic progressive supranuclear palsy syndrome in a patient with B-cell lymphoma. Parkinsonism Relat Disord 2005;11:187–91.
118. Peeters E, Vanacker P, Woodhall M, et al. Supranuclear gaze palsy in glycine receptor antibody-positive progressive encephalomyelitis with rigidity and myoclonus. Mov Disord 2012;27(14):1830–2.

119. Schlegel U, Clarenbach P, Cordt A, et al. Cerebral sarcoidosis presenting as supranuclear gaze palsy with hypokinetic rigid syndrome. Mov Disord 1989;4: 274–7.
120. Martino D, Chew NK, Mir P, et al. Atypical movement disorders in antiphospholipid syndrome. Mov Disord 2006;21:944–9.
121. Morris HR, Lees AJ. Primary antiphospholipid syndrome presenting as a corticobasal degeneration syndrome. Mov Disord 1999;14:530–2.

Medical and Surgical Treatment of Tremors

Susanne A. Schneider, MD, PhD*, Günther Deuschl, MD

KEYWORDS

• Tremor • Essential tremor • Dystonic tremor • Beta blocker • Primidone
• Topiramate • Deep brain stimulation

KEY POINTS

- Propranolol, primidone, and topiramate are the drugs of choice for essential arm tremor with a mean effect size of approximately 50%. In severe essential tremor, deep brain stimulation should be considered.
- There are only few data for dystonic tremor and tremor associated with dystonia. Anticholinergics are recommended, but controlled trials are needed.
- For head and voice tremor, consider botulinum toxin.
- Cerebellar tremor is often drug-refractory. Deep brain stimulation may be useful.
- Nonpharmacological approaches, such as orthoses or physical therapy, are not part of routine practice.
- Interesting new experimental treatments include noninvasive stereotactically guided lesioning using ultrasound, as recently described.

OVERVIEW: NATURE OF THE PROBLEM

Tremor is a hyperkinetic movement disorder characterized by rhythmic oscillations of one or more body parts. It most commonly affects the hands and arms. Other body parts including the legs, head, jaw, chin, palate, voice and trunk also may be affected. Tremor severity may range from asymptomatic or subtle to severe and most disabling. In fact, many patients with mild tremor do not have subjective impairment and may not

Disclosures: S.A. Schneider was supported by the Else Kröner-Fresenius-Stiftung (2013_A37), the Eva Luise und Horst Köhler Stiftung, and Novartis Pharma GmbH. She received royalties from Oxford University Press and an honorarium from Teva for lecturing. G. Deuschl has received lecture fees from UCB, Medtronic, and Desitin and has been serving as a consultant for Medtronic, Sapiens, Boston Scientific, and Britannica. He received royalties from Thieme publishers. He is a government employee and receives, through his institution, funding for his research from the German Research Council, the German Ministery of Education and Health, and Medtronic.
Department of Neurology, University-Hospital Schleswig-Holstein, Christian-Albrechts-University Kiel, Campus Kiel, Schittenhelmstr. 10, Kiel 24105, Germany
* Corresponding author.
E-mail address: s.schneider@neurologie.uni-kiel.de

Neurol Clin 33 (2015) 57–75
http://dx.doi.org/10.1016/j.ncl.2014.09.005 neurologic.theclinics.com

seek medical advice. In our population-based cohort study carried out in Germany, only 27% of patients ever consulted a doctor for their tremor.[1] In a North American study, only 8.3% of patients with tremor had been prescribed tremor medication.[2] On the other hand, the most severely affected cases may be unable to even eat or drink without help, and tremor may cause considerable impact on quality of life.[3,4]

DIFFERENT TYPES OF TREMOR

Different types of tremor are recognized. The diagnosis is based on the clinical history and the examination. There are no specific biological markers or diagnostic tests for primary tremor (ie, tremor without identifiable secondary cause).

The most common form of tremor is essential tremor (ET). With a prevalence of approximately 0.9%[5] in people older than 65 years, ET also accounts for one of the most common neurologic diseases. However, reported prevalence rates show broad variation for ET, ranging from 10 to 20,500 per 100,000, with an impressive variation factor of 2.050 between studies, and recruitment bias may lead to false results.[5,6] The vast majority of cases identified in large community studies have mild disease.[6]

Clinically, ET typically presents as postural arm tremor that may be accompanied by some tremor at rest or on intention as well as tremor of the head and voice in some, but there is little or no tremor in the lower limbs and torso.[7] Gross signs of ataxia, parkinsonism, and dystonia are by definition absent in ET.[7,8]

The most common cause of tremor at rest is parkinsonism, and these patients may have additional tremor on posture. The key feature of parkinsonism is, of course, bradykinesia and all patients with tremor should be carefully examined for its presence. A common form of kinetic (intention) tremor is cerebellar tremor, which may be due to a variety of underlying causes including strategic lesions in the context of multiple sclerosis.

Numerous studies have explored treatment responses in patients with tremor. Notably, most treatment studies have been conducted for ET, and these treatment algorithms may sometimes, in clinical practice, influence treatment of other tremor types due to lack of specific studies (ie, fragile x-associated tremor ataxia syndrome).[9] In this article, we review medical and surgical treatments options for common types of tremors.

It should be said that ET may cover different entities that are not separated by the current tremor investigation group (TRIG)- and movement disorders society (MDS) consensus criteria. This has to be kept in mind, as it may result in heterogeneity of study populations and results of treatment trials. There are thus recent efforts to better delineate and dissect these tremor forms,[10–12] and the Movement Disorders Society has commissioned a new task force on tremor to improve clinical practice and research into the field.

PATIENT EVALUATION OVERVIEW

Examination of a patient with tremor includes a full neurologic and medical examination. During the clinical examination, patients should be assessed at rest with the hands supported, when keeping the arms outstretched and when performing goal-directed movements (ie, rest tremor vs action tremor). Sometimes, tremor appears only after several seconds after a change in position, which is commonly seen in parkinsonian rest tremor (reemergent tremor). Tremor can be clinically further characterized according to the frequency (low, medium, or high frequency) and amplitude (small, medium, or high amplitude). The typical frequency of ET is 8 to 12 Hz; the typical frequency of Parkinson's disease tremor is 4 to 6 Hz. Furthermore, clinicians should observe which body parts are affected and whether the tremor in these regions is present constantly or intermittently (eg, only on distraction or when performing other tasks such as walking or counting). To exclude parkinsonism, patients should be carefully examined for signs of bradykinesia, which may contribute to impaired fine motor dexterity and motor coordination. Clinical signs for neuropathy, ataxia, dystonia, or central lesions may hint at specific tremors.

MANAGEMENT GOALS

With each patient, the aims for treatment have to be discussed. For most patients the treatment is symptomatic; treatment changes the course of the disease for only a few conditions and for only a very few tremor conditions a causal treatment is available (eg, Wilson disease). However, most patients will not tolerate side effects for long-term treatment. Treatment effects may be insufficient or contraindications may restrict treatment possibilities. Given that so many patients do not seek physicians' help tells us that just coping with tremor is the most popular handling of the problem. On the other hand, we need to seriously consider the problems of those who come to see us. The concerns of a banker and a farmer may be different. Even 2 farmers may have different requests. Invasive therapies, such as deep brain stimulation (DBS), should neither be indicated because we think the patient needs it nor should we uncritically accept the desire for these treatments of a patient with depression. On the other hand, possible bias against invasive therapies should not be guiding us to talk a patient into medication. The goal is to find the ideal management of tremor for each individual.

MEASUREMENTS OF TREMOR

Several rating scales have been developed to assess tremor severity. In a recent review by an MDS task force,[13] 5 of 7 identified and evaluated tremor rating scales were recommended for use. These include the Fahn-Tolosa-Marin (FTM), Bain and Findley Clinical Tremor Rating Scale, Bain and Findley Spirography Scale, version 2 of the washington heights-inwood genetic study of essential tremor (WHIGET) Tremor Rating Scale, and the rather recently developed the essential tremor rating assessment scale (TETRAS). Similarly, one of one activities of daily living (ADL)/disability scales (the Bain and Findley Tremor ADL Scale) and one quality-of-life scale (the Quality of Life in Essential Tremor Questionnaire [QUEST]), as well as one screening instrument (the WHIGET, version 1) were recommended by the committee after critical review.

Of these, the FTM tremor rating scale[14,15] incorporates evaluation of tremor (9 items, each rated 0 to 4), assessment of hand function (writing and pouring) (5 items), and ADLs (7 items). The new TETRAS scale[16] contains 9 performance items to rate action tremor in the head, face, voice, limbs, and trunk from 0 to 4 in half-point intervals. Head and limb tremor ratings are defined by specific amplitude ranges in centimeters.[16,17] Action tremor also can be reliably measured by assessment of spiral drawings[17] and the Bain and Findley Spirography Scale, which uses ratings from 0 to 10 for the assessment of Archimedes spirals (with samples shown in the original publication) is a useful tool. An assessment tool to objectively quantify is accelerometry, and there is good correlation between clinical ratings and log-transformed transducer measures of tremor, as predicted by the Weber-Fechner laws of psychophysics.[17] Considering minute-to-minute variations of tremor disorders, including ET,[18] in the future modern mobile applications[19,20] that allow long-duration monitoring may prove helpful.

PHARMACOLOGIC TREATMENT OPTIONS

As mentioned previously, most treatment studies have been conducted for ET. For the following section we chose to discuss limb, head, and voice tremor separately; followed by separate sections on dystonic tremor, orthostatic tremor, cerebellar tremor in the context of multiple sclerosis, Holmes and thalamic tremor, and finally functional (psychogenic) tremor.

TREATMENT OF LIMB TREMOR IN ESSENTIAL TREMOR

Numerous agents have been studied for potential benefit for ET over the years (**Fig. 1** for algorithm, and **Tables 1–3**) Many of these studies are, however, based on small patient numbers and relatively brief observation periods.

Two drugs, propranolol and primidone, appear to have sufficient Class I support for a Level A recommendation of efficacy and these are thus typically recommended as drugs of "first choice."[21–23] In addition, topiramate appears to be a reasonable choice. New drugs in the pipeline for ET tremor treatment include drugs analogous to alcohol (such as 1-octanol).[24,25]

Physicians should be aware that drugs used for tremor treatment in day-to-day practice may not always have approved indications, depending on the country, so when using medications "off label," published guidelines should be followed.

Propranolol and Other Beta-Blockers

Different beta-blockers, including propranolol,[26] metoprolol,[27,28] nadolol, atenolol, and sotalol, have been studied, mostly in crossover trials comparing propranolol (including long-acting suspensions) or other beta-blockers against placebo or

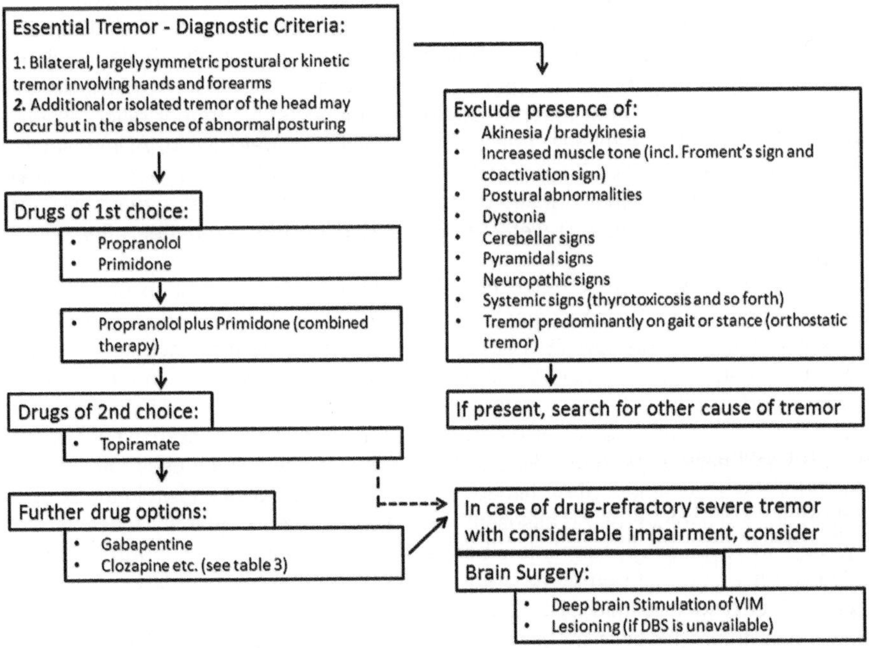

Fig. 1. Therapeutic algorithm for the treatment of essential tremor.

comparing beta-blockers in a head-to-head design or against other drugs (ie, gabapentin, primidone).

For propranolol, a literature search revealed 13 relevant double-blind placebo-controlled crossover trials[27,29–37] and 2 studies with a parallel design.[27,38] The average patient number recruited was 18. Short-term effects were studied over a mean duration of treatment (on stable dosages; 60–240 mg per day) of less than 3 weeks; whereas there are no randomized controlled trials (RCTs) on the long-term effects of propranolol in ET.

Improvement at the range of 60% to 70% was achieved and tremor amplitude was reduced to approximately 54% (range 32%–75%) measured by accelerometry.[27,29,30,32,34,35] Occasionally, response may be dramatic,[31] but there are no known predictors of response. Total daily dosages of 60 to 240 mg are adequate in most patients. Side effects of propranolol include bradycardia, syncope, fatigue, and erectile dysfunction, which are often dose limiting.

Other beta-blockers are likely efficacious, but none has been found to be superior to propranolol (**Fig. 2**).

Primidone

Six double-blind placebo-controlled crossover studies in ET were identified for primidone.[32,39–42] No study used a parallel design. Mean duration of treatment on stable dosages was 1 to 5 weeks. Data on long-term effects are scarce.[43,44] Benefit ranged around 60% for reduction in tremor amplitude.[32,39–42] Again, "dramatic response" has been described occasionally and at least 50% of patients experienced at least some benefit. Total daily dosages of 150 mg or less are often sufficient.

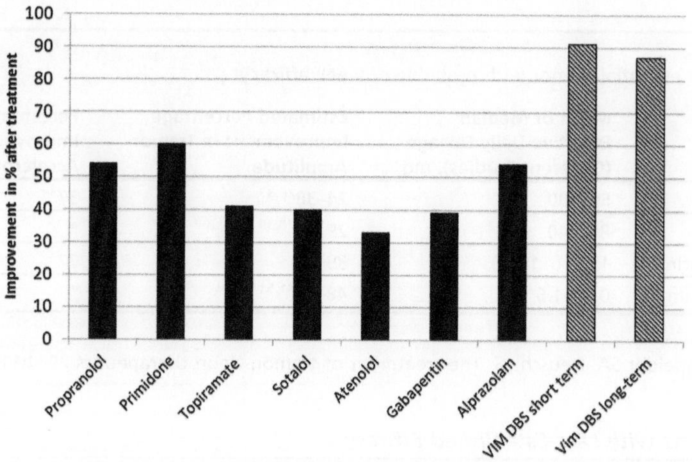

Fig. 2. The estimated percentage improvement of tremor amplitude of different interventions is shown. The values show the mean value of the studies reported here. Patients in the surgical studies usually have much higher tremor amplitudes. Tremor amplitude estimation is based on standard algorithms computed as change in tremor rating scale and change in tremor amplitude on accelerometry. (*From* Schneider SA, Deuschl G. The treatment of tremor. Neurotherapeutics 2014;11:128–38; with permission; *Data from* Elble RJ, Pullman SL, Matsumoto JY, et al. Tremor amplitude is logarithmically related to 4- and 5-point tremor rating scales. Brain 2006;129:2660–6; and Deuschl G, Raethjen J, Hellriegel H, et al. Treatment of patients with essential tremor. Lancet Neurol 2011;10:130.)

Side effects are common, including drowsiness, depression, and cognitive and behavioral effects. Acute toxic reactions to the first dose may occur, characterized by nausea, sedation, dizziness, and confusion, so that patients may refuse continuation of treatment. It is thus recommended to start on very low dosages (12.5 or 25 mg); although one study suggested that even a graduated titration schedule does not enhance tolerability.[45]

Table 1
Recommended drugs for essential tremor

Drug	Mean or Median Effective Daily Dosage	Estimated Percentage Improvement in Tremor Amplitude
Propranolol	40–240 (–320) mg/d	32–75
Primidone	<62,5–150 (–750) mg/d	42–76
Topiramate	100–333 mg	30–41

From Schneider SA, Deuschl G. The treatment of tremor. Neurotherapeutics 2014;11:129; with permission.

Topiramate

Four relevant studies[46–49] for topiramate were identified, including the largest tremor study[47] to date including more than 100 patients treated for 24 weeks in a multicenter, double-blind, placebo-controlled parallel-design trial. Target dose was 400 mg/d; the actual average final dose was 229 mg/d. Tremor ratings improved by approximately 30% (compared with 16% for placebo). Adverse events were common (32%), but similar to those seen with topiramate for other indications. Side effects include weight loss, paresthesias, and memory disturbances, as well as an increased risk of kidney stones.

Table 2
Drugs for essential tremor with probable or weak efficacy

Drug	Mean or Median Effective Daily Dosage (Different Studies), mg	Estimated Percentage Improvement in Tremor Amplitude	Percentage Improvement by Accelerometry
Atenolol	50–100	24–38[28,33]	37[34]
Sotalol	80–240	29–51[28,33]	[a]
Gabapentin	1200 (–1800)	39[50]	77
Alprazolam	0.75–1.5	48–60[41,51]	[a]

[a] No data.

From Schneider SA, Deuschl G. The treatment of tremor. Neurotherapeutics 2014;11:129; with permission.

Medications with Less-Established Efficacy

Numerous other agents have been reported, mostly based on small studies or single case reports, which makes conclusions difficult.

Botulinum Toxin for Essential Tremor Limb Tremor

There are 2 relevant published trials of botulinum toxin type A for treatment of limb tremor in ET.[52,53] This includes one RCT parallel-group study[52] using a 2-staged injection-pattern with low-dose injections into hand flexors and extensors followed by a higher dose 4 weeks later if patients were unresponsive to the initial dose.

Accelerometry revealed approximately 60% to 70% improvement of postural hand tremor, but there were no significant improvements in functional ratings. Eleven (92%) of 12 patients developed moderate nondisabling wrist or finger weakness. Another study in ET[53] compared low-dose (50 U) and high-dose (100 U) botulinum toxin with placebo in a 12-week randomized double-blind controlled trial in 133 patients. Postural and kinetic tremor improved, however, without consistent benefit on function. Dose-dependent weakness developed in 30% after low-dose and 70% after high-dose injections. Although botulinum toxin may be likely efficacious, side effects are often limiting and, in our experience, efficacy is at best modest.

Table 3
Drugs for essential tremor

Level C Possibly Effective (Daily Dosage of the Respective Studies)	Agents with Recommendations Against Use	Inadequate Evidence to Confirm or Exclude Efficacy (Level U, Inconclusive)
Clonazepam (0.5–4 mg)[54]	Acetazolamide[41,55]/ Methazolamide	Olanzapine[56]
Clozapine (18–75 mg)[57]	Amantadine[58]	Sodium oxybate[59]
Flunarizine (10 mg)[60]	Carisbamate[61]	T2000 (1,3-dimethoxymethyl-5, 5-diphenyl-barbituric acid)[62]
Gabapentin (1800 mg and 3600 mg)[63–65]	3,4-diaminopyridine[66]	Zonisamide[67–69]
Nadolol (120–240 mg)[70]	Isoniazid[71]	
Nimodipine (120 mg)[72]	Levetiracetam[14,65]	
Theophylline (150 mg/d)[73]	Mirtazapine[74]	
Botulinum toxin[52,53] (depending on injected muscles)	Nifedipine[75]	
	Pregabalin[76,77]	
	Progabide[58]	
	Trazodone[78]	
	Verapamil[75]	

From Schneider SA, Deuschl G. The treatment of tremor. Neurotherapeutics 2014;11:130; with permission.

TREATMENT OF DYSTONIC LIMB TREMOR

Only a few studies have focused on dystonic tremor (with no study specifically focusing on "tremor associated with dystonia"). We recently published a study of 25 patients with dystonic tremor and found that only 40% of patients had benefit from oral therapy. Anticholinergics (ie, trihexyphenidyl, range 3–6 mg/d) produced the best result; propranolol also produced some benefit.[79] Fasano and colleagues[80] recently presented a review of 487 patients with dystonic tremor published in 43 articles and concluded that drug efficacy is generally moderate (total improvement approximately 40%), depending on the distribution and type of tremor. Anticholinergics led to approximately 40% improvement. In comparison beta-blockers produced only approximately 20% improvement (1 report based on 1 patient!) for head/trunk tremor and 60% for limb tremor. Levodopa is only efficacious for tremor due to dopa-responsive dystonia. DBS of GPi, thalamus, or subthalamic area, however, leads to a marked improvement (approximately 50%–80%) of dystonic axial or appendicular tremors in most cases (**Fig. 3** for algorithm).

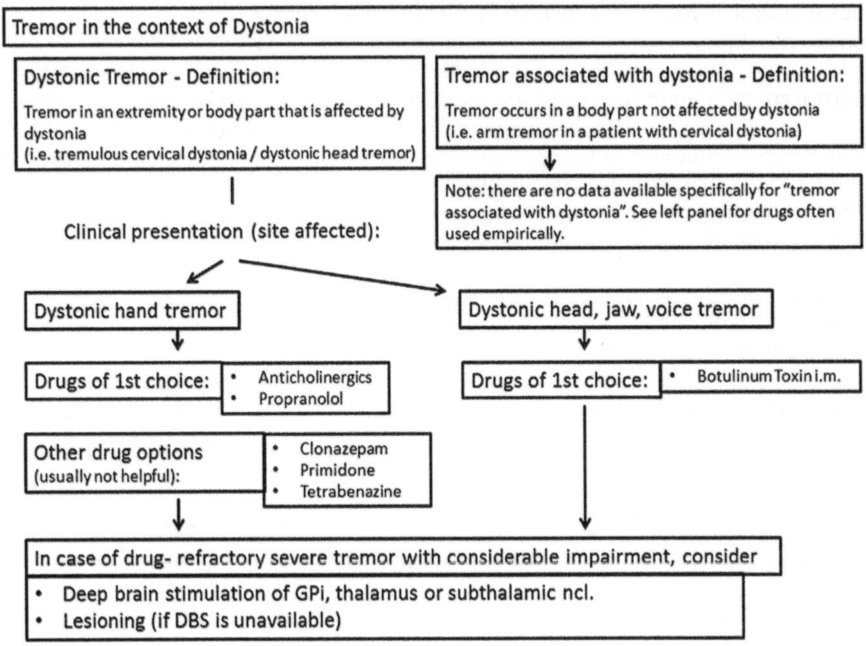

Fig. 3. Therapeutic algorithm for the treatment of dystonic tremor. i.m., intramuscular; ncl, nucleus.

TREATMENT OF PRIMARY WRITING TREMOR

Primary writing tremor is a condition in which tremor predominantly or only occurs during writing or also when adopting the hand position normally used for writing. More than half of the patients benefit from drug therapy (see Hai and colleagues[81] for review). Another option is botulinum toxin,[82] but there are no controlled trials. DBS for writing tremor also has been reported.

TREATMENT OF HEAD AND VOICE TREMOR IN ESSENTIAL TREMOR AND DYSTONIC TREMOR

Head and voice tremor may be a feature of both ET and dystonic tremor (present in 38% of patients with dystonia in one study[83]). Few studies have specifically addressed treatment of head and voice tremor. Oral therapy may be disappointing, but botulinum toxin injections often produce good benefit.[84,85] Ventralis intermedius (Vim)-DBS is an option for severe cases.[86,87]

Similarly, voice tremor may be a feature of both ET and dystonia (associated with dystonic limb or head tremor or as isolated dystonic voice tremor). Fewer than 50% patients with voice tremor respond to oral medication[88] and botulinum toxin may be helpful.[88]

TREATMENT OF ORTHOSTATIC TREMOR

A rare form of tremor is orthostatic tremor (OT). Patients report subjective unsteadiness when standing that is relieved by sitting or walking. Gabapentin (up to 2400 mg/d)[89–91] and clonazepam (0.25–3.5 mg/d, median 1 mg/d)[92,93] produce good results. If these fail, treatment is challenging: only 12% responded to alternative drugs in a large series.[94–96] Thalamic DBS was helpful in a few cases but less efficient than in other tremors.[97,98]

TREATMENT OF CEREBELLAR TREMOR RELATED TO MULTIPLE SCLEROSIS

Multiple sclerosis (MS) is commonly associated with cerebellar tremor,[99] which manifests as postural and kinetic arm tremor. The head, voice, and trunk also may be affected. The literature holds several small case series or single case descriptions reporting response to oral drugs,[100–103] but there is insufficient evidence to support or refute efficacy of any of these. Overall, oral treatment usually remains unsuccessful. A recent randomized placebo-controlled crossover study[104] assessed botulinum toxin for MS limb tremor, but the most potent treatment is surgery targeting the Vim of the thalamus.[105,106]

TREATMENT OF HOLMES TREMOR AND THALAMIC TREMOR

Holmes tremor due to lesions of the red nucleus is characterized by the combination of slow tremor at rest and on intention with an additional postural component in some. A combination of rest, postural and intention tremor, and dystonia also may be due to thalamic lesions (typically in the dorsolateral part) causing thalamic tremor. The 2 forms may be indistinguishable purely on clinical grounds, so thorough neuroimaging is helpful. Treatment is challenging in both conditions. Response to high dose of levodopa,[107] trihexyphenidyl (2–12 mg), clonazepam (0.5–4 mg), clozapine (<75 mg), or levetiracetam have been reported in single cases. DBS may be considered,[108–110] but placement of the electrode into the thalamic damaged area may be a challenge, so opting for 2 targets has been proposed.[111,112]

TREMOR IN PERIPHERAL NEUROPATHIES

Peripheral neuropathy may be another cause of tremor, mostly postural or kinetic in nature.[113] In inflammatory immunoglobulin M paraproteinemic neuropathies, for example, tremor is present in up to 80% of cases.[114,115] Oral tremor drugs may be helpful in individual cases[116,117] but usually fail, as shown in a recent series. Instead, improvement following intravenous immunoglobulin, rituximab, or CHOP-R chemotherapy prescribed as treatment of the underlying neuropathy has been reported.[114] Again, thalamic DBS may be considered for severe cases.[118–120]

TREATMENT OF FUNCTIONAL (PSYCHOGENIC) TREMOR

Psychogenic tremor is the most common form (55%) of all functional movement disorders. Suspicious features include a history of sudden onset and spontaneous remission and entrainment, distractibility, or the co-contraction sign on examination.[121] Tremor remission rates are rather low (20%–60%).[122–124] To improve the outcome, diagnostic delay should be avoided and treatment including symptom-focused cognitive-behavioral therapy approaches and physical interventions should be offered, best in a multidisciplinary setting.[125,126] Antidepressants[127] when there is a history of recent or current depression or anxiety may be helpful.

NONPHARMACOLOGIC TREATMENT OPTIONS

Several studies explored nonpharmacological treatment options for tremor and we refer the reader to an excellent review by O'Connor and Kini[128] for detailed reading. Briefly, different approaches have been studied, including the use of tremor-suppressing orthoses[129,130] (eg, externally applied devices, to suppress tremor using viscous materials, weighted splints, and vibration therapies). Physical therapy interventions include strength training,[131,132] resistance training,[133] or massage.[134] Several groups examined the effect of temperature change and limb cooling,[135,136] of limb weights,[137–139] or of vibration[140,141] on tremor. Finally, functional electrical[142,143] and transcranial magnetic[144] stimulation have been explored. In summary,[128] although there is potential in further developing these nonpharmacological treatments for tremor, there is currently insufficient evidence to recommend their use. The studies used mainly small numbers of probands, study periods were short, and long-term effectiveness has not been established. Some devices show promise, whereas others may not be feasible for continuous use.

SURGICAL TREATMENT OPTIONS: STEREOTACTIC SURGERY AND GAMMA KNIFE THALAMOTOMY

DBS of the thalamus (Vim), the posterior subthalamic area (PSA; radiatio paralemniscalis [a fiber bundle lying posterior to the subthalamic nucleus]), zona incerta (a band of gray matter lying dorsal to the subthalamic nucleus), as well as lesioning of these targets (ie, thalamotomy) have large treatment effects for upper limb tremor (including ET and other tremors).[23,145] Loss of tremor occurs gradually over months or years, producing a mean 0 to 10 satisfaction rating of more than 8 (10 = extremely satisfied and 0 = not satisfied).[146–151] Several articles have summarized the long-term results.[22,23] Notably, though, there are no double-blind placebo-controlled trials, also because true blinding is difficult.

The risks and side effects of thalamic DBS are well documented in the literature and include:

- Hardware complications: 25% of patients
- Paresthesias: 6%–36%
- Dysarthria: 3%–18%
- Ataxia: 6%
- Limb weakness: 4%–8%
- Balance disturbance: 3%–8%
- Dystonia: 2%–9%
- Perioperative complications (ie, intracerebral bleeding, ischemic stroke, infection)[152–154]

The mortality rate of DBS surgery was found to be 0.4%.[155]

There are only few controlled data for gamma knife thalamotomy. One study[156] used blinded rating but there are no placebo- (sham-) controlled trials. Two recent uncontrolled case series reported conflicting results, with efficacy and risks comparable to Vim-DBS in one,[157,158] but only mild benefit in the other.[156] Because there is a risk of long-term uncontrolled enlargement of the lesion,[156] we conclude that there is insufficient evidence to recommend the use of gamma knife thalamotomy in the treatment of tremor.

Experimental Approaches

Noninvasive magnetic resonance–guided focused ultrasound has most recently been proposed for treatment of disabling tremors. Ablative lesions were produced by stereotactically guided focused ultrasound energy in 4 patients with ET with immediate and sustained improvement in the range of 90%.[159] Another group[160] reported approximately 45% improvement using total tremor rating scales in 15 patients with

ET. This approach is currently experimental and larger studies are needed to validate safety and ascertain the efficacy. Transcranial magnetic stimulation also has been explored (also see section on Nonpharmacologic Treatment Options).[161]

SUMMARY

Treatment of tremor is challenging. The first step is to establish the correct diagnosis. For many tremors, controlled studies are lacking or the quality of existing trials do not satisfy modern standards. For ET, at least 3 drugs (propranolol, topiramate, primidone) have reasonable evidence to receive a Level A recommendation. But in general, only 50% of the patients respond to one of these. For many other drugs, there is insufficient evidence to recommend them for treatment of ET.

Other appendicular tremor types also show variable response to oral medication. Dystonic limb tremor may respond to anticholinergics. Gabapentin and clonazepam are often recommended for OT. Similarly, MS-tremor may respond to primidone or topiramate. Botulinum toxin improves head and voice tremor. Finally, patients with functional tremor may benefit from antidepressants, but should be best treated in a multidisciplinary setting.

For drug-refractory severe organic tremors, surgical treatments may be an option with usually good success, particularly for ET and probably dystonic tremor, whereas results are less promising for other tremors (MS-tremor, neuropathic tremor, thalamic and Holmes tremor) but still worth trying in severely handicapped patients when drugs have failed.

REFERENCES

1. Lorenz D, Poremba C, Papengut F, et al. The psychosocial burden of essential tremor in an outpatient- and a community-based cohort. Eur J Neurol 2011;18: 972–9.
2. Louis ED, Ford B, Wendt KJ, et al. Clinical characteristics of essential tremor: data from a community- based study. Mov Disord 1998;13:803–8.
3. Lorenz D, Schwieger D, Moises H, et al. Quality of life and personality in essential tremor patients. Mov Disord 2006;21:1114–8.
4. Troster AI, Pahwa R, Fields JA, et al. Quality of life in essential tremor questionnaire (QUEST): development and initial validation. Parkinsonism Relat Disord 2005;11:367–73.
5. Louis ED, Ferreira JJ. How common is the most common adult movement disorder? Update on the worldwide prevalence of essential tremor. Mov Disord 2010; 25:534–41.
6. Quinn NP, Schneider SA, Schwingenschuh P, et al. Tremor–some controversial aspects. Mov Disord 2011;26:18–23.
7. Deuschl G, Elble R. Essential tremor—neurodegenerative or nondegenerative disease towards a working definition of ET. Mov Disord 2009;24:2033–41.
8. Elble RJ. Tremor: clinical features, pathophysiology, and treatment. Neurol Clin 2009;27:679–95 v-vi.
9. Hall DA, O'Keefe JA. Fragile x-associated tremor ataxia syndrome: the expanding clinical picture, pathophysiology, epidemiology, and update on treatment. Tremor Other Hyperkinet Mov (N Y) 2012;2. pii:tre-02-56-352-1.
10. Elble RJ. Defining dystonic tremor. Curr Neuropharmacol 2013;11:48–52.
11. Schneider SA, Edwards MJ, Mir P, et al. Patients with adult-onset dystonic tremor resembling parkinsonian tremor have scans without evidence of dopaminergic deficit (SWEDDs). Mov Disord 2007;22:2210–5.

12. Deuschl G. Dystonic tremor. Rev Neurol (Paris) 2003;159:900–5.
13. Elble R, Bain P, Forjaz MJ, et al. Task force report: scales for screening and evaluating tremor: critique and recommendations. Mov Disord 2013;28: 1793–800.
14. Fahn S, Tolosa E, Marin C. Clinical rating scale for tremor. In: Jankovic J, Tolosa E, editors. Parkinson's disease and movement disorders. Baltimore (MD): Williams & Wilkins; 1993. p. 271–80.
15. Stacy MA, Elble RJ, Ondo WG, et al. Assessment of interrater and intrarater reliability of the Fahn-Tolosa-Marin tremor rating scale in essential tremor. Mov Disord 2007;22:833–8.
16. Elble R, Comella C, Fahn S, et al. The essential tremor rating assessment scale (TETRAS). Mov Disord 2008;23(Suppl 1):S1–6.
17. Elble RJ, Pullman SL, Matsumoto JY, et al. Tremor amplitude is logarithmically related to 4- and 5-point tremor rating scales. Brain 2006;129:2660–6.
18. Mostile G, Fekete R, Giuffrida JP, et al. Amplitude fluctuations in essential tremor. Parkinsonism Relat Disord 2012;18:859–63.
19. Daneault JF, Carignan B, Codere CE, et al. Using a smart phone as a standalone platform for detection and monitoring of pathological tremors. Front Hum Neurosci 2013;6:357.
20. Bhidayasiri R, Petchrutchatachart S, Pongthornseri R, et al. Low-cost, 3-dimension, office-based inertial sensors for automated tremor assessment: technical development and experimental verification. J Parkinsons Dis 2014; 4(2):273–82.
21. Ferreira JJ, Sampaio C. Essential tremor. Clin Evid (Online) 2007;2007. pii:1206.
22. Zesiewicz TA, Elble RJ, Louis ED, et al. Evidence-based guideline update: treatment of essential tremor: Report of the Quality Standards Subcommittee of the American Academy of Neurology. Neurology 2011;77(19):1752–5.
23. Deuschl G, Raethjen J, Hellriegel H, et al. Treatment of patients with essential tremor. Lancet Neurol 2011;10:148–61.
24. Nahab FB, Wittevrongel L, Ippolito D, et al. An open-label, single-dose, crossover study of the pharmacokinetics and metabolism of two oral formulations of 1-octanol in patients with essential tremor. Neurotherapeutics 2011;8: 753–62.
25. Haubenberger D, Nahab FB, Voller B, et al. Treatment of essential tremor with long-chain alcohols: still experimental or ready for prime time? Tremor Other Hyperkinet Mov (N Y) 2014;4. pii:tre-04-211-4673-2.
26. Winkler GF, Young RR. The control of essential tremor by propranolol. Trans Am Neurol Assoc 1971;96:66–8.
27. Calzetti S, Findely LJ, Gresty MA, et al. Effect of a single oral dose of propranolol on essential tremor: a double-blind controlled study. Ann Neurol 1983;13: 165–71.
28. Leigh PN, Jefferson D, Twomey A, et al. Beta-adrenoreceptor mechanisms in essential tremor; a double-blind placebo controlled trial of metoprolol, sotalol and atenolol. J Neurol Neurosurg Psychiatry 1983;46:710–5.
29. Baruzzi A, Procaccianti G, Martinelli P, et al. Phenobarbital and propranolol in essential tremor: a double-blind controlled clinical trial. Neurology 1983;33: 296–300.
30. Cleeves L, Findley LJ, Koller W. Lack of association between essential tremor and Parkinson's disease. Ann Neurol 1988;24:28.
31. Dupont E, Hansen HJ, Dalby MA. Treatment of benign essential tremor with propranolol. A controlled clinical trial. Acta Neurol Scand 1973;49:75–84.

32. Gorman G, Fairgrieve S, Birchall D, et al. Fragile X premutation presenting as essential tremor. J Neurol Neurosurg Psychiatry 2008;79:1195–6.
33. Jefferson D, Jenner P, Marsden CD. Beta-Adrenoreceptor antagonists in essential tremor. J Neurol Neurosurg Psychiatry 1979;42:904–9.
34. Larsen TA, Teravainen H, Calne DB. Atenolol vs. propranolol in essential tremor. A controlled, quantitative study. Acta Neurol Scand 1982;66:547–54.
35. Winkler GF, Young RR. Efficacy of chronic propranolol therapy in action tremors of the familial, senile or essential varieties. N Engl J Med 1974;290:984–8.
36. Murray TJ. Long-term therapy of essential tremor with propranolol. Can Med Assoc J 1976;115:892–4.
37. Sweet RD, Blumberg J, Lee JE, et al. Propranolol treatment of essential tremor. Neurology 1974;24:64–7.
38. Tolosa ES, Loewenson RB. Essential tremor: treatment with propranolol. Neurology 1975;25:1041–4.
39. Findley LJ, Calzetti S. Double-blind controlled study of primidone in essential tremor: preliminary results. Br Med J (Clin Res Ed) 1982;285:608.
40. Findley LJ, Cleeves L, Calzetti S. Primidone in essential tremor of the hands and head: a double blind controlled clinical study. J Neurol Neurosurg Psychiatry 1985;48:911–5.
41. Gunal DI, Afsar N, Bekiroglu N, et al. New alternative agents in essential tremor therapy: double-blind placebo-controlled study of alprazolam and acetazolamide. Neurol Sci 2000;21(5):315–7.
42. Sasso E, Perucca E, Calzetti S. Double-blind comparison of primidone and phenobarbital in essential tremor. Neurology 1988;38(5):808–10.
43. Koller WC, Vetere-Overfield B. Acute and chronic effects of propranolol and primidone in essential tremor. Neurology 1989;39:1587–8.
44. Martinez-Martin P, Serrano-Duenas M, Forjaz MJ, et al. Two questionnaires for Parkinson's disease: are the PDQ-39 and PDQL equivalent? Qual Life Res 2007;16:1221–30.
45. O'Suilleabhain PE, Matsumoto JY. Time-frequency analysis of tremors. Brain 1998;121(Pt 11):2127–34.
46. Connor GS. A double-blind placebo-controlled trial of topiramate treatment for essential tremor. Neurology 2002;59:132–4.
47. Ondo WG, Jankovic J, Connor GS, et al. Topiramate in essential tremor: a double-blind, placebo-controlled trial. Neurology 2006;66:672–7.
48. Frima N, Grunewald RA. A double-blind, placebo-controlled, crossover trial of topiramate in essential tremor. Clin Neuropharmacol 2006;29:94–6.
49. Connor GS, Edwards K, Tarsy D. Topiramate in essential tremor: findings from double-blind, placebo-controlled, crossover trials. Clin Neuropharmacol 2008; 31:97–103.
50. Schneider SA, Deuschl G. The treatment of tremor. Neurotherapeutics 2014;11: 128–38.
51. Huber SJ, Paulson GW. Efficacy of alprazolam for essential tremor. Neurology 1988;38:241–3.
52. Jankovic J, Schwartz K, Clemence W, et al. A randomized, double-blind, placebo-controlled study to evaluate botulinum toxin type A in essential hand tremor. Mov Disord 1996;11:250–6.
53. Brin MF, Lyons KE, Doucette J, et al. A randomized, double masked, controlled trial of botulinum toxin type A in essential hand tremor. Neurology 2001;56:1523–8.
54. Thompson C, Lang A, Parkes JD, et al. A double-blind trial of clonazepam in benign essential tremor. Clin Neuropharmacol 1984;7:83–8.

55. Pahwa R, Busenbark K, Gray C, et al. Identical twins with similar onset of Parkinson's disease: a case report. Neurology 1993;43:1159–61.
56. Yetimalar Y, Irtman G, Kurt T, et al. Olanzapine versus propranolol in essential tremor. Clin Neurol Neurosurg 2005;108:32–5.
57. Ceravolo R, Salvetti S, Piccini P, et al. Acute and chronic effects of clozapine in essential tremor. Mov Disord 1999;14:468–72.
58. Mondrup K, Dupont E, Pedersen E. The effect of the GABA-agonist, progabide, on benign essential tremor. A controlled clinical trial. Acta Neurol Scand 1983; 68:248–52.
59. Frucht SJ, Houghton WC, Bordelon Y, et al. A single-blind, open-label trial of sodium oxybate for myoclonus and essential tremor. Neurology 2005;65: 1967–9.
60. Biary N, al Deeb SM, Langenberg P. The effect of flunarizine on essential tremor. Neurology 1991;41:311–2.
61. Elble RJ, Biondi DM, Ascher S, et al. Carisbamate in essential tremor: brief report of a proof of concept study. Mov Disord 2010;25:634–8.
62. Melmed C, Moros D, Rutman H. Treatment of essential tremor with the barbiturate T2000 (1,3-dimethoxymethyl-5,5-diphenyl-barbituric acid). Mov Disord 2007;22:723–7.
63. Ondo W, Hunter C, Vuong KD, et al. Gabapentin for essential tremor: a multiple-dose, double-blind, placebo-controlled trial. Mov Disord 2000;15:678–82.
64. Pahwa R, Lyons K, Hubble JP, et al. Double-blind controlled trial of gabapentin in essential tremor. Mov Disord 1998;13:465–7.
65. Gironell A, Kulisevsky J, Barbanoj M, et al. A randomized placebo-controlled comparative trial of gabapentin and propranolol in essential tremor. Arch Neurol 1999;56:475–80.
66. Lorenz D, Hagen K, Ufer M, et al. No benefit of 3,4-diaminopyridine in essential tremor: a placebo-controlled crossover study. Neurology 2006;66:1753–5.
67. Handforth A, Martin FC, Kang GA, et al. Zonisamide for essential tremor: an evaluator-blinded study. Mov Disord 2009;24:437–40.
68. Morita S, Miwa H, Kondo T. Effect of zonisamide on essential tremor: a pilot crossover study in comparison with arotinolol. Parkinsonism Relat Disord 2005;11:101–3.
69. Ondo WG. Zonisamide for essential tremor. Clin Neuropharmacol 2007;30: 345–9.
70. Koller WC. Nadolol in essential tremor. Neurology 1983;33:1076–7.
71. Hallett M, Ravits J, Dubinsky RM, et al. A double-blind trial of isoniazid for essential tremor and other action tremors. Mov Disord 1991;6:253–6.
72. Fukuda M, Barnes A, Simon ES, et al. Thalamic stimulation for parkinsonian tremor: correlation between regional cerebral blood flow and physiological tremor characteristics. Neuroimage 2004;21:608–15.
73. Mally J, Stone TW. Efficacy of an adenosine antagonist, theophylline, in essential tremor: comparison with placebo and propranolol. J Neurol Sci 1995;132: 129–32.
74. Pahwa R, Lyons KE. Mirtazapine in essential tremor: a double-blind, placebo-controlled pilot study. Mov Disord 2003;18:584–7.
75. Topaktas S, Onur R, Dalkara T. Calcium channel blockers and essential tremor. Eur Neurol 1987;27:114–9.
76. Ferrara JM, Kenney C, Davidson AL, et al. Efficacy and tolerability of pregabalin in essential tremor: a randomized, double-blind, placebo-controlled, crossover trial. J Neurol Sci 2009;285:195–7.

77. Zesiewicz TA, Sullivan KL, Hinson V, et al. Multisite, double-blind, randomized, controlled study of pregabalin for essential tremor. Mov Disord 2013; 28:249–50.
78. Koller WC. Tradozone in essential tremor. Probe of serotoninergic mechanisms. Clin Neuropharmacol 1989;12:134–7.
79. Schwingenschuh P, Ruge D, Edwards MJ, et al. Distinguishing SWEDDs patients with asymmetric resting tremor from Parkinson's disease: a clinical and electrophysiological study. Mov Disord 2010;25:560–9.
80. Fasano A, Bove F, Lang AE. The treatment of dystonic tremor: a systematic review. J Neurol Neurosurg Psychiatry 2014;85(7):759–69.
81. Hai C, Yu-ping W, Hua W, et al. Advances in primary writing tremor. Parkinsonism Relat Disord 2010;16:561–5.
82. Papapetropoulos S, Singer C. Treatment of primary writing tremor with botulinum toxin type A injections: report of a case series. Clin Neuropharmacol 2006;29: 364–7.
83. Godeiro-Junior C, Felicio AC, Aguiar PC, et al. Head tremor in patients with cervical dystonia: different outcome? Arq Neuropsiquiatr 2008;66:805–8.
84. Pahwa R, Busenbark K, Swanson-Hyland EF, et al. Botulinum toxin treatment of essential head tremor. Neurology 1995;45:822–4.
85. Wissel J, Masuhr F, Schelosky L, et al. Quantitative assessment of botulinum toxin treatment in 43 patients with head tremor. Mov Disord 1997;12:722–6.
86. Obwegeser AA, Uitti RJ, Turk MF, et al. Thalamic stimulation for the treatment of midline tremors in essential tremor patients. Neurology 2000;54:2342–4.
87. Limousin P, Speelman JD, Gielen F, et al. Multicentre European study of thalamic stimulation in parkinsonian and essential tremor. J Neurol Neurosurg Psychiatry 1999;66:289–96.
88. Gurey LE, Sinclair CF, Blitzer A. A new paradigm for the management of essential vocal tremor with botulinum toxin. Laryngoscope 2013;123(10): 2497–501.
89. Rodrigues JP, Edwards DJ, Walters SE, et al. Blinded placebo crossover study of gabapentin in primary orthostatic tremor. Mov Disord 2006;21:900–5.
90. Evidente VG, Adler CH, Caviness JN, et al. Effective treatment of orthostatic tremor with gabapentin. Mov Disord 1998;13:829–31.
91. Onofrj M, Thomas A, Paci C, et al. Gabapentin in orthostatic tremor: results of a double-blind crossover with placebo in four patients. Neurology 1998;51:880–2.
92. FitzGerald PM, Jankovic J. Orthostatic tremor: an association with essential tremor. Mov Disord 1991;6:60–4.
93. McManis PG, Sharbrough FW. Orthostatic tremor: clinical and electrophysiologic characteristics. Muscle Nerve 1993;16:1254–60.
94. Rodrigues JP, Edwards DJ, Walters SE, et al. Gabapentin can improve postural stability and quality of life in primary orthostatic tremor. Mov Disord 2005;20: 865–70.
95. Hellriegel H, Raethjen J, Deuschl G, et al. Levetiracetam in primary orthostatic tremor: a double-blind placebo-controlled crossover study. Mov Disord 2011; 26:2431–4.
96. Gerschlager W, Münchau A, Katzenschlager R, et al. Natural history and syndromic associations of orthostatic tremor: a review of 41 patients. Mov Disord 2004;19:788–95.
97. Espay AJ, Duker AP, Chen R, et al. Deep brain stimulation of the ventral intermediate nucleus of the thalamus in medically refractory orthostatic tremor: preliminary observations. Mov Disord 2008;23:2357–62.

98. Guridi J, Rodriguez-Oroz MC, Arbizu J, et al. Successful thalamic deep brain stimulation for orthostatic tremor. Mov Disord 2008;23:1808–11.
99. Alusi SH, Aziz TZ, Glickman S, et al. Stereotactic lesional surgery for the treatment of tremor in multiple sclerosis: a prospective case-controlled study. Brain 2001;124:1576–89.
100. Sechi GP, Zuddas M, Piredda M, et al. Treatment of cerebellar tremors with carbamazepine: a controlled trial with long-term follow-up. Neurology 1989;39:1113–5.
101. Schroeder A, Linker RA, Lukas C, et al. Successful treatment of cerebellar ataxia and tremor in multiple sclerosis with topiramate: a case report. Clin Neuropharmacol 2010;33:317–8.
102. Naderi F, Javadi SA, Motamedi M, et al. The efficacy of primidone in reducing severe cerebellar tremors in patients with multiple sclerosis. Clin Neuropharmacol 2012;35:224–6.
103. Schniepp R, Jakl V, Wuehr M, et al. Treatment with 4-aminopyridine improves upper limb tremor of a patient with multiple sclerosis: a video case report. Mult Scler 2013;19:506–8.
104. Van Der Walt A, Sung S, Spelman T, et al. A double-blind, randomized, controlled study of botulinum toxin type A in MS-related tremor. Neurology 2012;79:92–9.
105. Schuurman PR, Bosch DA, Merkus MP, et al. Long-term follow-up of thalamic stimulation versus thalamotomy for tremor suppression. Mov Disord 2008;23:1146–53.
106. Hooper AK, Okun MS, Foote KD, et al. Venous air embolism in deep brain stimulation. Stereotact Funct Neurosurg 2009;87:25–30.
107. Boelmans K, Gerloff C, Munchau A. Long-lasting effect of levodopa on Holmes' tremor. Mov Disord 2012;27:1097–8.
108. Diederich NJ, Verhagen ML, Bakay RA, et al. Ventral intermediate thalamic stimulation in complex tremor syndromes. Stereotact Funct Neurosurg 2008;86:167–72.
109. Kudo M, Goto S, Nishikawa S, et al. Bilateral thalamic stimulation for Holmes' tremor caused by unilateral brainstem lesion. Mov Disord 2001;16:170–4.
110. Nikkhah G, Prokop T, Hellwig B, et al. Deep brain stimulation of the nucleus ventralis intermedius for Holmes (rubral) tremor and associated dystonia caused by upper brainstem lesions. Report of two cases. J Neurosurg 2004;100:1079–83.
111. Lim DA, Khandhar SM, Heath S, et al. Multiple target deep brain stimulation for multiple sclerosis related and poststroke Holmes' tremor. Stereotact Funct Neurosurg 2007;85:144–9.
112. Foote KD, Okun MS. Ventralis intermedius plus ventralis oralis anterior and posterior deep brain stimulation for posttraumatic Holmes tremor: two leads may be better than one: technical note. Neurosurgery 2005;56:E445 [discussion: E445].
113. Bain PG, Britton TC, Jenkins IH, et al. Tremor associated with benign IgM paraproteinaemic neuropathy. Brain 1996;119(Pt 3):789–99.
114. Saifee TA, Schwingenschuh P, Reilly MM, et al. Tremor in inflammatory neuropathies. J Neurol Neurosurg Psychiatry 2013;84:1282–7.
115. Dalakas MC, Teravainen H, Engel WK. Tremor as a feature of chronic relapsing and dysgammaglobulinemic polyneuropathies. Incidence and management. Arch Neurol 1984;41:711–4.
116. Alonso-Navarro H, Fernandez-Diaz A, Martin-Prieto M, et al. Tremor associated with chronic inflammatory demyelinating peripheral neuropathy: treatment with pregabalin. Clin Neuropharmacol 2008;31:241–4.

117. Coltamai L, Magezi DA, Croquelois A. Pregabalin in the treatment of neuropathic tremor following a motor axonal form of Guillain-Barre syndrome. Mov Disord 2010;25:517–9.
118. Ruzicka E, Jech R, Zarubova K, et al. VIM thalamic stimulation for tremor in a patient with IgM paraproteinaemic demyelinating neuropathy. Mov Disord 2003;18:1192–5.
119. Weiss D, Govindan RB, Rilk A, et al. Central oscillators in a patient with neuropathic tremor: evidence from intraoperative local field potential recordings. Mov Disord 2011;26:323–7.
120. Breit S, Wachter T, Schols L, et al. Effective thalamic deep brain stimulation for neuropathic tremor in a patient with severe demyelinating neuropathy. J Neurol Neurosurg Psychiatry 2009;80:235–6.
121. Kenney C, Diamond A, Mejia N, et al. Distinguishing psychogenic and essential tremor. J Neurol Sci 2007;263(1–2):94–9.
122. Edwards MJ, Talelli P, Rothwell JC. Clinical applications of transcranial magnetic stimulation in patients with movement disorders. Lancet Neurol 2008;7:827–40.
123. Gupta A, Lang AE. Psychogenic movement disorders. Curr Opin Neurol 2009;22:430–6.
124. Roper LS, Saifee TA, Parees I, et al. How to use the entrainment test in the diagnosis of functional tremor. Pract Neurol 2013;13:396–8.
125. Edwards MJ, Bhatia KP. Functional (psychogenic) movement disorders: merging mind and brain. Lancet Neurol 2012;11:250–60.
126. Dallocchio C, Arbasino C, Klersy C, et al. The effects of physical activity on psychogenic movement disorders. Mov Disord 2010;25:421–5.
127. Voon V, Lang AE. Antidepressant treatment outcomes of psychogenic movement disorder. J Clin Psychiatry 2005;66:1529–34.
128. O'Connor RJ, Kini MU. Non-pharmacological and non-surgical interventions for tremor: a systematic review. Parkinsonism Relat Disord 2011;17:509–15.
129. Espay AJ, Hung SW, Sanger TD, et al. A writing device improves writing in primary writing tremor. Neurology 2005;64:1648–50.
130. Gallego JA, Rocon E, Belda-Lois JM, et al. A neuroprosthesis for tremor management through the control of muscle co-contraction. J Neuroeng Rehabil 2013;10:36.
131. Bilodeau M, Keen DA, Sweeney PJ, et al. Strength training can improve steadiness in persons with essential tremor. Muscle Nerve 2000;23:771–8.
132. Keogh JW, Morrison S, Barrett R. Strength and coordination training are both effective in reducing the postural tremor amplitude of older adults. J Aging Phys Act 2010;18:43–60.
133. Sequeira G, Keogh JW, Kavanagh JJ. Resistance training can improve fine manual dexterity in essential tremor patients: a preliminary study. Arch Phys Med Rehabil 2012;93:1466–8.
134. Craig LH, Svircev A, Haber M, et al. Controlled pilot study of the effects of neuromuscular therapy in patients with Parkinson's disease. Mov Disord 2006;21:2127–33.
135. Cooper C, Evidente VG, Hentz JG, et al. The effect of temperature on hand function in patients with tremor. J Hand Ther 2000;13:276–88.
136. Feys P, Helsen W, Liu X, et al. Effects of peripheral cooling on intention tremor in multiple sclerosis. J Neurol Neurosurg Psychiatry 2005;76:373–9.
137. Hewer RL, Cooper R, Morgan MH. An investigation into the value of treating intention tremor by weighting the affected limb. Brain 1972;95:579–90.

138. Meshack RP, Norman KE. A randomized controlled trial of the effects of weights on amplitude and frequency of postural hand tremor in people with Parkinson's disease. Clin Rehabil 2002;16:481–92.
139. McGruder J, Cors D, Tiernan AM, et al. Weighted wrist cuffs for tremor reduction during eating in adults with static brain lesions. Am J Occup Ther 2003;57: 507–16.
140. Feys P, Helsen WF, Verschueren S, et al. Online movement control in multiple sclerosis patients with tremor: effects of tendon vibration. Mov Disord 2006; 21:1148–53.
141. King LK, Almeida QJ, Ahonen H. Short-term effects of vibration therapy on motor impairments in Parkinson's disease. NeuroRehabilitation 2009;25:297–306.
142. Javidan M, Elek J, Prochazka A. Attenuation of pathological tremors by functional electrical stimulation. II: Clinical evaluation. Ann Biomed Eng 1992;20:225–36.
143. Gillard DM, Cameron T, Prochazka A, et al. Tremor suppression using functional electrical stimulation: a comparison between digital and analog controllers. IEEE Trans Rehabil Eng 1999;7:385–8.
144. Brittain JS, Probert-Smith P, Aziz TZ, et al. Tremor suppression by rhythmic transcranial current stimulation. Curr Biol 2013;23:436–40.
145. Chopra A, Klassen BT, Stead M. Current clinical application of deep-brain stimulation for essential tremor. Neuropsychiatr Dis Treat 2013;9:1859–65.
146. Wardell K, Blomstedt P, Richter J, et al. Intracerebral microvascular measurements during deep brain stimulation implantation using laser Doppler perfusion monitoring. Stereotact Funct Neurosurg 2007;85:279–86.
147. Pilitsis JG, Metman LV, Toleikis JR, et al. Factors involved in long-term efficacy of deep brain stimulation of the thalamus for essential tremor. J Neurosurg 2008; 109:640–6.
148. Pahwa R, Lyons KE, Wilkinson SB, et al. Long-term evaluation of deep brain stimulation of the thalamus. J Neurosurg 2006;104:506–12.
149. Zhang K, Bhatia S, Oh MY, et al. Long-term results of thalamic deep brain stimulation for essential tremor. J Neurosurg 2010;112:1271–6.
150. Koller WC, Lyons KE, Wilkinson SB, et al. Long-term safety and efficacy of unilateral deep brain stimulation of the thalamus in essential tremor. Mov Disord 2001;16:464–8.
151. Kumar R, Lozano AM, Sime E, et al. Long-term follow-up of thalamic deep brain stimulation for essential and parkinsonian tremor. Neurology 2003;61:1601–4.
152. Baizabal-Carvallo JF, Kagnoff MN, Jimenez-Shahed J, et al. The safety and efficacy of thalamic deep brain stimulation in essential tremor: 10 years and beyond. J Neurol Neurosurg Psychiatry 2014;85(5):567–72.
153. Baizabal Carvallo JF, Mostile G, Almaguer M, et al. Deep brain stimulation hardware complications in patients with movement disorders: risk factors and clinical correlations. Stereotact Funct Neurosurg 2012;90(5):300–6.
154. DiLorenzo DJ, Jankovic J, Simpson RK, et al. Neurohistopathological findings at the electrode-tissue interface in long-term deep brain stimulation: systematic literature review, case report, and assessment of stimulation threshold safety. Neuromodulation 2014;17(5):405–18.
155. Voges J, Hilker R, Botzel K, et al. Thirty days complication rate following surgery performed for deep-brain-stimulation. Mov Disord 2007;22:1486–9.
156. Lim SY, Hodaie M, Fallis M, et al. Gamma knife thalamotomy for disabling tremor: a blinded evaluation. Arch Neurol 2010;67:584–8.
157. Kondziolka D, Ong JG, Lee JY, et al. Gamma knife thalamotomy for essential tremor. J Neurosurg 2008;108:111–7.

158. Young RF, Li F, Vermeulen S, et al. Gamma knife thalamotomy for treatment of essential tremor: long-term results. J Neurosurg 2010;112:1311–7.
159. Lipsman N, Schwartz ML, Huang Y, et al. MR-guided focused ultrasound thalamotomy for essential tremor: a proof-of-concept study. Lancet Neurol 2013;12: 462–8.
160. Elias WJ, Huss D, Voss T, et al. A pilot study of focused ultrasound thalamotomy for essential tremor. N Engl J Med 2013;369:640–8.
161. Popa T, Russo M, Vidailhet M, et al. Cerebellar rTMS stimulation may induce prolonged clinical benefits in essential tremor, and subjacent changes in functional connectivity: an open label trial. Brain Stimul 2013;6:175–9.

Diagnosis and Treatment of Dystonia

H.A. Jinnah, MD, PhD[a,b,c,*], Stewart A. Factor, DO[a]

KEYWORDS

• Blepharospasm • Botulinum toxin • Cervical dystonia • Deep brain stimulation
• Focal hand dystonia • Meige syndrome • Oromandibular dystonia
• Spasmodic dysphonia

KEY POINTS

- The dystonias are a large group of heterogeneous conditions characterized by excessive muscle contractions leading to abnormal postures and/or repetitive movements.
- A careful evaluation is needed for all patients with dystonia to identify uncommon subtypes in which specific etiology-based treatments can dramatically alter the course of the disorder.
- Botulinum toxins are the treatment of first choice for most focal and segmental dystonias, and may be used also to target specific problematic regions in patients with broader involvement.
- Deep brain stimulation and other surgical procedures are available when oral medications and botulinum toxins provide inadequate relief of symptoms.

Videos of various dystonias accompany this article at http://www.neurologic.theclinics.com/

INTRODUCTION

The dystonias are a group of disorders defined by specific types of abnormal movements. The essential feature is overactivity of muscles needed for movement. This overactivity can be expressed as excessive force in the primary muscles used for a movement, overflow activation of additional muscles that are not required for a

Disclosures: See last page of article.

[a] Department of Neurology, Emory University School of Medicine, 6300 Woodruff Memorial Research Building, 101 Woodruff Circle, Emory University, Atlanta, GA 30322, USA; [b] Department of Human Genetics, Emory University School of Medicine, 6300 Woodruff Memorial Research Building, 101 Woodruff Circle, Emory University, Atlanta, GA 30322, USA; [c] Department of Pediatrics, Emory University School of Medicine, 6300 Woodruff Memorial Research Building, 101 Woodruff Circle, Emory University, Atlanta, GA 30322, USA
* Corresponding author. Department of Neurology, Emory University School of Medicine, 6300 Woodruff Memorial Research Building, 101 Woodruff Circle, Emory University, Atlanta, GA 30322.
E-mail address: hjinnah@emory.edu

Neurol Clin 33 (2015) 77–100
http://dx.doi.org/10.1016/j.ncl.2014.09.002
neurologic.theclinics.com

movement, or coactivation of muscles that antagonize the primary muscles. The clinical expression of dystonia is determined by the severity and distribution of muscles involved. In mild cases, dystonic movements appear merely as exaggerations of specific actions. In moderate cases, the movements are more clearly abnormal with a quality that is cramped, stiff, or twisting. In more severe cases, dystonic movements appear as persistent odd postures or fixed deformities.

Dystonic movements are often slow, but they sometimes may be rapid or jerky.[1,2] Sometimes the movements may resemble tremor.[3–5] They tend to be patterned or stereotyped in individual cases. A recent consensus work group provided the following formal definition for the dystonias[6]:

> *Dystonia is a movement disorder characterized by sustained or intermittent muscle contractions causing abnormal, often repetitive movements, postures, or both. Dystonic movements are typically patterned, twisting, and may be tremulous. Dystonia is often initiated or worsened by voluntary action and associated with overflow muscle activation.*

Virtually any region of the body may be affected, alone or in various combinations. The dystonias may emerge at any age; and once they begin, they rarely remit. Some remain relatively static, whereas others are progressive or intermittent. Dystonia may occur in isolation, or it may be combined with other clinical problems. The many different clinical manifestations are classified according to 4 dimensions (**Table 1**), including the region of the body affected, the age at onset, temporal aspects, and whether there are associated clinical problems.[6] Each of these dimensions has implications for diagnosis and treatment.

In addition to the widely varying clinical manifestations of the dystonias, there also are many different causes.[7] Some dystonias are inherited, others are acquired (**Table 2**). Some dystonias have no apparent pathology in the nervous system, whereas others are associated with defects that can be detected by neuroimaging or postmortem histopathological studies. At the molecular level, multiple genes have been discovered for rare subtypes of dystonia,[8,9] and they are involved in diverse biochemical processes.[9–11] At the anatomic level, several brain regions have been implicated, leading to the concept that dystonia does not arise from dysfunction of

Table 1
Classification of the dystonias according to clinical features

Dimension for Classification	Subgroups
Age at onset	Infancy (birth to 2 y) Childhood (3–12 y) Adolescence (13–20 y) Early adulthood (21–40 y) Late adulthood (40 y and older)
Body distribution	Focal (1 isolated region) Segmental (2 or more contiguous regions) Multifocal (2 or more noncontiguous regions) Hemidystonia (half the body) Generalized (trunk plus 2 other sites)
Temporal pattern	Disease course (static vs progressive) Short-term variation (persistent, action-specific, diurnal, paroxysmal)
Associated features	Isolated (with or without tremor) Combined (with other neurologic or systemic features)

Table 2
Classification of the dystonias according to etiology

Dimension for Classification	Subgroups
Nervous system pathology	Degenerative Structural (typically static) No evidence for degenerative or structural lesions
Heritability	Inherited (eg, autosomal dominant, autosomal recessive, mitochondrial) Acquired (eg, brain injury, drugs/toxins, vascular, neoplastic)
Idiopathic	Sporadic Familial

a single brain region, but rather from dysfunction of a motor network.[12–14] Physiologically, many forms of dystonia have evidence for impaired inhibitory processes in the nervous system, abnormal sensory feedback, and/or maladaptive neural plasticity.[15–17] Determining how these diverse processes relate to one another to produce the motor syndrome we know as dystonia is a major current focus of research.[11,18]

DIAGNOSIS

Because there are so many different clinical manifestations and causes, there are no simple algorithms for diagnosis that address all dystonias. A shotgun approach in which all possible disorders are evaluated in a "dystonia test battery" is not recommended. Available genetic test batteries are very expensive, they include only a small fraction of known causes, and the probability of finding a positive result in sporadic cases with dystonia is less than 1%. Another strategy sometimes recommended follows a "red flag" approach in which diagnostic testing is guided by the identification of telltale clinical features, such as a corneal Kayser-Fleischer ring or liver disease in Wilson disease.[19,20] This strategy is not ideal, because most dystonic disorders lack red flags. Another strategy sometimes recommended is to test only for disorders in which there are specific treatments that target underlying etiologies, such as Wilson disease in which copper-lowering therapies are life saving. This strategy also is untenable, because recent progress in dystonia research has led to a long list of treatable disorders that grows every year (**Table 3**).

A more methodical strategy for diagnosis is shown in **Fig. 1**. Once a diagnosis of dystonia is suspected based on clinical phenomenology, the first step is to rule out disorders that may mimic dystonia (pseudodystonia), such as those due to orthopedic, neuromuscular, or psychogenic processes. The next step is to delineate the clinical syndrome according to the 4 dimensions used for clinical classification (see **Table 1**). A careful delineation of the syndromic pattern, along with neuroimaging characteristics, is important because it aids in narrowing down the long list of potential etiologies for more targeted diagnostic testing.[7]

For patients with isolated dystonia, the laboratory workup depends on the age at onset, the body distribution, and whether there are affected family members. In adults with focal or segmental dystonia only, no diagnostic tests are required because they usually are unrevealing.[18,21] In adults with hemidystonia or generalized dystonia, neuroimaging is useful because the likelihood of disclosing a structural cause is higher. In sporadic adult-onset isolated dystonias, the chance of finding a genetic cause is less than 1% to 2%, so genetic testing usually is not cost-effective, unless there are other affected family members. The diagnostic approach in younger

Table 3
Disorders with dystonia that have specific disease-modifying therapies

Disorder	Typical Age at Onset[a]	Typical Characteristics of Dystonia	Other Typical Clinical Features[b]	Treatment
Abetalipoproteinemia (Bassen-Kornzweig)	Childhood to early adulthood	Progressive oromandibular or generalized dystonia	Ataxia, chorea, retinitis pigmentosa, fat malabsorption	Vitamin E, reduced-fat diet
Aromatic amino acid decarboxylase deficiency	Infancy	Generalized dystonia	Developmental delay, hypotonia, oculogyric crises, autonomic dysfunction	Dopamine agonists, monoamine oxidase inhibitors
Ataxia with vitamin E deficiency	Childhood to early adulthood	Rare patients present with dystonia instead of ataxia	Ataxia, neuropathy	Vitamin E
Autoimmune movement disorders	Any age	Focal or generalized dystonia	Systemic signs of autoimmune disease	Address autoimmune process
Biotinidase deficiency	Infancy	Generalized dystonia	Developmental delay, encephalopathy, seizures, sensory defects, skin rash	Biotin
Cerebral folate deficiency	Early childhood to adolescence	Progressive dystonia	Developmental delay, neuropsychiatric syndromes, seizures	Folinic acid
Cerebrotendinous xanthomatosis	Late childhood to adulthood	Oromandibular or limb dystonia	Neurocognitive defects, spasticity, myoclonus, tendon xanthomas	Chenodeoxycholic acid
Cobalamin deficiencies (inherited subtypes A–G)	Infancy	Generalized dystonia	Developmental delay, ataxia, spasticity, seizures, bone marrow defects	Cobalamin derivatives and/or protein restriction
CoEnzyme Q10 deficiency	Any age	Some cases present with dystonia and ataxia	Varied phenotypes, most often progressive ataxia or encephalopathy	Coenzyme Q10
Cerebral creatine deficiency type 3	Infancy	Generalized dystonia	Developmental delay, myopathy	Creatine
Dopa-responsive dystonia, classic	Early childhood to late adulthood	Generalized dystonia	Parkinsonism	Levodopa

Dopa-responsive dystonia, complicated	Infancy to adolescence	Generalized dystonia	Hypokinetic-rigid syndrome, oculogyric crises, autonomic dysfunction	Levodopa, 5-hydroxytryptophan, and/or tetrahydrobiopterin
Dystonia with brain manganese accumulation	Childhood	Progressive generalized dystonia	Parkinsonism, liver disease, polycythemia	Chelation therapy
Galactosemia	Childhood to early adulthood	Mild focal or generalized dystonia	Ataxia, tremor, food intolerance	Lactose restriction
GLUT1 deficiency	Childhood to adolescence	Paroxysmal exertional dystonia	Developmental delay, seizures	Ketogenic diet
Glutaric aciduria type 1	Early childhood to early adulthood	Static generalized dystonia following encephalopathic crisis	Developmental delay, encephalopathic crisis	Avoid or treat aggressively any intercurrent illness, lysine restriction
Homocystinuria	Childhood	Generalized or paroxysmal dystonia	Neurocognitive dysfunction, myopia, ectopic lens	Methionine restriction
Guanidinoacetate methyltransferase deficiency	Infancy	Progressive generalized dystonia	Developmental delay, seizures	Arginine restriction, creatine and ornithine
Maple syrup urine disease	Childhood	Focal or paroxysmal dystonia	Neonatal encephalopathy, ataxia	Leucine restriction ± thiamine
Methylmalonic aciduria	Childhood	Static generalized dystonia after encephalopathic crisis	Developmental delay, encephalopathic crisis, renal insufficiency, pancytopenia	Avoid or treat aggressively any intercurrent illness, protein restriction
Molybdenum cofactor deficiency (sulfite oxidase)	Adolescence	Rare patients present with dystonia and parkinsonism	Developmental delay, encephalopathy, seizures	Cyclic pyranopterin monophosphate

(*continued on next page*)

Table 3
(*continued*)

Disorder	Typical Age at Onset[a]	Typical Characteristics of Dystonia	Other Typical Clinical Features[b]	Treatment
Niemann Pick type C	Early childhood to early adulthood	Progressive generalized dystonia	Dementia, ataxia, spasticity, seizures, supranuclear gaze palsy	N-butyl-deoxynojirimycin (Miglustat)
Paraneoplastic movement disorders	Any age	Rapidly progressive focal or generalized dystonia	Malignancy, often occult	Address underlying malignancy
Propionic aciduria	Early childhood to adolescence	Static generalized dystonia after encephalopathic crisis	Developmental delay, encephalopathic crisis, optic atrophy, pancytopenia	Avoid or treat aggressively any intercurrent illness, protein restriction
Pyruvate dehydrogenase deficiency	Infancy	Progressive generalized or paroxysmal dystonia	Developmental delay, seizures	Thiamine, ketogenic diet, dichloroacetate
Rapid-onset dystonia-parkinsonism	Early childhood to late adulthood	Bulbar or generalized dystonia after encephalopathic crisis	Psychomotor disability	Avoid or treat aggressively any intercurrent illness, protein restriction
Wilson disease	Early childhood to late adulthood	Progressive generalized dystonia	Neurocognitive dysfunction, liver disease, Kayser-Fleischer rings	Zinc, tetrathiomolybdate

[a] For most childhood-onset disorders, rare patients may present instead in adulthood.
[b] Some associated clinical features may be attenuated or absent in atypical cases.

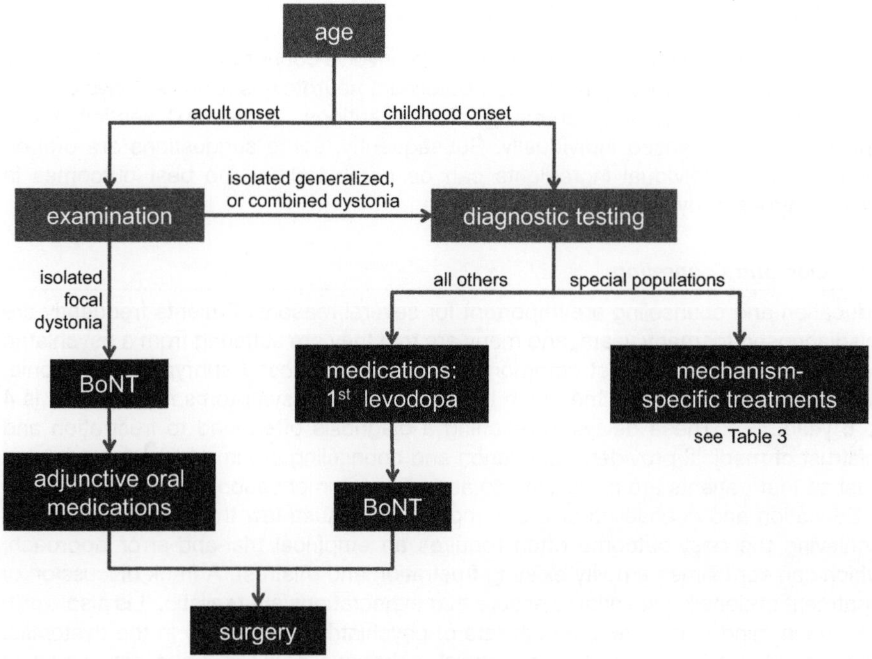

Fig. 1. Methodical strategy for diagnosis of dystonia.

individuals with isolated dystonia is quite different, because there is a much higher likelihood of disclosing a cause.[7] Neuroimaging is important for all early-onset cases, regardless of body distribution. Genetic testing for early-onset isolated dystonias should target the *TOR1A* gene for DYT1 dystonia and the *THAP1* gene for DYT6 dystonia.

For all patients in whom dystonia is combined with other neurologic or systemic features, some additional workup is warranted, regardless of the age at onset or body distribution. The laboratory workup depends on the nature of the associated features and the age at onset. A recent review summarized more than 100 different disorders in which dystonia may be combined with other features, organized in 18 tables according to the associated clinical features and age at onset.[7] Neuroimaging is useful in virtually all combined dystonias, because it can provide important diagnostic clues. Genetic testing for DYT1 and DYT6 dystonia is not useful in combined dystonia syndromes. Instead, laboratory testing is driven by the syndromic pattern. For example, dystonia combined with parkinsonism leads to a relatively small list of disorders for more targeted diagnostic testing.[22–24]

When a specific etiology cannot be determined, it is important to follow patients and revise the diagnosis as additional clinical features are recognized. Many combined dystonic disorders may present first with what appears to be isolated dystonia, and additional clinical features may develop over the following months or years. One of the most common examples is idiopathic Parkinson disease and related parkinsonian syndromes, in which 10% to 15% of patients may present first with isolated dystonia of an arm or leg.[25–30] It is not until other clinical features emerge that the diagnosis becomes more obvious. Another example that should always be considered is Wilson's disease, because treatments are life-saving.

TREATMENT

There are many different treatment options that involve counseling and education, oral medications, intramuscular injection of botulinum neurotoxins (BoNTs), physical and occupational therapy, and neurosurgical interventions. In the next section, these options are summarized individually. Subsequently, some suggestions are offered for how these individual ingredients can be combined for the best outcomes in different types of dystonia.

Education and Counseling

Education and counseling are important for several reasons. Patients frequently are misdiagnosed for many years, and many are told they are suffering from a psychiatric problem. Even for the most common and readily diagnosed subtypes of dystonia, such as cervical dystonia, the mean time from onset of symptoms to diagnosis is 4 to 6 years.[31–33] These delays in reaching a diagnosis often lead to frustration and mistrust of medical providers. Education and counseling are important for regaining trust so that patients are more likely to accept recommendations.

Education and counseling also are important because few therapies are curative. Achieving the best outcome often requires an empirical trial-and-error approach, which can sometimes amplify existing frustration and mistrust. A frank discussion of treatment options is essential to ensure that expectations are realistic. It is also worth bearing in mind that there is a high rate of psychiatric comorbidity in the dystonias, including depression, anxiety, and social withdrawal.[34–37] An open discussion of how these factors may influence overall quality of life is important.

Finally, many patients learn about their medical diagnoses and treatment options via the Internet, which is not always a reliable source of information. Educating patients about the most reliable online sources of information can help to avoid misunderstandings. **Table 4** provides a summary of some Internet sites where information is regularly updated, and other educational and research opportunities are available to patients. Most of these groups also provide informational brochures, newsletters, and local patient support group meetings where patients can obtain new information.

Table 4
Online educational resources for patients

Organization	Internet Address
American Dystonia Society	dystoniasociety.org
Bachmann-Strauss Dystonia & Parkinson Foundation	dystonia-parkinsons.org
Benign Essential Blepharospasm Research Foundation	blepharospasm.org
Dystonia Coalition	dystoniacoalition.org
Dystonia Ireland	dystonia.ie
Dystonia Medical Research Foundation	dystonia-foundation.org
Dystonia Medical Research Foundation, Canada	dystoniacanada.org
Global Dystonia Registry	globaldystoniaregistry.org
National Institute of Neurologic Disorders and Stroke	ninds.nih.gov/disorders/dystonias
National Spasmodic Dysphonia Association	dysphonia.org
National Spasmodic Torticollis Association	torticollis.org
ST/Dystonia	spasmodictorticollis.org
The Dystonia Society (UK)	dystonia.org.uk

Physical and Occupational Therapy

Patients frequently ask about the value of exercise and physical therapy, because they seem intuitively helpful for addressing abnormal muscle activity and pain. Although many patients seem to appreciate physical therapy, benefits often are temporary, and there are no large-scale double-blind studies that demonstrate objective benefits to justify regular application.

Several investigators have sought to demonstrate objective improvements using specific methods based on theories regarding the pathophysiology of dystonia. For example, the theory that dystonia results from maladaptive neural plasticity[15,38,39] has led to attempts to re-train normal patterns of activity via "constraint-induced" movement training to limit abnormal movements while reinforcing normal ones,[40,41] "sensorimotor retuning" with intensive exercises,[42] "slow-down" therapy,[43] active exercise,[44] and electromyography-biofeedback.[45,46] Theories regarding maladaptive plasticity also have led to the opposing strategy of attempting to erase abnormal plasticity via lengthy periods of immobilization.[47] Theories relating the pathophysiology of dystonia to defects in sensory processes or sensorimotor integration[48] have led to attempts to alter sensory feedback as a treatment strategy. Various methods have been exploited, including modification of sensory inputs,[49,50] "kinesogenic taping,"[51] transcutaneous electrical nerve stimulation,[52] and augmentation of somatosensory discrimination by Braille training.[53]

Despite the enthusiasm for physical therapy in dystonia, systematic reviews have concluded that there is insufficient evidence to recommend any particular strategy.[45,46] There are several reasons for the lack of clear guidelines. First, most of the studies have been quite small with outcomes that often were not reproducible, and the larger studies frequently demonstrated wide response variations among patients. Second, the reported benefits often have been quite small, transient, or subjective. The modest benefits of individual techniques have led to attempts to combine treatments using "multimodal" strategies, further obscuring the value of specific interventions. Third, there is a tradition in physical therapy to customize procedures according to the needs of individual patients. As a result, large studies using uniform protocols are scarce. Double-blind and placebo-controlled studies are rare also in part because of the difficulty in designing an appropriate control group to rule out nonspecific placebo effects. Finally, many of the methods are cumbersome and time consuming, limiting enthusiasm for clinical application.

Enthusiasm for specific strategies also is blunted by concerns that some well-intentioned designs may be harmful. For example, significant improvements have been reported for patients with hand dystonia after 4 to 6 weeks of immobilization with a rigid splint.[54,55] However, broad adoption has been limited by the long duration of splinting, side effects of hand clumsiness, and weakness after splinting, and concerns that prolonged immobilization can trigger more severe fixed dystonia, sometimes as part of the complex regional pain syndrome.[56] Similarly, transcutaneous electrical nerve stimulation has been reported to be helpful in some patients,[52] yet detrimental to others.[57] Despite these limitations, the available studies have provided some promising suggestions that deserve further exploration and development before more general recommendations can be formulated.[58]

In the absence of solid evidence to guide more specific recommendations, it seems reasonable to incorporate general physical therapy methods according to patient preferences. These may include regular stretching exercises to mitigate against contractures, muscle relaxation methods to attenuate pulling and pain, and strengthening of antagonist muscles to balance abnormal postures. Various assistive devices also are available to allow more significantly disabled patients to function more independently.

Oral Medications

There are multiple articles summarizing oral medications for dystonia,[59–63] including 2 systematic evidence-based reviews.[64,65] None of the commonly used drugs has been subject to large-scale, double-blinded, placebo-controlled trials. None of them has been approved by the Food and Drug Administration for treatment of dystonia. Much of the evidence supporting the use of these drugs comes from small controlled trials, nonblinded trials, retrospective reviews, and anecdotal experience (**Table 5**).

Acetylcholine-related drugs

One of the most frequently prescribed classes of medications for the dystonias include anticholinergics, such as trihexyphenidyl, benztropine, biperiden, ethopropazine, orphenadrine, and procyclidine. These drugs are thought to work by blocking muscarinic acetylcholine receptors in the basal ganglia.[66] Their use is supported by multiple retrospective studies,[67] and one prospective, double-blind trial of trihexyphenidyl that showed clinically significant improvements in 71% of patients on a mean dose of 30 mg daily.[68] However, this study included only 31 patients with predominantly isolated dystonia, and a mean age of 19 years. Similar studies of children with dystonia associated with cerebral palsy showed that a significant proportion may worsen with anticholinergics.[69] There are no prospective double-blind, placebo-controlled trials of anticholinergics for older adults, who are less likely to tolerate their many side effects.[70,71]

Despite the limited and sometimes conflicting information, anticholinergics remain in broad use because they seem to be at least partly effective for many types of dystonia, regardless of the underlying etiology. Trihexyphenidyl must be started at a low dose, for example 2 mg twice daily. It can be increased by 2 mg every few days until benefits are observed or side effects emerge. Effective dosages range from 6 to 40 mg daily, divided across 3 to 4 doses. Typical side effects include memory loss, confusion, restlessness, depression, dry mouth, constipation, urinary retention, blurry vision, or worsening of narrow-angle glaucoma.

Dopamine-related drugs

Medications that augment or suppress dopaminergic transmission in the basal ganglia may be extraordinarily helpful in select populations of patients with dystonia. Augmenting dopamine transmission with levodopa is dramatically effective in dopa-responsive dystonia, which is most often caused by mutations in the *GCH1* gene

Table 5
Commonly used oral medications for dystonia

Class of Medication	Examples
Anticholinergics	Benztropine, biperiden, ethopropazine, orphenadrine, procyclidine, trihexyphenidyl
Dopaminergics	Levodopa, pramipexole, ropinirole, tetrabenazine
GABAergics	Alprazolam, baclofen, chlordiazepoxide, clonazepam, diazepam
Muscle "relaxants"	Baclofen, benzodiazepines, carisoprodol, chlorzoxazone, cyclobenzaprine, metaxalone, methocarbamol, orphenadrine
Others	Carbamazepine, cannabidiol, cyproheptadine, gabapentin, lithium, mexiletine, nabilone, riluzole, tizanidine, zolpidem

encoding the enzyme GTP-cyclohydrolase.[72,73] Many patients respond to dosages as low as half of a 25/100-mg tablet of carbidopa/levodopa twice daily, although others require larger dosages.[72] For an adequate trial of levodopa, the dose should be increased slowly to 1000 mg in an adult (or 20 mg/kg for children) divided across 3 daily doses for 1 month before concluding it will not be effective. In addition to levodopa, patients with classical dopa-responsive dystonia respond to dopamine agonists and drugs that block dopamine metabolism, such as monoamine oxidase inhibitors.

Levodopa is also at least partially effective in other disorders affecting dopamine synthesis that are caused by deficiency of tyrosine hydroxylase, sepiapterin reductase, and others.[74] It also may be effective in some other rare disorders, such as the dystonia in some cases of spinocerebellar ataxia type 3[75] or variant forms of ataxia telangiectasia,[76] and for dystonia in Parkinson disease. Aside from these specific populations, levodopa and dopamine agonists are not broadly useful for other types of dystonia, such as the more common adult-onset isolated focal or segmental dystonias.[77]

Medications that suppress dopaminergic transmission also may be useful for specific subgroups of patients. Although dopamine receptor antagonists have been used with variable success in small unblinded studies, their use is generally discouraged because the risk for development of acute dystonic reactions and tardive syndromes may lead to diagnostic confusion and increased disability. However, depletion of dopamine with tetrabenazine does not carry these same risks, and it may be useful for some patients with dystonia, particularly those with tardive dystonia.[78–80] It can be started at half of a 25-mg tablet daily, and titrated up by a half tablet every 3 to 5 days, to a target of 25 to 100 mg daily. Dose-limiting side effects include drowsiness, parkinsonism, depression, insomnia, nervousness, anxiety, and akathisia.

Gamma-aminobutyric acid–related drugs

Another frequently prescribed group of medications is the benzodiazepines such as alprazolam, chlordiazepoxide, clonazepam, and diazepam. They are thought to work by amplifying transmission through gamma-aminobutyric acid (GABA) receptors. There are no large double-blind and controlled studies of the benzodiazepines in dystonia. Their use is supported by multiple small or retrospective studies. Anecdotal experience suggests they may be most useful for suppressing phasic aspects of dystonia, such as blinking in blepharospasm or tremor-dominant forms of dystonia.[67,81,82] They also appear to be useful in the paroxysmal dyskinesias, where dystonia can be a prominent feature.[83] Common side effects include sedation, impaired mentation and coordination, and depression. There also is a risk for tachyphylaxis and dependency, so abrupt discontinuation or sudden large decreases in doses should be avoided.

Baclofen is a GABA receptor agonist that also is often used in dystonia. There are no controlled studies to guide recommendations for its use, but several retrospective studies and anecdotal reports suggest it is most often useful in childhood-onset dystonias, especially those with coexisting spasticity of the lower limbs.[67,84] Some adults also may benefit, but most do not. Effective oral dosages range from 30 to 120 mg daily divided across 3 to 4 doses. Common side effects include sedation, nausea, impaired mentation, dizziness, and loss of muscle tone. Abrupt discontinuation or sudden large decreases in doses can be associated with withdrawal reactions that include delirium and seizures.

Baclofen also can be delivered intrathecally via chronically implanted minipumps, where it may be useful in a subpopulation of patients with dystonia.[85–87] Here again, it has been most often used in children where dystonia is combined with spasticity, especially in the lower limbs. The side effects are similar to those listed previously for oral administration, with additional complications related to the implanted device. These complications include pump malfunction, catheter obstruction or leaks, or infection of the equipment.

Muscle relaxants

Many patients request "muscle relaxants" because they seem intuitively useful for overactive and sore muscles. This is a broad category of medications with diverse mechanisms of action that include baclofen and benzodiazepines described previously, along with carisoprodol, chlorzoxazone, cyclobenzaprine, metaxalone, methocarbamol, and orphenadrine. There are no formal studies to guide recommendations for the use of these drugs in dystonia, and responses vary widely. Nevertheless, many patients seem to derive at least partial benefits, especially those with pain from uncontrolled muscle pulling.

Other medications

A wide variety of other drugs have been advocated for specific forms of dystonia, generally based on small and nonblinded studies or anecdotal experiences. For example, carbamazepine and other anticonvulsants seem particularly useful for dystonic spasms in paroxysmal kinesigenic dyskinesia,[88–90] and alcohol is useful in the myoclonus-dystonia syndrome.[91] Mexiletine and intravenous lidocaine may be helpful in some cases.[92,93] Other options suggested for specific populations include amphetamines, cannabidiol, cyproheptadine, gabapentin, lithium, nabilone, riluzole, tizanidine, and zolpidem.

Botulinum Neurotoxins

Medical BoNTs are derived from a neurotoxic protein produced by the bacterium *Clostridium botulinum*. The bacterial toxin causes a paralytic disorder known as botulism, but medical-grade BoNT is purified and attenuated so that local intramuscular injections can suppress overactive muscles. There are 7 distinct serotypes: A to G. Type A is marketed as onabotulinumtoxinA (Botox), abobotulinumtoxinA (Dysport), and incobotulinumtoxinA (Xeomin). Type B is marketed as rimabotulinumtoxinB (Myobloc). Their safety and efficacy have been the subject of multiple previous summaries, including several systematic evidence-based reviews.[64,94,95] They are effective for many types of dystonia, significantly reducing abnormal movements and associated disability, and improving overall quality of life.

Many detailed resources are available for application of the BoNTs, including target muscle selection, dosing, and the use of ancillary procedures for localization, such as electromyography and ultrasound.[96,97] The technical details associated with administration of BoNTs will not be reviewed here. Instead, the focus is on practical issues faced by physicians who may refer patients for BoNT treatments, and on some of the most common questions regarding their application. The first important issue involves the type of dystonia. The BoNTs are considered the treatment of first choice for most focal and segmental dystonias, including blepharospasm, cervical dystonia, oromandibular and laryngeal dystonias, limb dystonias, and others. The benefits from injections usually emerge after 2 to 7 days, and they last for approximately 3 to 4 months.[98] Most patients return for treatments 3 to 4 times yearly. BoNTs also can be valuable for patients with broader patterns of dystonia, where they are often underutilized. For these patients, the goal is to target the muscles that cause the most discomfort. For example, patients with dyskinetic cerebral palsy often have generalized dystonia with prominent involvement of the neck, and treatment with BoNT can alleviate this discomfort and reduce the risk of acquired myelopathy.[99]

The BoNTs are dramatically effective for most focal dystonias, but it can be challenging to get good results with certain subtypes. Some patients with blepharospasm have coexisting apraxia of eyelid opening, which is more difficult to treat with BoNT.[100] Injections into the pretarsal portion of the orbicularis oculi muscles may improve outcomes in these cases.[101,102] Among patients with cervical dystonia, those with prominent anterocollis can be more difficult to treat.[103] Deep injections into prevertebral muscles have been advocated,[104,105] although responses vary. For laryngeal dystonias, spasmodic adductor dysphonia responds more predictably than spasmodic abductor dysphonia.[106,107] Oromandibular and lingual dystonias can sometimes be challenging to treat, although good outcomes can be achieved in experienced hands.[108–112] Because there are so many small muscles that work together for coordinated activities, it can be difficult to achieve satisfactory outcomes for hand dystonias. Some patients enjoy dramatic benefits with very small doses, but achieving the right dose to avoid weakness or involvement of nearby muscles can be difficult to balance.[113]

Another important issue involves side effects. There are no deleterious long-term side effects even after decades of treatment, apart from a small risk of developing resistance due to antibodies that neutralize the BoNT protein. However, the development of immunologically mediated resistance is rare with current preparations of BoNT.[114,115] The short-term side effects depend mostly on local diffusion from the sites of injection. For blepharospasm, the most common side effects are ptosis, local hematoma formation, tearing, and, rarely, blurry vision or diplopia. For cervical dystonia, the most common side effects are dysphagia, excessive neck muscle weakness, and, occasionally, dry mouth. For laryngeal dystonias, the most common side effects are hoarseness or hypophonia, and rarely dysphagia and aspiration. For limb dystonias, the most common side effects involve excessive weakening, or weakness of nearby muscles. Systemic side effects are unusual, but a few patients complain of a flulike syndrome for 3 to 5 days after their treatments.

A third issue involves the selection of a specific product. Many articles have summarized differences among the BoNTs regarding efficacy, side effects, and formulations. However, there are few scientifically rigorous comparisons, and the similarities are more striking than the differences (**Table 6**). The choice of product depends largely on the experience and preferences of individual providers.

Surgical Interventions

Multiple surgical interventions are available for the treatment of the dystonias. Typically, these more invasive approaches are reserved for patients who fail more conservative therapies. The most common intervention involves neuromodulation of brain activity via an implanted electrical impulse generator that is connected to an electrical lead in the brain, although focal ablation of select brain areas and peripheral approaches that target nerves or muscles can be applied in some circumstances.

Neuromodulation

Neuromodulation is synonymous with deep brain stimulation (DBS). The term neuromodulation is increasingly preferred because some targets may not be "deep" and "stimulation" implies a mechanism that has not been established. Several extensive reviews on neuromodulation have been published recently,[116–118] including a whole issue of the journal *Movement Disorders* (volume 26, supplement 1, 2011). Here, the

Table 6
Comparison of the most common botulinum toxin formulations

Characteristic	OnabotulinumtoxinA (Botox)	AbobotulinumtoxinA (Dysport)	IncobotulinumtoxinA (Xeomin)	RimabotulinumtoxinB (Myobloc)
FDA-approved indications for dystonia	Blepharospasm, cervical dystonia	Cervical dystonia	Blepharospasm, cervical dystonia	Cervical dystonia
Preparation	Vacuum dried	Freeze dried	Powder	Liquid
Available dose sizes (units)	100, 200	300, 500	50, 100	1000, 2500, 5000
Storage	Refrigerate	Refrigerate	Room temperature	Refrigerate
Approximate dose equivalency[a]	1	2.5–3	1	40

Abbreviation: FDA, Food and Drug Administration.
[a] As the first FDA-approved botulinum neurotoxin, onabotulinumtoxinA was arbitrarily defined as having a strength of 1. The relative strengths of the others are compared against this value.

focus is on practical issues of relevance to any physician who may counsel patients regarding these options. The issues include patient selection for best outcomes, long-term expectations, and some ongoing debates.

Some patients with dystonia respond quite well to neuromodulation, whereas others derive no benefit. Many years of experience have provided some important insights into several factors that predict responses.[118,119] Patients with isolated generalized dystonia syndromes (previously "primary" dystonia) tend to respond most consistently, with the most objective blinded studies showing improvements in standardized dystonia rating scales of 40% to 60%.[120,121] Among this patient population, best outcomes appear to be associated with younger ages, shorter disease durations, and those who have the common *TOR1A* mutation for DYT1 dystonia. There is insufficient evidence to predict outcomes for the more recently discovered genes, including the *THAP1* gene for DYT6. Patients with fixed contractures or scoliosis do not do so well as those with more a more mobile syndrome.

Patients with isolated focal and segmental dystonias also appear to respond well to neuromodulation, although perhaps less predictably than those with isolated generalized dystonia. This group includes patients with relatively localized or segmental patterns involving the neck, face, trunk, or limbs. Patients with dystonic syndromes that are combined with other neurologic features (previously "dystonia plus" or "secondary" dystonias) respond variably. Some subtypes consistently respond very well, for example myoclonus dystonia and tardive dystonia. Others have a consistently poor outcome (eg, degenerative disorders) or are less predictable (eg, cerebral palsy). One of the reasons for the poor outcomes in some populations is that it is difficult to detect a stable benefit for progressive degenerative disorders, or for disorders in which dystonia is combined with other motor defects, such as spasticity, that are not expected to improve with neuromodulation. These populations should be considered for surgery only by very experienced centers after careful counseling, ideally as part of a methodical study aimed at elucidating risk/benefit profiles.

The long-term outcomes of neuromodulation are good,[122–124] with benefits sustained for many years, and some studies reporting good outcomes even after 10 years.[125] Ongoing access to an experienced center to adjust stimulator settings and address potential complications is essential. Benefits from surgery can be delayed for weeks or even months, requiring frequent visits to adjust stimulator settings for optimal outcomes. Return visits also should be anticipated every 2 to 4 years for battery replacement. In one study of 47 cases with DYT1 dystonia followed by a very experienced multidisciplinary neuromodulation center for more than 10 years, 8.5% had delayed postoperative infection of equipment requiring antibiotics and/or equipment removal, 8.5% had malfunction of equipment, such as impulse generator failure or lead defects, and 4.3% required revisions of lead location.[125] These observations indicate that close follow-up by an experienced team is essential for long-term maintenance therapy. This requirement for return visits presents a barrier for some patients who may live far from experienced providers.

There are several unresolved questions that the counseling physician may be asked to address. One is the ideal surgical target.[116,118] The internal segment of the globus pallidus is the traditional target used by most centers. However, observations that patients with dystonia sometimes develop bradykinesia in unaffected body regions or gait failure have led to interest in other targets, such as the subthalamic nucleus. On the other hand, neuromodulation of the subthalamic nucleus has been associated with dyskinesias, weight gain, and psychiatric changes. Others have targeted various regions of the thalamus, usually for focal hand dystonia and those with prominent tremor.[126–128] The "ideal" target remains unknown. Whether this target varies according to the subtype of dystonia also remains uncertain. As a result, the selection of targets often is driven by the opinions of individual centers.

Another unresolved question involves the expected outcomes for patients with dystonias combined with other neurologic features (previously "secondary" dystonias). Aside from tardive dystonia and myoclonus dystonia, there is insufficient information to counsel interested patients regarding expectations. The lack of information should not be viewed as an absolute contraindication for surgery, but patients must be clearly informed about the chances for failure.

Ablative approaches

Making controlled focal lesions in specific parts of the brain was the most common surgical procedure conducted for patients with dystonia before neuromodulation became more popular.[129] Lesions were made in a variety of locations, most notably the thalamus, globus pallidus, and cerebellum. Neuromodulation rapidly became more popular because it is more readily tunable, and because it is reversible in the event that intolerable side effects develop. However, neuromodulation has its own risk of complications related to the hardware, and it is expensive. Therefore, there is still a role for ablative procedures in some circumstances.[116,129]

Ablative procedures may be useful in developing countries where the cost of equipment for neuromodulation and requirements for regular follow-up are prohibitive. Ablations also are useful for patients with a body habitus that presents a high risk for hardware-related complications, such as those with severe dystonia and fixed contractions, or very young or otherwise small patients. They may be offered to patients who suffer repeated hardware infections, or merely do not wish to have chronically implanted hardware. They also may be appropriate as palliative procedures for patients with severe illness who cannot tolerate surgery to install and maintain the hardware, and for some progressive neurodegenerative disorders.

Peripheral surgeries

Another category of surgeries often offered to patients with dystonia before BoNTs and neuromodulation became more popular involved directly sectioning or destroying overactive muscles or the nerves controlling them. These procedures are far less commonly used today, but they are still offered by some centers. They are covered briefly here for physicians encountering patients who may ask about them.

Selective peripheral denervation may be offered to patients with cervical dystonia who fail oral agents and botulinum toxins. The procedure involves extraspinal sectioning of nerves to specific muscles, so best outcomes are seen for patients with a limited number of muscles involved (eg, pure torticollis or pure laterocollis). Success rates are reported from 60% to 90%.[130–135] Side effects may include permanent somatosensory loss or dysesthesia in an isolated region of the neck, cosmetic changes associated with scaring or muscle atrophy, muscle weakness, decreased range of motion and dysphagia. Abnormal movements may reemerge after several weeks or years, a phenomenon that may reflect reinnervation or progression of the underlying disorder.

A variety of procedures are offered to patients with blepharospasm too. They include orbicularis myectomy, frontalis suspension, surgical shortening of the levator palpebrae, and removal of redundant eyelid skin.[136–138] None of these procedures has been subject to rigorous trials, so they usually are offered only to patients who fail botulinum toxins. Included are patients who are resistant to the toxins, and those with coexisting apraxia of eyelid opening that may respond poorly to the toxins.

There also are several procedures in use for patients with laryngeal dystonia.[139,140] Patients with spasmodic dysphonia may undergo thyroplasty to modify the cartilaginous structure of the larynx or thyroarytenoid myectomy. The most common approach involves sectioning the recurrent laryngeal nerve to the thyroarytenoid and annealing the stump to the ansa cervicalis. Complications can include transient or permanent voice impediment, dysphagia, and return of symptoms requiring reoperation.

STRATEGIES FOR COMBINING THERAPIES FOR SPECIFIC POPULATIONS

Because there are so many different clinical manifestations and causes of the dystonias, it is not feasible to devise a universal treatment algorithm for all subtypes that combines the various medical and surgical options outlined previously. Although treatment plans must be individualized, there are some useful guiding principles. The first step is to delineate the diagnosis (see **Fig. 1**). The diagnostic subtype is important for the application of some types of treatments that target underlying etiologic mechanisms and substantially modify the course of the disease (see **Table 3**). The next step involves counseling to address expectations from treatment and any psychiatric comorbidities.

For most patients in whom disease-modifying therapies are not yet available, treatments are symptomatic. For late-onset focal or segmental dystonia, BoNTs are the treatment of first choice. Because symptoms may wax and wane in severity, an oral agent may be offered as adjunctive therapy to use when needed. When BoNTs and oral medications are not adequate, patients with focal and segmental dystonias may undergo more invasive surgical approaches.

For adults with generalized dystonia and all early-onset dystonias, regardless of body distribution, where diagnostic testing does not reveal a cause with etiology-based treatments, a trial of levodopa is mandatory to address the possibility of dopa-responsive dystonia. There are no data to guide the exact age cutoff at which a levodopa trial is essential, but many providers proceed with a levodopa trial for any patient with isolated dystonia who is younger than 40 years. Following this trial, other oral agents also may be attempted. BoNT may be offered to those in whom one particular region of the body creates the most disability, and surgical interventions are offered when oral agents and BoNT provide insufficient benefits. In many cases, multiple treatment options are combined.

SUMMARY

The treatment of patients with dystonia has improved dramatically over recent years. There is a rapidly growing list of specific subtypes with specific treatments that target the underlying etiology. This list is expected to continue to grow, as more is learned about the underlying causes for dystonia. There are 4 widely available BoNT preparations. They are highly effective in the treatment of focal and segmental dystonias, and can be of benefit in patients with broader distributions too. Neuromodulation of the brain and peripheral surgeries that target nerve or muscles also can be very useful when more conservative methods fail. Knowing how to mix and match these various treatment modalities for specific populations can be challenging, but significant benefits can be achieved in the vast majority of patients (Videos 1–8).

DISCLOSURES

H.A. Jinnah has received in the past 3 years research grant support from the National Institutes of Health (NIH), Ipsen Pharmaceuticals, Merz Pharmaceuticals, Psyadon Pharmaceuticals, the Atlanta Clinical & Translational Science Institute, the Emory

University Research Council, the Lesch-Nyhan Syndrome Children's Research Foundation, the Dystonia Medical Research Foundation, the Bachmann-Strauss Dystonia & Parkinson's Foundation, and the Benign Essential Blepharospasm Research Foundation. He is principal investigator for the Dystonia Coalition, which receives most of its support through NIH grant NS065701 from the Office of Rare Diseases Research in the National Center for Advancing Translational Sciences and National Institute of Neurologic Disorders and Stroke. The Dystonia Coalition receives additional material or administrative support from industry sponsors (Allergan Inc, Ipsen Biopharm, Medtronics Inc, and Merz Pharmaceuticals) as well as private foundations (The American Dystonia Society, The Bachmann-Strauss Dystonia and Parkinson Foundation, BeatDystonia, The Benign Essential Blepharospasm Foundation, Dystonia Europe, Dystonia Ireland, The Dystonia Medical Research Foundation, The Dystonia Society, The Foundation for Dystonia Research, The National Spasmodic Dysphonia Association, and The National Spasmodic Torticollis Association). Dr H.A. Jinnah serves on the Scientific Advisory Boards for Cure Dystonia Now, the Dystonia Medical Research Foundation, Tyler's Hope for a Dystonia Cure, the Lesch-Nyhan Syndrome Children's Research Foundation, and Lesch-Nyhan Action France.

SUPPLEMENTARY DATA

Supplementary data related to this article can be found online at http://dx.doi.org/10.1016/j.ncl.2014.09.002

REFERENCES

1. Fahn S. The varied clinical expressions of dystonia. Neurol Clin 1984;2:541–54.
2. Fahn S. Clinical variants of idiopathic torsion dystonia. J Neurol Neurosurg Psychiatry 1989;(Suppl):96–100.
3. Elble RJ. Defining dystonic tremor. Curr Neuropharmacol 2013;11:48–52.
4. Erro R, Rubio-Agusti I, Saifee TA, et al. Rest and other types of tremor in adult-onset primary dystonia. J Neurol Neurosurg Psychiatry 2014;85:965–8.
5. Defazio G, Gigante AF, Abbruzzese G, et al. Tremor in primary adult-onset dystonia: prevalence and associated clinical features. J Neurol Neurosurg Psychiatry 2013;84:404–8.
6. Albanese A, Bhatia K, Bressman SB, et al. Phenomenology and classification of dystonia: a consensus update. Mov Disord 2013;28:863–73.
7. Fung VS, Jinnah HA, Bhatia K, et al. Assessment of the patient with dystonia: an update on dystonia syndromes. Mov Disord 2013;28:889–98.
8. LeDoux MS. The genetics of dystonias. Adv Genet 2012;79:35–85.
9. Lohmann K, Klein C. Genetics of dystonia: what's known? what's new? what's next? Mov Disord 2013;28:899–905.
10. LeDoux MS, Dauer WT, Warner T. Emerging molecular pathways for dystonia. Mov Disord 2013;15:968–81.
11. Thompson VB, Jinnah HA, Hess EJ. Convergent mechanisms in etiologically-diverse dystonias. Expert Opin Ther Targets 2011;15:1387–403.
12. Neychev VK, Gross R, Lehericy S, et al. The functional neuroanatomy of dystonia. Neurobiol Dis 2011;42:185–201.
13. Lehericy S, Tijssen MA, Vidailhet M, et al. The anatomical basis of dystonia: current view using neuroimaging. Mov Disord 2013;28:944–57.
14. Prudente CN, Hess EJ, Jinnah HA. Dystonia as a network disorder: what is the role of the cerebellum? Neuroscience 2014;260:23–35.

15. Quartarone A, Hallett M. Emerging concepts in the physiological basis of dystonia. Mov Disord 2013;28:958–67.
16. Kojovic M, Parees I, Kassavetis P, et al. Secondary and primary dystonia: pathophysiological differences. Brain 2013;136:2038–49.
17. Hallett M. Pathophysiology of dystonia. J Neural Transm Suppl 2006;70:485–8.
18. Jinnah HA, Berardelli A, Comella C, et al. The focal dystonias: current views and challenges for future research. Mov Disord 2013;7:926–43.
19. Stamelou M, Lai SC, Aggarwal A, et al. Dystonic opisthotonus: a "red flag" for neurodegeneration with brain iron accumulation syndromes? Mov Disord 2013;28:1325–9.
20. Schneider SA, Aggarwal A, Bhatt MH, et al. Severe tongue protrusion dystonia: clinical syndromes and possible treatment. Neurology 2006;67:940–3.
21. Evatt ML, Freeman A, Factor S. Adult-onset dystonia. Handb Clin Neurol 2011; 100:481–511.
22. Schneider SA, Bhatia KP. Secondary dystonia—clinical clues and syndromic associations. Eur J Neurol 2010;17(Suppl 1):52–7.
23. Schneider SA, Bhatia KP, Hardy J. Complicated recessive dystonia parkinsonism syndromes. Mov Disord 2009;24:490–9.
24. Garcia-Cazorla A, Wolf NI, Serrano M, et al. Inborn errors of metabolism and motor disturbances in children. J Inherit Metab Dis 2009;32:618–29.
25. Stamelou M, Alonso-Canovas A, Bhatia KP. Dystonia in corticobasal degeneration: a review of the literature on 404 pathologically proven cases. Mov Disord 2012;27:696–702.
26. Wickremaratchi MM, Knipe MD, Sastry BS, et al. The motor phenotype of Parkinson's disease in relation to age at onset. Mov Disord 2011;26:457–63.
27. Lalli S, Albanese A. The diagnostic challenge of primary dystonia: evidence from misdiagnosis. Mov Disord 2010;25:1619–26.
28. McKeon A, Matsumoto JY, Bower JH, et al. The spectrum of disorders presenting as adult-onset focal lower extremity dystonia. Parkinsonism Relat Disord 2008;14:613–9.
29. Tolosa E, Compta Y. Dystonia in Parkinson's disease. J Neurol 2006; 253(Suppl 7):7–13.
30. Jankovic J. Dystonia and other deformities in Parkinson's disease. J Neurol Sci 2005;229:1–3.
31. Tiderington E, Goodman EM, Rosen AR, et al. How long does it take to diagnose cervical dystonia? J Neurol Sci 2013;335:72–4.
32. Jog M, Chouinard S, Hobson D, et al. Causes for treatment delays in dystonia and hemifacial spasm: a Canadian survey. Can J Neurol Sci 2011;38:704–11.
33. Charles PD, Adler CH, Stacy M, et al. Cervical dystonia and pain: characteristics and treatment patterns from CD PROBE (Cervical Dystonia Patient Registry for Observation of OnabotulinumtoxinA Efficacy). J Neurol 2014;261:1309–19.
34. Zurowski M, Marsh L, McDonald W. Psychiatric comorbidities in dystonia: emerging concepts. Mov Disord 2013;28:914–20.
35. Kuyper DJ, Parra V, Aerts S, et al. Nonmotor manifestations of dystonia: a systematic review. Mov Disord 2011;26:1206–17.
36. Fabbrini G, Berardelli I, Moretti G, et al. Psychiatric disorders in adult-onset focal dystonia: a case-control study. Mov Disord 2010;25:459–65.
37. Lewis L, Butler A, Jahanshahi M. Depression in focal, segmental and generalized dystonia. J Neurol 2008;255:1750–5.
38. Peterson DA, Sejnowski TJ, Poizner H. Convergent evidence for abnormal striatal synaptic plasticity in dystonia. Neurobiol Dis 2010;37:558–73.

39. Quartarone A, Siebner HR, Rothwell JC. Task-specific hand dystonia: can too much plasticity be bad for you? Trends Neurosci 2006;29:192–9.
40. Candia V, Schafer T, Taub E, et al. Sensory motor retuning: a behavioral treatment for focal hand dystonia of pianists and guitarists. Arch Phys Med Rehabil 2002;83:1342–8.
41. Uswatte G, Taub E. Constraint-induced movement therapy: a method for harnessing neuroplasticity to treat motor disorders. Prog Brain Res 2013;207: 379–401.
42. Zeuner KE, Shill HA, Sohn YH, et al. Motor training as treatment in focal hand dystonia. Mov Disord 2005;20:335–41.
43. Sakai N. Slow-down exercise for the treatment of focal hand dystonia in pianists. Med Probl Perform Art 2006;21:25–8.
44. Boyce MJ, Canning CG, Mahant N, et al. Active exercise for individuals with cervical dystonia: a pilot randomized controlled trial. Clin Rehabil 2012;27: 226–35.
45. Delnooz CC, Horstink MW, Tijssen MA, et al. Paramedical treatment in primary dystonia: a systematic review. Mov Disord 2009;24:2187–98.
46. De Pauw J, Van der Velden K, Meirte J, et al. The effectiveness of physiotherapy for cervical dystonia: a systematic literature review. J Neurol 2014;261:1857–65.
47. Cogiamanian F, Barbieri S, Priori A. Novel nonpharmacologic perspectives for the treatment of task-specific focal hand dystonia. J Hand Ther 2009;22:156–61.
48. Tinazzi M, Fiorio M, Fiaschi A, et al. Sensory functions in dystonia: insights from behavioral studies. Mov Disord 2009;24:1427–36.
49. Karnath HO, Konczak J, Dichgans J. Effect of prolonged neck muscle vibration on lateral head tilt in severe spasmodic torticollis. J Neurol Neurosurg Psychiatry 2000;69:658–60.
50. Leis AA, Dimitrijevic MR, Delapasse JS, et al. Modification of cervical dystonia by selective sensory stimulation. J Neurol Sci 1992;110:79–89.
51. Pelosin E, Avanzino L, Marchese R, et al. Kinesiotaping reduces pain and modulates sensory function in patients with focal dystonia: a randomized cross-over pilot study. Neurorehabil Neural Repair 2013;27:722–31.
52. Tinazzi M, Farina S, Bhatia K, et al. TENS for the treatment of writer's cramp dystonia: a randomized, placebo-controlled study. Neurology 2005;64:1946–8.
53. Zeuner KE, Bara-Jimenez W, Noguchi PS, et al. Sensory training for patients with focal hand dystonia. Ann Neurol 2002;51:593–8.
54. Pesenti A, Barbieri S, Priori A. Limb immobilization for occupational dystonia: a possible alternative treatment for selected patients. Adv Neurol 2004;94: 247–54.
55. Priori A, Pesenti A, Cappellari A, et al. Limb immobilization for the treatment of focal occupational dystonia. Neurology 2001;57:405–9.
56. Okun MS, Nadeau SE, Rossi F, et al. Immobilization dystonia. J Neurol Sci 2002; 201:79–83.
57. Meunier S, Bleton JP, Mazevet D, et al. TENS is harmful in primary writing tremor. Clin Neurophysiol 2011;122:171–5.
58. van den Dool J, Visser B, Koelman JH, et al. Cervical dystonia: effectiveness of a standardized physical therapy program; study design and protocol of a single blind randomized controlled trial. BMC Neurol 2013;13:85.
59. Jankovic J. Medical treatment of dystonia. Mov Disord 2013;28:1001–12.
60. Jankovic J. Treatment of dystonia. Lancet Neurol 2006;5:864–72.
61. Bhidayasiri R, Tarsy D. Treatment of dystonia. Expert Rev Neurother 2006;6: 863–86.

62. Goldman JG, Comella CL. Treatment of dystonia. Clin Neuropharmacol 2003;26: 102–8.
63. Cloud LJ, Jinnah HA. Treatment strategies for dystonia. Expert Opin Pharmacother 2010;11:5–15.
64. Albanese A, Barnes MP, Bhatia KP, et al. A systematic review on the diagnosis and treatment of primary (idiopathic) dystonia and dystonia plus syndromes: report of an EFNS/MDS-ES task force. Eur J Neurol 2006;13:433–44.
65. Balash Y, Giladi N. Efficacy of pharmacological treatment of dystonia: evidence-based review including meta-analysis of the effect of botulinum toxin and other cure options. Eur J Neurol 2004;11:361–70.
66. Pisani A, Bernardi G, Ding J, et al. Re-emergence of striatal cholinergic interneurons in movement disorders. Trends Neurosci 2007;30:545–53.
67. Greene P, Shale H, Fahn S. Experience with high dosages of anticholinergic and other drugs in the treatment of torsion dystonia. Adv Neurol 1988;50:547–56.
68. Burke RE, Fahn S, Marsden CD. Torsion dystonia: a double-blind, prospective trial of high-dosage trihexyphenidyl. Neurology 1986;36:160–4.
69. Sanger TD, Bastian A, Brunstrom J, et al. Prospective open-label clinical trial of trihexyphenidyl in children with secondary dystonia due to cerebral palsy. J Child Neurol 2007;22:530–7.
70. Fahn S. High dosage anticholinergic therapy in dystonia. Neurology 1983;33: 1255–61.
71. Taylor AE, Lang AE, Saint-Cyr JA, et al. Cognitive processes in idiopathic dystonia treated with high-dose anticholinergic therapy: implications for treatment strategies. Clin Neuropharmacol 1991;14:62–77.
72. Nygaard TG, Marsden CD, Fahn S. Dopa-responsive dystonia: long-term treatment response and prognosis. Neurology 1991;41:174–81.
73. Segawa M, Nomura Y, Nishiyama N. Dopa-responsive dystonia. In: Stacey MA, editor. Handbook of dystonia. New York: Informa Healthcare, Inc; 2008. p. 219–44.
74. Kurian MA, Gissen P, Smith M, et al. The monoamine neurotransmitter disorders: an expanding range of neurological syndromes. Lancet Neurol 2011; 10:721–33.
75. Wilder-Smith E, Tan EK, Law HY, et al. Spinocerebellar ataxia type 3 presenting as an L-DOPA responsive dystonia phenotype in a Chinese family. J Neurol Sci 2003;213:25–8.
76. Charlesworth G, Mohire MD, Schneider SA, et al. Ataxia telangiectasia presenting as dopa-responsive cervical dystonia. Neurology 2013;81:1148–51.
77. Lang AE. Dopamine agonists and antagonists in the treatment of idiopathic dystonia. Adv Neurol 1988;50:561–70.
78. Chen JJ, Ondo WG, Dashtipour K, et al. Tetrabenazine for the treatment of hyperkinetic movement disorders: a review of the literature. Clin Ther 2012;34: 1487–504.
79. Jankovic J, Beach J. Long-term effects of tetrabenazine in hyperkinetic movement disorders. Neurology 1997;48:358–62.
80. Jankovic J, Orman J. Tetrabenazine therapy of dystonia, chorea, tics, and other dyskinesias. Neurology 1988;38:391–4.
81. Fasano A, Bove F, Lang AE. The treatment of dystonic tremor: a systematic review. J Neurol Neurosurg Psychiatry 2014;85:759–69.
82. Jankovic J, Ford J. Blepharospasm and orofacial-cervical dystonia: clinical and pharmacological findings in 100 patients. Ann Neurol 1983;13:402–11.
83. Strzelczyk A, Burk K, Oertel WH. Treatment of paroxysmal dyskinesias. Expert Opin Pharmacother 2011;12:63–72.

84. Greene P. Baclofen in the treatment of dystonia. Clin Neuropharmacol 1992;15: 276–88.
85. Walker RH, Danisi FO, Swope DM, et al. Intrathecal baclofen for dystonia: benefits and complications during six years of experience. Mov Disord 2000; 15:1242–7.
86. Albright AL, Barry MJ, Shafron DH, et al. Intrathecal baclofen for generalized dystonia. Dev Med Child Neurol 2001;43:652–7.
87. Hou JG, Ondo W, Jankovic J. Intrathecal baclofen for dystonia. Mov Disord 2001;16:1201–2.
88. Houser MK, Soland VL, Bhatia KP, et al. Paroxysmal kinesigenic choreoathetosis: a report of 26 patients. J Neurol 1999;246:120–6.
89. Fahn S, Marsden CD. The paroxysmal dyskinesias. In: Marsden CD, Fahn S, editors. Movement disorders 3. Oxford (United Kingdom): Butterworth-Heinemann; 1994. p. 310–47.
90. Demirkiran M, Jankovic J. Paroxysmal dyskinesias: clinical features and classification. Ann Neurol 1995;38:571–9.
91. Kinugawa K, Vidailhet M, Clot F, et al. Myoclonus-dystonia: an update. Mov Disord 2009;24:479–89.
92. Lucetti C, Nuti A, Gambaccini G, et al. Mexiletine in the treatment of torticollis and generalized dystonia. Clin Neuropharmacol 2000;23:186–9.
93. Ohara S, Hayashi R, Momoi H, et al. Mexiletine in the treatment of spasmodic torticollis. Mov Disord 1998;13:934–40.
94. Hallett M, Benecke R, Blitzer A, et al. Treatment of focal dystonias with botulinum neurotoxin. Toxicon 2009;54:628–33.
95. Simpson DM, Blitzer A, Brashear A, et al. Assessment: botulinum neurotoxin for the treatment of movement disorders (an evidence-based review): report of the Therapeutics and Technology Assessment Subcommittee of the American Academy of Neurology. Neurology 2008;70:1699–706.
96. Truong D, Dressler D, Hallet M, et al. Manual of botulinum toxin. Cambridge (United Kingdom): Cambridge University Press; 2009.
97. Jost W, Valerius KP. Pictorial atlas of botulinum toxin injection: dosage, localization, application. Berlin: Quintessence Publishing Company; 2008.
98. Marsh WA, Monroe DM, Brin MF, et al. Systematic review and meta-analysis of the duration of clinical effect of onabotulinumtoxinA in cervical dystonia. BMC Neurol 2014;14:91.
99. Vidailhet M. Treatment of movement disorders in dystonia-choreoathetosis cerebral palsy. Handb Clin Neurol 2013;111:197–202.
100. Rana AQ, Shah R. Combination of blepharospasm and apraxia of eyelid opening: a condition resistant to treatment. Acta Neurol Belg 2012;112:95–6.
101. Aramideh M, Ongerboer de Visser BW, Brans JW, et al. Pretarsal application of botulinum toxin for treatment of blepharospasm. J Neurol Neurosurg Psychiatry 1995;59:309–11.
102. Esposito M, Fasano A, Crisci C, et al. The combined treatment with orbital and pretarsal botulinum toxin injections in the management of poorly responsive blepharospasm. Neurol Sci 2013;35:397–400.
103. Waln O, Ledoux MS. Blepharospasm plus cervical dystonia with predominant anterocollis: a distinctive subphenotype of segmental craniocervical dystonia? Tremor Other Hyperkinet Mov (N Y) 2011;2011(1). pii: 33.
104. Glass GA, Ku S, Ostrem JL, et al. Fluoroscopic, EMG-guided injection of botulinum toxin into the longus colli for the treatment of anterocollis. Parkinsonism Relat Disord 2009;15:610–3.

105. Bhidayasiri R. Treatment of complex cervical dystonia with botulinum toxin: involvement of deep-cervical muscles may contribute to suboptimal responses. Parkinsonism Relat Disord 2011;17(Suppl 1):S20–4.
106. Blitzer A. Spasmodic dysphonia and botulinum toxin: experience from the largest treatment series. Eur J Neurol 2010;17(Suppl 1):28–30.
107. Watts CC, Whurr R, Nye C. Botulinum toxin injections for the treatment of spasmodic dysphonia. Cochrane Database Syst Rev 2004;(3):CD004327.
108. Esper CD, Freeman A, Factor SA. Lingual protrusion dystonia: frequency, etiology and botulinum toxin therapy. Parkinsonism Relat Disord 2010;16:438–41.
109. Charles PD, Davis TL, Shannon KM, et al. Tongue protrusion dystonia: treatment with botulinum toxin. South Med J 1997;90:522–5.
110. Singer C, Papapetropoulos S. A comparison of jaw-closing and jaw-opening idiopathic oromandibular dystonia. Parkinsonism Relat Disord 2006;12:115–8.
111. Blitzer A, Brin MF, Greene PE, et al. Botulinum toxin injection for the treatment of oromandibular dystonia. Ann Otol Rhinol Laryngol 1989;98:93–7.
112. Gonzalez-Alegre P, Schneider RL, Hoffman H. Clinical, etiological, and therapeutic features of jaw-opening and jaw-closing oromandibular dystonias: a decade of experience at a single treatment center. Tremor Other Hyperkinet Mov (N Y) 2014;4:231.
113. Lungu C, Karp BI, Alter K, et al. Long-term follow-up of botulinum toxin therapy for focal hand dystonia: outcome at 10 years or more. Mov Disord 2011;26:750–3.
114. Naumann M, Boo LM, Ackerman AH, et al. Immunogenicity of botulinum toxins. J Neural Transm 2013;120:275–90.
115. Brin MF, Comella CL, Jankovic J, et al. Long-term treatment with botulinum toxin type A in cervical dystonia has low immunogenicity by mouse protection assay. Mov Disord 2008;23:1353–60.
116. Moro E, Gross RE, Krauss JK. What's new in surgical treatments for dystonia? Mov Disord 2013;28:1013–20.
117. Vidailhet M, Jutras MF, Grabli D, et al. Deep brain stimulation for dystonia. J Neurol Neurosurg Psychiatry 2012;84:1029–40.
118. Mills KA, Starr PA, Ostrem JL. Neuromodulation for dystonia: target and patient selection. Neurosurg Clin N Am 2014;25:59–75.
119. Andrews C, Aviles-Olmos I, Hariz M, et al. Which patients with dystonia benefit from deep brain stimulation? A metaregression of individual patient outcomes. J Neurol Neurosurg Psychiatry 2010;81:1383–9.
120. Vidailhet M, Vercueil L, Houeto JL, et al. Bilateral deep-brain stimulation of the globus pallidus in primary generalized dystonia. N Engl J Med 2005;352: 459–67.
121. Kupsch A, Benecke R, Muller J, et al. Pallidal deep-brain stimulation in primary generalized or segmental dystonia. N Engl J Med 2006;355:1978–90.
122. Tagliati M, Krack P, Volkmann J, et al. Long-term management of DBS in dystonia: response to stimulation, adverse events, battery changes, and special considerations. Mov Disord 2011;26(Suppl 1):S54–62.
123. Volkmann J, Wolters A, Kupsch A, et al. Pallidal deep brain stimulation in patients with primary generalised or segmental dystonia: 5-year follow-up of a randomised trial. Lancet Neurol 2012;11:1029–38.
124. Reese R, Gruber D, Schoenecker T, et al. Long-term clinical outcome in Meige syndrome treated with internal pallidum deep brain stimulation. Mov Disord 2011;26:691–8.
125. Panov F, Gologorsky Y, Connors G, et al. Deep brain stimulation in DYT1 dystonia: a 10-year experience. Neurosurgery 2013;73:86–93.

126. Morishita T, Foote KD, Haq IU, et al. Should we consider Vim thalamic deep brain stimulation for select cases of severe refractory dystonic tremor. Stereotact Funct Neurosurg 2010;88:98–104.
127. Goto S, Shimazu H, Matsuzaki K, et al. Thalamic Vo-complex vs pallidal deep brain stimulation for focal hand dystonia. Neurology 2008;70:1500–1.
128. Fukaya C, Katayama Y, Kano T, et al. Thalamic deep brain stimulation for writer's cramp. J Neurosurg 2007;107:977–82.
129. Gross R. What happened to posteroventral pallidotomy for Parkinson's disease and dystonia? Neurotherapeutics 2008;5:281–93.
130. Arce CA. Selective denervation in cervical dystonia. In: Stacey MA, editor. Handbook of dystonia. New York: Informa Healthcare USA, Inc; 2007. p. 381–92.
131. Bertrand CM. Selective peripheral denervation for spasmodic torticollis: surgical technique, results, and observations in 260 cases. Surg Neurol 1993;40:96–103.
132. Munchau A, Palmer JD, Dressler D, et al. Prospective study of selective peripheral denervation for botulinum toxin resistant patients with cervical dystonia. Brain 2001;124:769–83.
133. Cohen-Gadol AA, Ahlskog JE, Matsumoto JY, et al. Selective peripheral denervation for the treatment of intractable spasmodic torticollis: experience with 168 patients at the Mayo clinic. J Neurosurg 2003;98:1247–54.
134. Chen X, Ma A, Liang J, et al. Selective denervation and resection of cervical muscles in the treatment of spasmodic torticollis: long-term follow-up results in 207 cases. Stereotact Funct Neurosurg 2000;75:96–102.
135. Braun V, Richter HP. Selective peripheral denervation for spasmodic torticollis: 13 year experience with 155 patients. J Neurosurg 2002;97:207–12.
136. Georgescu D, Vagefi MR, McMullan TF, et al. Upper eyelid myectomy in blepharospasm with associated apraxia of lid opening. Am J Ophthalmol 2008;145:541–7.
137. Grivet D, Robert PY, Thuret G, et al. Assessment of blepharospasm surgery using an improved disability scale: study of 138 patients. Ophthal Plast Reconstr Surg 2005;21:230–4.
138. Pariseau B, Worley MW, Anderson RL. Myectomy for blepharospasm 2013. Curr Opin Ophthalmol 2013;24:488–93.
139. Ludlow CL. Treatment for spasmodic dysphonia: limitations of current approaches. Curr Opin Otolaryngol Head Neck Surg 2009;17:160–5.
140. Ludlow CL, Adler CH, Berke GS, et al. Research priorities in spasmodic dysphonia. Otolaryngol Head Neck Surg 2008;139:495–505.

Huntington Disease

Pathogenesis and Treatment

Praveen Dayalu, MD[a,*], Roger L. Albin, MD[a,b]

KEYWORDS

• Huntington • Chorea • Huntingtin • Polyglutamine • Striatum • Pathogenesis
• Neurodegeneration • Treatment

KEY POINTS

- Huntington disease (HD) is an autosomal dominant inherited neurodegenerative disease characterized by progressive motor, behavioral, and cognitive decline, ultimately culminating in death.
- Mutant huntingtin protein alters neuronal function via multiple intracellular mechanisms. Striatal neurons in particular are selectively vulnerable to these toxic effects, and degenerate in a sequence, which helps explain the evolution of chorea and other motor features.
- Although there is currently no direct treatment of HD, chorea and psychiatric symptoms often respond to pharmacotherapy. A better understanding of HD pathogenesis, as well as more sophisticated clinical trials using newer biomarkers, may lead to meaningful therapeutic advances.

OVERVIEW

Huntington disease (HD) is an autosomal dominant inherited neurodegenerative disease characterized by progressive motor, behavioral, and cognitive decline, resulting in death within 15 to 20 years after diagnosis.[1] In the United States and Canada, approximately 30,000 people carry the diagnosis and an estimated 150,000 more are at risk. HD is most prevalent in people of European descent; approximately 10 to 15 per 100,000.[2,3] Men and women are equally at risk. Median age of diagnosis approximates 40 years, with a wide range in age of onset. Onset before age 20 years or after age 65 years is rare. The combination of typical midlife onset and dominant inheritance affects entire families across the social scale, and devastates the lives of patients, at-risk individuals, and genetically normal family members alike. Management options at this time are limited, and there is still no therapy to slow down the inexorable loss of function.

The authors have nothing to disclose.
[a] Department of Neurology, University of Michigan, 1500 East Medical Center Drive, Ann Arbor, MI 48109, USA; [b] Neuroscience Research, Veterans Affairs Medical Center, 2215 Fuller Road, Ann Arbor, MI 48105, USA
* Corresponding author.
E-mail address: pravd@med.umich.edu

Neurol Clin 33 (2015) 101–114
http://dx.doi.org/10.1016/j.ncl.2014.09.003 neurologic.theclinics.com

The pathologic mutation consists of an expanded CAG repeat in the *huntingtin* gene (HTT) on chromosome 4, encoding the huntingtin (htt) protein,[4] resulting in an excessively long polyglutamine stretch near the N-terminus of this protein. In the general population, there are on average 17 to 20 CAG repeats in the HTT gene.[5] With 40 or more repeats, a person develops HD with 100% certainty, but with repeats of 36 to 39, there is incomplete penetrance. CAG repeat lengths of 6 to 26 do not cause disease and are thus considered normal. The intermediate range, from 27 to 35 repeats, does not cause HD, with a few reported exceptions.[6] It is notable that all alleles of 27 repeats and higher are unstable and prone to expand in future generations, particularly when transmitted by a male parent. Although most patients with HD have an affected parent, up to 10% of cases may result from new expansions into the disease range.[7,8] The appearance of earlier and more severe symptoms in successive generations caused by intergenerational repeat expansion is known as anticipation.

This article highlights the current knowledge of pathogenesis and treatment. It begins with a review of the clinical features.

CLINICAL FEATURES

The typical clinical triad in HD is (1) a progressive motor disorder; (2) progressive cognitive disturbance culminating in dementia; and (3) psychiatric disturbances including depression, anxiety, apathy, obsessive-compulsive behaviors, outbursts, addictions, and occasionally psychosis. Weight loss is a common feature. Note that a diagnosis of HD is made only when the characteristic motor features are apparent. By convention, gene-positive individuals without motor features are considered premanifest, even though there is an accumulation of subclinical and imaging anomalies in such individuals (discussed later).

Motor Disorder

Although chorea is only a small part of motor dysfunction in HD, it remains its most recognizable feature. Chorea often begins as fleeting, suppressible, random fidgety movements, seen best in the distal extremities. With time, chorea becomes more overt, involving larger and more proximal muscles. Most patients with chorea are not aware of the extent of their involuntary movements; some deny them altogether. Particularly violent chorea is indistinguishable from ballism and may result in exhaustion or falls.

Saccadic eye movement abnormalities occur early and persist throughout the disease. Saccades are slow to initiate, often requiring a head movement or a blink to break fixation; saccade velocity may slow.[9]

Ataxia of speech, limbs, or gait can occur as the disease advances. Dystonia, which is a more sustained posturing or twisting, is common. Bradykinesia is common in HD and refers to slowness and reduced scaling of movement, such as diminished facial expression; reduced spontaneous gesturing; small, hesitant finger taps; reduced arm swing; and small steps.

There is considerable heterogeneity in motor findings from patient to patient. Juvenile patients with HD may lack chorea and present with bradykinesia and rigidity; this is known as the Westphal variant of HD. Even within the disease course of an individual patient with HD, the motor abnormalities evolve: chorea early in the disease may give way to superimposed dystonia as the disease progresses,[10] culminating in striking bradykinesia, rigidity, and poor postural reflexes in late stages.

Progressive motor failure is a major cause of life-ending complications. Dysphagia contributes to weight loss and aspiration, and falls and serious injuries become increasingly common.

Cognitive Disorder

Dementia is an underappreciated facet of HD, and is especially serious because it develops in the prime of life, disrupting social and occupational functions. Initial difficulties affect multitasking, focus, short-term memory, and learning new skills. A recent large-scale prospective observational analysis of premanifest persons[11] showed declines in several measures, including working memory, attention, and verbal fluency, consistent with prior smaller studies. These deficits were worse for subjects approaching their expected motor onset. By the time of diagnosis, most subjects with HD have cognitive impairment clearly evident on neuropsychological testing.

Over many years, cognitive impairment eventually progresses to frank dementia. Unlike Alzheimer dementia, HD dementia is largely subcortical, marked by slow thought processes and executive dysfunction, and problems with attention and sequencing.[12,13] Although impaired, episodic memory is better preserved than in Alzheimer dementia, as is language function.

Individuals with HD often show striking lack of insight into their own cognitive and motor symptoms, even when these are obvious to others.[14] This lack of insight may reflect dysfunction of striatal neurons receiving prominent frontal lobe inputs.

Psychiatric Disorder

For many patients with HD and their families, behavioral problems are the most vexing. These problems range from affective illness to anxiety disorders to delusional behavior and, rarely, hallucinations.[15,16] Psychiatric features and their severity vary greatly, and do not correlate with chorea or dementia.[15]

Most patients experience some behavioral symptoms before their diagnosis[17–19]; most common are depression, obsessive-compulsive behaviors, irritability, and outbursts.[17,18] Personality changes may occur for years before the diagnosis, although this may be apparent to families only in retrospect.

Up to 50% of patients are depressed at some point in the disease.[20] Apathy is also common, although it is more difficult to treat. Compulsive behaviors in HD may resemble the cognitive rigidity and perseveration typical of frontal lobe disorders, and probably reflect striatal dysfunction.

There is a high rate of suicide in gene-positive individuals, both before and after diagnosis.[21,22]

PATHOGENESIS

This article reviews HD pathogenesis in a progressively reductionist sequence: (1) considerations pertaining to the organism and the brain as a whole, (2) a discussion of striatal disorders specifically, and (3) a review of genetic and molecular pathogenesis. Clinical correlations are provided where possible.

HUNTINGTON DISEASE PATHOGENESIS AT THE WHOLE-BRAIN AND ORGANISM LEVELS

The htt protein is expressed by neurons throughout the central nervous system (CNS) without dramatic regional differences. Despite this, there is a regional pattern to HD on pathology.[23] Although classically described as a striatal degeneration, widespread brain degeneration is apparent in late-stage autopsies. Gross striatal atrophy is prominent, but thinning of the cortical mantle and low brain weights and volumes are documented well. Careful studies reveal neuronal loss in many regions, including the neocortex, cerebellum, hippocampus, substantia nigra, and brainstem nuclei. There is also diffuse loss of cerebral white matter. These findings correlate well with the many clinical deficits in advanced HD, including pyramidal signs, ataxia, dysarthria, dysphagia, incoordination, and dementia.

Recent work has helped clinicians to better understand HD pathogenesis at the whole-brain and regional levels. Volumetric MRI analyses, performed in ongoing large prospective studies of at-risk individuals, reveal that the most clearly measurable and progressive atrophy affects the striatum and global cerebral white matter.[24,25] These changes occur well before the earliest typical motor features. Cortical atrophy also occurs in asymptomatic subjects,[26–28] changing quantitatively over short intervals (2–3 years), consistent with histopathologic findings of early neocortical degeneration.[23] There is interest in developing such MRI analyses as biomarkers for use in future clinical trials with premanifest subjects.

Weight loss is common in HD, even in the earliest manifest stages.[29] At least some of this might be attributed to hyperkinesia. However, disordered somatic and brain development caused by mutant htt might occur even as early as early life. In a comparison study of at-risk children, those with an expanded allele had modestly lower weight and body mass index, and a smaller head circumference, than those with normal allelles.[30] In another study of premanifest adults who underwent predictive testing, a subtle reduction in intracranial volume was shown for expansion-positive individuals versus their expansion-negative counterparts.[31] If confirmed, such results would be consistent with a purported role for htt in development and metabolism, along with its broad expression in human tissue (discussed later).

The mechanisms for selective involvement of the striatum have been best studied, and are described next.

HUNTINGTON DISEASE PATHOGENESIS AT THE STRIATAL LEVEL

Disproportionate striatal degeneration early in the disease was described decades ago.[32] Within the striatum, neurodegeneration progresses in caudal to rostral and dorsal to ventral gradients. Initial explorations of HD striatal disorders suggested loss of intrinsic gamma-aminobutyric acid (GABA)ergic and cholinergic neurons with relative sparing of extrinsic dopaminergic terminals. PET imaging research in HD has shown declines in striatal neurotransmitter markers (particularly dopamine receptors) that occur very early.[33–35] The striatum receives massive glutamatergic input from the cortex and thalamus, and has been shown to be particularly susceptible to the postulated excitotoxic effects.[36–38]

Intrinsic striatal neurons are differentially affected. There are 2 major populations: (1) aspiny interneurons whose projection arbors are restricted to the striatum, and (2) GABAergic medium spiny projection neurons whose primary axons synapse in targets downstream of the striatum. The best studied aspiny neurons are cholinergic, which are virtually spared in HD.[39] However, striatal choline acetyltransferase levels decline markedly, suggesting significant striatal cholinergic interneuron dysfunction, even in the absence of degeneration. At least 1 other population of striatal interneurons, those cocontaining somatostatin and neuropeptide Y and expressing high levels of nitric oxide synthase, are spared in HD. Recent work has identified progressive depletion of parvalbuminergic interneurons; this is a possible explanation for the emergence of dystonia as HD advances.[40]

Subpopulations of medium spiny projection neurons are defined by their primary projection targets, coexpressed neuropeptides, and neurotransmitter receptors. Segregated pools of these neurons project to the external segment of the globus pallidus (GPe), internal segment of the globus pallidus (GPi), substantia nigra dopaminergic pars compacta, and substantia nigra GABAergic pars reticulata (SNr). Striato-GPe neurons express enkephalins, dopamine D2 receptors, and adenosine A2a receptors, whereas the other striatal projection neuron pools tend to express tachykinins and dopamine D1 receptors. Examination of postmortem HD material suggests a sequential pattern in degeneration of striatal projection neuron subpopulations. The early changes seem to be loss of striato-GPe neurons and perhaps striato-SNr neurons,[41–43] whereas striato-GPi neurons are spared until late.

This temporal order of neuronal loss correlates broadly with features of the natural history of HD. Because basal ganglia inputs to the superior colliculus come from SNr, the early loss of striato-SNr projection neurons correlates well with early saccadic abnormalities. The evolution of involuntary movements in HD also has neuropathologic correlates. Initial degeneration of striato-GPe neurons results in inhibition of the subthalamic nucleus. Diminished subthalamic activity is associated with chorea. In many patients, disease progression is associated with gradual worsening of chorea, which then peaks in intensity and gradually declines, only to be accompanied by worsening dystonia and bradykinesia. In these later stages, there is generalized loss of striatal projection neurons and probably neurons within other nuclei of the basal ganglia.[44] In one study of a marker of striosomal striatal projection neurons in a broad spectrum of HD postmortem specimens there was a correlation between disordered mood and striosomal disorders.[45]

The ultimate cause of HD neurodegeneration, regardless of regional patterns, is the expanded HTT gene and its transcribed product.

HUNTINGTON DISEASE PATHOGENESIS AT THE GENE AND PROTEIN LEVEL

The htt protein is very large (359 kD) and expressed widely in the CNS and in other tissues. In neurons, it is found largely in somatodendritic and axonal cytoplasm, and interacts with many other proteins. Htt is essential for early neuronal development, but its precise functions in adults are unclear.

There is a wide range of age of onset and symptom features in HD. CAG repeat length is a major factor, correlating inversely with age of onset.[46–49] For unclear reasons, the rarer highly expanded repeats (>60) result in uniformly young age of onset. However, for the more common smaller repeat lengths (<45) there is much larger variance in age of onset. Other genetic and environmental factors, as yet unknown, must also contribute to age of onset. Repeat length also influences motor phenotype, because early-onset disease is more likely to present with prominent dystonia and bradykinesia, although this may reflect the impact of the mutant allele on developing brains.

It is unclear whether repeat length influences the rate of disease progression. Although some studies have found no correlation,[47] other studies have.[50] Age may have been a confounder; a more recent analysis showed a stronger correlation between longer repeats and faster decline after adjusting for age.[51] Familial aggregation of certain symptoms (eg, psychosis) occurs in HD and this likely reflects genetic modifiers.

An expanded allele of intermediate length (27–35 repeats) may not be benign. A prospective observational study showed that such individuals, who were unaware of their own allele status, had a higher rate of apathy and suicidal ideation compared with subjects with normal repeat lengths.[52] Cases have been reported of a syndrome indistinguishable from manifest HD in individuals whose repeat length was within this intermediate range.[6]

Most evidence points to a toxic gain-of-function role for mutant htt (mhtt) in causing the disease, although some loss of function may contribute. There is emerging evidence of abnormal transcription of the expanded HTT allele. Aberrant splicing may produce a truncated mRNA that only codes for exon 1, which contains the polyglutamine domain.[53] Even when the full mutant protein is transcribed and translated, protease activity can lead to the formation of shorter N-terminal fragments containing the mutant polyglutamine expansion.[54] Posttranslational modification may modify toxicity, via phosphorylation, acetylation, and conformational changes.[55]

Regardless of how these short mhtt fragments are formed, they are likely toxic as individual molecules or as oligomers. Larger aggregates become visible in the cytoplasm or nucleus,[56] although these may be compensatory or incidental rather than pathogenic. Studies of animal models as well as human brain tissue have identified several key mechanisms whereby mhtt fragments could be toxic to the cell (summarized in **Box 1**)[55,57]:

1. Transcriptional interference. Mhtt can enter the nucleus, and is thought to directly perturb gene transcription. Altered transcription has been shown for multiple other genes,[58,59] notably neurotransmitter receptors and ion channels,[60,61] and BDNF.[62]
2. Cytoskeletal disruption. Htt has many interactions with cytoplasmic proteins, some of which function closely with the microtubule system, and thus may regulate vesicular transport.[63,64] Mutant htt could cause such trafficking to fail.
3. Protein mishandling. Directly or indirectly, mhtt may overwhelm the neuron's ability to tag and clear degraded and misfolded proteins via the ubiquitin-proteosome[65,66] and autophagy-lysosome[67,68] systems.
4. Altered mitochondrial dynamics. Messenger RNA levels of numerous mitochondria-associated proteins are altered in HD brains.[69] Mhtt seems to reduce the transcription of PGC-alpha, itself a key transcription regulator that activates many genes important in the structure and function of mitochondria.[70,71] Neurons in regions most affected by mhtt show altered high-energy phosphate stores, including reduced ATP levels[72] and evidence of oxidative stress.[73] Brain metabolic

Box 1
Key intracellular mechanisms for neurodegeneration in HD, and the likely role of the disease mutation therein. See text for details and citations

HD Pathogenetic Mechanism	Explanation	Role of Disease Mutation
Transcription interference	Critical neuronal proteins and transcription factors are overexpressed or underexpressed	Gain of function and haploinsufficiency
Cytoskeletal disruption	Impaired trafficking of organelles and vesicles within the neuron	Gain of function and haploinsufficiency
Protein mishandling	Ubiquitin-proteosome and autophagy-lysosome systems cannot effectively tag and clear aggregated and misfolded proteins	Gain of function
Altered mitochondrial dynamics	Mitochondrial function is impaired, resulting in imbalance of cellular metabolites, and oxidative stress	Gain of function
Excitotoxicity and disturbed calcium homeostasis	Excess NMDA receptor sensitivity to glutamatergic input, and increased calcium permeability, promote cell death	Gain of function

Abbreviation: NMDA, *N*-methyl-D-aspartate.

deficits have been shown in patients with HD via magnetic resonance spectroscopy and increased cerebrospinal fluid lactate levels.[74]

5. Excitotoxicity and disordered calcium signaling. Numerous studies have implicated glutamatergic stimulation of *N*-methyl-D-aspartate (NMDA) receptors as a proximate cause in HD neurodegeneration, particularly within the striatum.[36–38] Mhtt directly sensitizes NMDA receptors via the NR2B subunit.[75,76] Mhtt also seems to interact with the inositol triphosphate receptor type 1, which is a major calcium channel in neuronal membranes.[77] These changes result in excessive calcium influx, stressing the neuron and ultimately pushing it toward apoptosis and death.[36,75,77]

Given strong experimental evidence for all these mechanisms, it is highly possible that pleiotropic toxic effects of mutant htt are responsible for neuronal degeneration. Different mechanisms may be more important in different neuronal populations. Other potential mechanisms, such as aberrant cholesterol metabolism and even RNA toxicity, have been proposed. A better understanding of these complex cellular events, including their timing in a person's life, their sequence, and their associated feedbacks, may be forthcoming. This understanding will enable clinicians to better understand the selective vulnerability of different brain regions and cell populations, and better explain the clinical features and course; most importantly, it may lead to the development of more effective therapies. For example, major ongoing multicenter trials are testing coenzyme Q10 and high-dose creatine; compounds that support mitochondrial function and might delay disease progression.

Many of the themes described earlier are common to other forms of neurodegeneration, including Parkinson disease and Alzheimer disease. However, in HD there is a clearly established starting point: the mutation of a single gene. Studying the pathogenesis of HD may therefore help clinicians to improve not only the lives of those who have it but also the lives of those who have other brain degenerations.

MANAGEMENT

HD has no cure. Furthermore, there is no known therapy that slows the degeneration or the rate of clinical decline. This unmet need is a major area of HD research. Some symptoms can be treated pharmacologically, and others can only be addressed via nonpharmacologic supportive measures (summarized in **Table 1**).

Symptomatic Pharmacotherapy

HD symptoms respond variably to medications. In general, psychiatric symptoms are perhaps the most amenable to pharmacotherapy. Of motor symptoms, chorea is the most readily responsive. Cognitive symptoms and dementia are the least responsive.

Many patients with chorea are not aware of their involuntary movements or are not impaired by chorea. In these cases, reassurance and education (especially of family members) is important. When chorea does require treatment because it affects a patient's quality of life, function, or safety, it responds best to medications that reduce dopaminergic neurotransmission. In the past, dopamine receptor blockers have been most commonly prescribed. Examples include haloperidol, risperidone, and olanzapine. These agents have the advantage of augmenting treatment of depression, and helping with irritability, outbursts, and psychosis. A disadvantage is that typical and atypical antipsychotics increase the risk of sudden cardiac death.[78] The other major option for chorea is the dopamine-depleting agent tetrabenazine, which reduces chorea in a dose-dependent manner.[79] However, this agent depletes other catecholamines, including serotonin and norepinephrine, so it is best avoided in individuals

Table 1
Frequently used interventions, both pharmacologic and nonpharmacologic, in the management of the commonest HD symptoms and complications. See text for details and citations

HD Symptom or Complication	Therapeutic Intervention
Chorea	Dopamine depletion (tetrabenazine) Dopamine receptor blockers Amantadine
Parkinsonism and rigidity	Levodopa (juvenile HD)
Dysarthria	Speech therapy
Dysphagia	Speech and swallow therapy Dietary modification
Gait impairment and falls	Physical therapy Assistive devices Home modification
Depression	SSRIs Other antidepressants
Anxiety	SSRIs Buspirone
Obsessive-compulsive behaviors	SSRIs
Outbursts and impulsivity	Antipsychotics Mood-stabilizing anticonvulsants
Delusions and hallucinations	Antipsychotics
Apathy	Structured routine and cues
Cognitive dysfunction and dementia	Structured routine and cues
Weight loss	High-calorie supplements Dietary consultation
Caregiver burden and family stress	Social work services Individual and family therapy Respite care

Abbreviation: SSRI, selective serotonin reuptake inhibitor.

with significant depression or anxiety. Tetrabenazine may worsen dysphagia. All of these therapies may worsen gait and bradykinesia, or cause somnolence.

Other medications (eg, amantadine) have been reported as modestly beneficial for chorea.[80,81] Bradykinesia and rigidity in younger onset individuals can respond to dopaminergic agents used in parkinsonism.[82] Myoclonus, which is rare in HD and is sometimes mistaken for chorea, can respond to valproic acid.[83]

There is a lack of clinical trials for psychiatric treatments in HD specifically.[84] Most experts agree that depression in HD often responds well to antidepressants; most commonly selective serotonin reuptake inhibitor (SSRIs). Obsessive-compulsive behaviors, anxiety, and irritability may also respond to SSRIs. Mood stabilizers such as valproate and carbamazepine may help with emotional lability and impulsivity. Buspirone may help with anxiety. Antipsychotics, both typical and atypical, may help with psychosis, delusions, and agitation, but doses should be maintained at a minimum to reduce the risk of extrapyramidal side effects. Apathy is the target of an ongoing clinical trial of bupropion.[85]

Thus far, limited trials of cognitive enhancing agents used primarily in Alzheimer disease, such as memantine,[86] rivastigmine,[87] and donepezil,[88] have shown only questionable benefit.

Deep brain stimulation has been performed on isolated subjects with severe chorea in HD.[89,90] Follow-up reports indicate benefit for chorea, but it is not always sustained, and there is no evidence of benefit for other motor and cognitive-behavioral symptoms.

Nonpharmacologic Management

Comprehensive care in HD draws from a range of professionals: primary care physicians, neurologists, psychiatrists, geneticists, physical and occupational therapists, speech pathologists, nutritionists, social workers, and counselors. Nondrug interventions are a critical part of HD management.[91]

Physical and occupational therapy are important in HD care. Gait assist devices (such as walkers) and home safety improvements (eg, hazard removal, grab-bars, shower chairs) are also valuable. Speech therapists can evaluate and palliate dysarthria and dysphagia; options include exercises and food consistency modifications. Distractions should be minimized during mealtimes so that patients can concentrate on the mechanics of eating and swallowing. Dietary consultation can be a valuable adjunct in dealing with weight loss; high-calorie supplements are often used.

Behavioral symptoms such as apathy and cognitive problems such as executive dysfunction can be ameliorated via structured daily schedules, cues, and regular routines. Daytime respite care may provide a social outlet for patients and relieve caregiver burden. Family members of all ages struggle with the interpersonal, financial, and social stresses of this disease, so clinicians must remember the value of social work services, as well as individual or family counseling services. Even in advanced HD, clinicians must assume that a patient's recognition and comprehension are preserved; severe dysarthria, rigidity, and bradykinesia can make patients appear more cognitively impaired than they really are, leading to frustration and a loss of dignity. Clinicians and family members must avoid talking over the patient.

The efficacy of many nonpharmacologic interventions is often limited by the patient's cognitive and behavioral status. As with many aspects of HD, the burden of maximizing benefits from supportive interventions is placed on caregivers.

SUMMARY

HD is a relentlessly progressive inherited polyglutamine neurodegeneration causing severe cognitive, motor, and psychiatric disability in the prime of life. It is fatal in most cases. Although many of its clinical characteristics can be explained by pathology of the striatum, and its connections to the frontal lobes, HD is no longer simply considered a basal ganglia disorder. Subtle but measurable markers of global brain degeneration emerge even before the motor symptoms manifest, as revealed by volumetric imaging and cognitive batteries. In retrospect, this is not surprising, given the wide expression of the htt protein, and its many important interactions within the neuron.

Current treatment is limited to symptomatic pharmacotherapy for behavioral disturbance and chorea, and other supportive care. A major goal of current research is to identify disease-modifying therapy. Improved understanding of the genetic and molecular pathogenesis may lead to newer drug candidates with greater chances of success.

REFERENCES

1. Roos R, Hermans J, Vegtervandervlis M, et al. Duration of illness in Huntington's disease is not related to age at onset. J Neurol Neurosurg Psychiatr 1993;56(1): 98–100.

2. Evans SJ, Douglas I, Rawlins MD, et al. Prevalence of adult Huntington's disease in the UK based on diagnoses recorded in general practice records. J Neurol Neurosurg Psychiatr 2013;84(10):1156–60.
3. Fisher ER, Hayden MR. Multisource ascertainment of Huntington disease in Canada: prevalence and population at risk. Mov Disord 2014;29(1):105–14.
4. Macdonald ME, Ambrose CM, Duyao MP, et al. A novel gene containing a trinucleotide repeat that is expanded and unstable on Huntington's disease chromosomes. Cell 1993;72(6):971–83.
5. Kremer B, Goldberg P, Andrew SE, et al. A worldwide study of the Huntington's disease mutation: the sensitivity and specificity of measuring CAG repeats. N Engl J Med 1994;330(20):1401–6.
6. Ha AD, Jankovic J. Exploring the correlates of intermediate CAG repeats in Huntington disease. Postgrad Med 2011;123(5):116–21.
7. Almqvist EW, Elterman DS, MacLeod PM, et al. High incidence rate and absent family histories in one quarter of patients newly diagnosed with Huntington disease in British Columbia. Clin Genet 2001;60(3):198–205.
8. Falush D, Almqvist EW, Brinkmann RR, et al. Measurement of mutational flow implies both a high new-mutation rate for Huntington disease and substantial underascertainment of late-onset cases. Am J Hum Genet 2001;68(2):373–85.
9. Lasker AG, Zee DS, Hain TC, et al. Saccades in Huntington's disease: initiation defects and distractibility. Neurology 1987;37(3):364–70.
10. Feigin A, Kieburtz K, Bordwell K, et al. Functional decline in Huntington's disease. Mov Disord 1995;10(2):211–4.
11. Paulsen JS, Smith MM, Long JD, PREDICT HD Investigators, Huntington Study Group. Cognitive decline in prodromal Huntington disease: implications for clinical trials. J Neurol Neurosurg Psychiatr 2013;84(11):1233–9.
12. Rohrer D, Salmon DP, Wixted JT, et al. The disparate effects of Alzheimer's disease and Huntington's disease on semantic memory. Neuropsychology 1999;13(3):381–8.
13. Paulsen JS, Butters N, Sadek JR, et al. Distinct cognitive profiles of cortical and subcortical dementia in advanced illness. Neurology 1995;45(5):951–6.
14. Hoth KF, Paulsen JS, Moser DJ, et al. Patients with Huntington's disease have impaired awareness of cognitive, emotional, and functional abilities. J Clin Exp Neuropsychol 2007;29(4):365–76.
15. Paulsen JS, Ready RE, Hamilton JM, et al. Neuropsychiatric aspects of Huntington's disease. J Neurol Neurosurg Psychiatr 2001;71(3):310–4.
16. Caine ED, Shoulson I. Psychiatric syndromes in Huntington's disease. Am J Psychiatry 1983;140(6):728–33.
17. Duff K, Paulsen JS, Beglinger LJ, et al, Predict-HD Investigators. Psychiatric symptoms in Huntington's disease before diagnosis: the predict-HD study. Biol Psychiatry 2007;62(12):1341–6.
18. Kirkwood SC, Siemers E, Viken R, et al. Longitudinal personality changes among presymptomatic Huntington disease gene carriers. Neuropsychiatry Neuropsychol Behav Neurol 2002;15(3):192–7.
19. Kirkwood SC, Siemers E, Viken RJ, et al. Evaluation of psychological symptoms among presymptomatic HD gene carriers as measured by selected MMPI scales. J Psychiatr Res 2002;36(6):377–82.
20. Paulsen JS, Nehl C, Hoth KF, et al. Depression and stages of Huntington's disease. J Neuropsychiatry Clin Neurosci 2005;17(4):496–502.
21. Lipe H, Schultz A, Bird TD. Risk-factors for suicide in Huntington's disease: a retrospective case-controlled study. Am J Med Genet 1993;48(4):231–3.

22. Almqvist EW, Bloch M, Brinkman R, et al, Int Huntington Dis Collaborative Group. A worldwide assessment of the frequency of suicide, suicide attempts, or psychiatric hospitalization after predictive testing for Huntington disease. Am J Hum Genet 1999;64(5):1293–304.
23. Vonsattel JP, DiFiglia M. Huntington disease. J Neuropathol Exp Neurol 1998; 57(5):369–84.
24. Aylward EH, Nopoulos PC, Ross CA, et al. Longitudinal change in regional brain volumes in prodromal Huntington disease. J Neurol Neurosurg Psychiatr 2011; 82(4):405–10.
25. Tabrizi SJ, Scahill RI, Owen G, et al. Predictors of phenotypic progression and disease onset in premanifest and early-stage Huntington's disease in the TRACK-HD study: analysis of 36-month observational data. Lancet Neurol 2013;12(7):637–49.
26. Tabrizi SJ, Langbehn DR, Leavitt BR, et al. Biological and clinical manifestations of Huntington's disease in the longitudinal TRACK-HD study: Cross-sectional analysis of baseline data. Lancet Neurol 2009;8(9):791–801.
27. Rosas HD, Liu AK, Hersch S, et al. Regional and progressive thinning of the cortical ribbon in Huntington's disease. Neurology 2002;58(5):695–701.
28. Rosas HD, Hevelone ND, Zaleta AK, et al. Regional cortical thinning in preclinical Huntington disease and its relationship to cognition. Neurology 2005;65(5): 745–7.
29. Djousse L, Knowlton B, Cupples L, et al. Weight loss in early stage of Huntington's disease. Neurology 2002;59(9):1325–30.
30. Lee JK, Mathews K, Schlaggar B, et al. Measures of growth in children at risk for Huntington disease. Neurology 2012;79(7):668–74.
31. Nopoulos PC, Aylward EH, Ross CA, et al. Smaller intracranial volume in prodromal Huntington's disease: evidence for abnormal neurodevelopment. Brain 2011; 134:137–42.
32. Vonsattel JP, Myers RH, Stevens TJ, et al. Neuropathological classification of Huntington's disease. J Neuropathol Exp Neurol 1985;44(6):559–77.
33. Weeks RA, Piccini P, Harding AE, et al. Striatal D1 and D2 dopamine receptor loss in asymptomatic mutation carriers of Huntington's disease. Ann Neurol 1996;40(1):49–54.
34. van Oostrom JC, Maguire RP, Verschuuren-Bemelmans CC, et al. Striatal dopamine D2 receptors, metabolism, and volume in preclinical Huntington disease. Neurology 2005;65(6):941–3.
35. Ginovart N, Lundin A, Farde L, et al. PET study of the pre- and post-synaptic dopaminergic markers for the neurodegenerative process in Huntington's disease. Brain 1997;120:503–14.
36. Zeron MM, Hansson O, Chen NS, et al. Increased sensitivity to N-methyl-D-aspartate receptor-mediated excitotoxicity in a mouse model of Huntington's disease. Neuron 2002;33(6):849–60.
37. Heng MY, Detloff PJ, Wang PL, et al. In vivo evidence for NMDA receptor-mediated excitotoxicity in a murine genetic model of Huntington disease. J Neurosci 2009;29(10):3200–5.
38. Fan MMY, Raymond LA. N-methyl-D-aspartate (NMDA) receptor function and excitotoxicity in Huntington's disease. Prog Neurobiol 2007;81(5–6):272–93.
39. Ferrante RJ, Beal MF, Kowall NW, et al. Sparing of acetylcholinesterase-containing striatal neurons in Huntington's disease. Brain Res 1987;411(1):162–6.
40. Reiner A, Shelby E, Wang H, et al. Striatal parvalbuminergic neurons are lost in Huntington's disease: implications for dystonia. Mov Disord 2013;28(12):1691–9.

41. Deng YP, Albin RL, Penney JB, et al. Differential loss of striatal projection systems in Huntington's disease: a quantitative immunohistochemical study. J Chem Neuroanat 2004;27(3):143–64.
42. Albin RL, Reiner A, Anderson KD, et al. Preferential loss of striato-external pallidal projection neurons in presymptomatic Huntington's disease. Ann Neurol 1992;31(4):425–30.
43. Reiner A, Albin RL, Anderson KD, et al. Differential loss of striatal projection neurons in Huntington disease. Proc Natl Acad Sci U S A 1988;85(15):5733–7.
44. Albin RL, Reiner A, Anderson KD, et al. Striatal and nigral neuron subpopulations in rigid Huntington's disease: implications for the functional-anatomy of chorea and rigidity-akinesia. Ann Neurol 1990;27(4):357–65.
45. Tippett LJ, Waldvogel HJ, Thomas SJ, et al. Striosomes and mood dysfunction in Huntington's disease. Brain 2007;130:206–21.
46. Stine OC, Pleasant N, Franz ML, et al. Correlation between the onset age of Huntington's disease and length of the trinucleotide repeat in it-15. Hum Mol Genet 1993;2(10):1547–9.
47. Kieburtz K, Macdonald M, Shih C, et al. Trinucleotide repeat length and progression of illness in Huntington's disease. J Med Genet 1994;31(11):872–4.
48. Andrew SE, Goldberg YP, Kremer B, et al. The relationship between trinucleotide (CAG) repeat length and clinical-features of Huntington's disease. Nat Genet 1993;4(4):398–403.
49. Ashizawa T, Wong LJC, Richards CS, et al. CAG repeat size and clinical presentation in Huntington's disease. Neurology 1994;44(6):1137–43.
50. Marder K, Sandler S, Lechich A, et al. Relationship between CAG repeat length and late-stage outcomes in Huntington's disease. Neurology 2002;59(10):1622–4.
51. Rosenblatt A, Kumar BV, Mo A, et al. Age, CAG repeat length, and clinical progression in Huntington's disease. Mov Disord 2012;27(2):272–6.
52. Killoran A, Biglan KM, Jankovic J, et al. Characterization of the Huntington intermediate CAG repeat expansion phenotype in PHAROS. Neurology 2013;80(22):2022–7.
53. Sathasivam K, Neueder A, Gipson TA, et al. Aberrant splicing of HTT generates the pathogenic exon 1 protein in Huntington disease. Proc Natl Acad Sci U S A 2013;110(6):2366–70.
54. Landles C, Sathasivam K, Weiss A, et al. Proteolysis of mutant huntingtin produces an exon 1 fragment that accumulates as an aggregated protein in neuronal nuclei in Huntington disease. J Biol Chem 2010;285(12):8808–23.
55. Ross CA, Tabrizi SJ. Huntington's disease: from molecular pathogenesis to clinical treatment. Lancet Neurol 2011;10(1):83–98.
56. DiFiglia M, Sapp E, Chase KO, et al. Aggregation of huntingtin in neuronal intranuclear inclusions and dystrophic neurites in brain. Science 1997;277(5334):1990–3.
57. Shoulson I, Young AB. Milestones in Huntington disease. Mov Disord 2011;26(6):1127–33.
58. Steffan JS, Kazantsev A, Spasic-Boskovic O, et al. The Huntington's disease protein interacts with p53 and CREB-binding protein and represses transcription. Proc Natl Acad Sci U S A 2000;97(12):6763–8.
59. Kuhn A, Goldstein DR, Hodges A, et al. Mutant huntingtin's effects on striatal gene expression in mice recapitulate changes observed in human Huntington's disease brain and do not differ with mutant huntingtin length or wild-type huntingtin dosage. Hum Mol Genet 2007;16(15):1845–61.

60. Cha JH, Kosinski CM, Kerner JA, et al. Altered brain neurotransmitter receptors in transgenic mice expressing a portion of an abnormal human Huntington disease gene. Proc Natl Acad Sci U S A 1998;95(11):6480–5.
61. Hodges A, Strand AD, Aragaki AK, et al. Regional and cellular gene expression changes in human Huntington's disease brain. Hum Mol Genet 2006;15(6):965–77.
62. Zuccato C, Ciammola A, Rigamonti D, et al. Loss of huntingtin-mediated BDNF gene transcription in Huntington's disease. Science 2001;293(5529):493–8.
63. Caviston JP, Holzbaur EL. Huntingtin as an essential integrator of intracellular vesicular trafficking. Trends Cell Biol 2009;19(4):147–55.
64. Caviston JP, Ross JL, Antony SM, et al. Huntingtin facilitates dynein/dynactin-mediated vesicle transport. Proc Natl Acad Sci U S A 2007;104(24):10045–50.
65. Bennett EJ, Shaler TA, Woodman B, et al. Global changes to the ubiquitin system in Huntington's disease. Nature 2007;448(7154):704–8.
66. Wang J, Wang C, Orr A, et al. Impaired ubiquitin-proteasome system activity in the synapses of Huntington's disease mice. J Cell Biol 2008;180(6):1177–89.
67. Wong YC, Holzbaur EL. The regulation of autophagosome dynamics by huntingtin and HAP1 is disrupted by expression of mutant huntingtin, leading to defective cargo degradation. J Neurosci 2014;34(4):1293–305.
68. Martinez-Vicente M, Talloczy Z, Wong E, et al. Cargo recognition failure is responsible for inefficient autophagy in Huntington's disease. Nat Neurosci 2010;13(5):567–76.
69. Shirendeb U, Reddy AP, Manczak M, et al. Abnormal mitochondrial dynamics, mitochondrial loss and mutant huntingtin oligomers in Huntington's disease: implications for selective neuronal damage. Hum Mol Genet 2011;20(7):1438–55.
70. Weydt P, Pineda VV, Torrence AE, et al. Thermoregulatory and metabolic defects in Huntington's disease transgenic mice implicate PGC-1 alpha in Huntington's disease neurodegeneration. Cell Metab 2006;4(5):349–62.
71. Cui L, Jeong H, Borovecki F, et al. Transcriptional repression of PGC-alpha by mutant huntingtin leads to mitochondrial dysfunction and neurodegeneration. Cell 2006;127(1):59–69.
72. Mochel F, Durant B, Meng X, et al. Early alterations of brain cellular energy homeostasis in Huntington disease models. J Biol Chem 2012;287(2):1361–70.
73. Browne SE, Bowling AC, MacGarvey U, et al. Oxidative damage and metabolic dysfunction in Huntington's disease: selective vulnerability of the basal ganglia. Ann Neurol 1997;41(5):646–53.
74. Koroshetz WJ, Jenkins BG, Rosen BR, et al. Energy metabolism defects in Huntington's disease and effects of coenzyme Q(10). Ann Neurol 1997;41(2):160–5.
75. Chen N, Luo T, Wellington C, et al. Subtype-specific enhancement of NMDA receptor currents by mutant huntingtin. J Neurochem 1999;72(5):1890–8.
76. Zeron M, Chen N, Moshaver A, et al. Mutant huntingtin enhances excitotoxic cell death. Mol Cell Neurosci 2001;17(1):41–53.
77. Tang T, Slow E, Lupu V, et al. Disturbed Ca2+ signaling and apoptosis of medium spiny neurons in Huntington's disease. Proc Natl Acad Sci U S A 2005;102(7):2602–7.
78. Ray WA, Chung CP, Murray KT, et al. Atypical antipsychotic drugs and the risk of sudden cardiac death. N Engl J Med 2009;360(3):225–35.
79. Marshall FJ, Walker F, Frank S, et al. Tetrabenazine as antichorea therapy in Huntington disease: a randomized controlled trial. Neurology 2006;66(3):366–72.
80. Metman LV, Morris MJ, Farmer C, et al. Huntington's disease - a randomized, controlled trial using the NMDA-antagonist amantadine. Neurology 2002;59(5):694–9.

81. O'Suilleabhain P, Dewey RB. A randomized trial of amantadine in Huntington disease. Arch Neurol 2003;60(7):996–8.
82. Jongen PJ, Renier WO, Gabreels FJ. Seven cases of huntington's disease in childhood and levodopa induced improvement in the hypokinetic – Rigid form. Clin Neurol Neurosurg 1980;82(4):251–61.
83. Saft C, Lauter T, Kraus PH, et al. Dose-dependent improvement of myoclonic hyperkinesia due to valproic acid in eight Huntington's disease patients: a case series. BMC Neurol 2006;6:11.
84. Mestre TA, Ferreira JJ. An evidence-based approach in the treatment of Huntington's disease. Parkinsonism Relat Disord 2012;18(4):316–20.
85. Gelderblom H, Fischer W, McLean T, et al. ACTION-HD: a randomized, double-blind, placebo-controlled prospective crossover trial investigating the efficacy and safety of bupropion in Huntington's disease. Neurotherapeutics 2013;10(1): 180–1.
86. Beister A, Kraus P, Kuhn W, et al. The N-methyl-D-aspartate antagonist memantine retards progression of Huntington's disease. J Neural Transm Suppl 2004;(68):117–22.
87. de Tommaso M, Difruscolo O, Sciruicchio V, et al. Two years' follow-up of rivastigmine treatment in Huntington disease. Clin Neuropharmacol 2007;30(1):43–6.
88. Cubo E, Shannon KM, Tracy D, et al. Effect of donepezil on motor and cognitive function in Huntington disease. Neurology 2006;67(7):1268–71.
89. Biolsi B, Cif L, El Fertit H, et al. Long-term follow-up of Huntington disease treated by bilateral deep brain stimulation of the internal globus pallidus. J Neurosurg 2008;109(1):130–2.
90. Kang GA, Heath S, Rothlind J, et al. Long-term follow-up of pallidal deep brain stimulation in two cases of Huntington's disease. J Neurol Neurosurg Psychiatr 2011;82(3):272–7.
91. Nance MA. Comprehensive care in Huntington's disease - a physician's perspective. Brain Res Bull 2007;72(2–3):175–8.

Tics and Tourette Syndrome

Christos Ganos, MD[a,b,1], Davide Martino, PhD[c,d,*,1]

KEYWORDS

• Gilles de la Tourette syndrome • Tics • Functional anatomy • Tic pathophysiology • Tic treatment

KEY POINTS

- The prevalence of Gilles de la Tourette syndrome (GTS) is approximately 0.8% between the ages of 6 and 18 years.
- GTS is complicated by psychiatric comorbidities (attention-deficit/hyperactivity disorder [ADHD], obsessive-compulsive disorder, anxiety/depressive disorders, autism spectrum disorders) in about 90% of cases.
- Secondary tic disorders are less frequent than primary tic disorders and should be suspected in older onset (>20 years) and associated neurologic abnormalities.
- GTS is associated with abnormal trajectories of cortico-subcortical and corticocortical circuits regulating motor control.
- Management of GTS rests first on psychoeducational intervention.
- α-2-Agonists (clonidine and guanfacine) are first-line medications for the treatment of tics in the United States and Canada and may be more effective in patients with GTS and ADHD compared with GTS alone. Antipsychotic medications (mostly risperidone, haloperidol, pimozide, fluphenazine, aripiprazole) are also effective, but with a less favorable side-effect profile.

Continued

Financial Disclosures: C. Ganos has received research support from the Deutsche Forschungsgemeinschaft (MU1692/2-1 and GA2031/1-1) and travel grants from Actelion, Ipsen, Pharm Allergan, and Merz Pharmaceuticals; Nil (D. Martino).

[a] Sobell Department of Motor Neuroscience and Movement Disorders, UCL Institute of Neurology, 33 Queen Square, London WC1N 3BG, UK; [b] Department of Neurology, University Medical Center Hamburg-Eppendorf (UKE), Martinistraße 52 D, Hamburg 20246, Germany; [c] Neurology Department, King's College Hospital NHS Foundation Trust, 9th Floor, Ruskin Wing, Denmark Hill, London SE5 9RS, UK; [d] Department of Neurology, Queen Elizabeth Hospital, Lewisham & Greenwich NHS Trust, Stadium Road, London SE18 4QH, UK
[1] Author Contributions: Drafting/revising the article for content, including medical writing for content; acquisition of data; and study supervision or coordination.
* Corresponding author. Department of Neurology, King's College Hospital NHS Foundation Trust, 9th Floor, Ruskin Wing, Denmark Hill, London SE5 9RS, UK.
E-mail address: davidemartino@nhs.net

Neurol Clin 33 (2015) 115–136
http://dx.doi.org/10.1016/j.ncl.2014.09.008 neurologic.theclinics.com

Continued

- Behavioral treatment, particularly habit reversal training and the comprehensive behavioral intervention for tics, is more effective than supportive psychotherapy in reducing tic severity in both children and adults.
- Deep brain stimulation (mainly of the centromedian/parafascicularis thalamic nuclei and globus pallidus internus) should be restricted to adult drug-refractory GTS patients who are significantly disabled by their tics. More evidence of efficacy and harmonization of patient selection criteria is required.

Video of multiple tics accompanies this article at http://www.neurologic.theclinics.com/

THE CLINICAL DEFINITION

Tics are the defining feature of Gilles de la Tourette syndrome (GTS). According to DSM-5 criteria, the presence of motor and vocal (or phonic) tics manifesting before the age of 18 for more than 12 months in the absence of secondary causes warrants diagnosis of GTS.[1] Together with the more common persistent (chronic) motor or vocal (phonic) tic disorder and provisional tic disorder, GTS is classified as a primary tic disorder. GTS is a common disorder in nearly all studied cultures; it affects more boys than girls, and its prevalence in children and adolescents has been estimated to be up to 0.8%.[2] However, although tics are the mainstay of the GTS diagnostic criteria and the emblematic feature of the disorder, in most cases neuropsychiatric comorbidities complicate clinical presentations and may negatively impact the developmental profiles of patients even more than tics.[3,4] Here, the current state of knowledge on the movement disorder and neuropsychiatric profile of GTS is presented, providing a synthesis on prevailing pathophysiologic models and reviewing contemporary treatment strategies.

THE MOVEMENT DISORDER OF TICS

Tics resemble voluntary actions and share most of their neurophysiologic properties,[5,6] but appear repetitive, seemingly uncontrollable, out of context, and exaggerated. Any single movement can be a tic. Hence, among hyperkinesias such as tremor, myoclonus, or chorea, tics possess the greatest phenomenological variability reflecting the complete range of human motor behavior.

Tics are divided into simple, if they affect single muscle groups, and complex, if they resemble goal-directed behavior but lack obvious purpose.[7] Tics are further arbitrarily categorized as motor if they lead to movement or vocal (or phonic) if they lead to the generation of sounds.[7] Finally, tics can be clonic or dystonic (ie, lasting longer, leading to sustained abnormal posture or movement) (Video 1).[7] Tics that largely interfere with the execution of normal motor behavior have been labeled "blocking" tics.[7] In rare cases, blocking tics have been described to lead to a complete interruption of ongoing motor activity.

Conscious awareness of tics is facilitated in most cases by an unpleasant preceding sensation known as the "premonitory urge."[8] The exact phenomenological qualities of the premonitory urge have not been well characterized; however, it is most commonly described as an *urge to move* or an *impulse to tic*, but may be also experienced as specific bodily sensations such as *pressure/fullness*, *ache*, or *itch*.[8,9] It has been suggested that awareness of the premonitory urge develops a few years after the appearance of tics,[10] but prospective evidence is missing.

The temporal and spatial occurrence of tics is not random. First, tics usually occur in bouts interspersed by tic-free intervals.[11] Second, tic manifestation across body parts appears to follow a rostrocaudal gradient. Tics affecting craniocervical areas are far more common than tics of the trunk or feet, particularly in children. Interestingly, the distribution of premonitory urges across body parts is also not random; however, it may diverge from that of tics.[8]

Tics can be completely or partially inhibited under volition by most patients, further aiding their distinction from other hyperkinesias where voluntary inhibition is inefficient. However, the extent of tic inhibition and the temporal capacity to maintain it differ between patients. Tic inhibition *on demand* was suggested to be facilitated by the premonitory urge; however, this notion has been challenged by a recent study, which revealed that the capacity of tic inhibition and the extent of premonitory urges are unrelated.[12] Tic inhibition may be enhanced through motivational modulation.[13] On the other hand, increased awareness and habituation to specific urges may enhance the ability to inhibit tics, and this has been exploited in behavioral treatment approaches for tics.[14] However, current knowledge suggests that mechanisms underlying premonitory urges and voluntary inhibition of tics differ.

Paliphenomena, echophenomena, and coprophenomena are additional typical features in GTS. Although not specific to GTS, with the exception of coprophenomena, these are classified by convention as complex tics. Paliphenomena indicate the repetition and echophenomena indicate the imitation of movements and vocalizations,[15] while coprophenomena denote the unintentional performance of obscene and socially inappropriate gestures.[16]

THE NEUROPSYCHIATRIC SPECTRUM

Despite the emblematic and defining character of tics in GTS, only a minority of patients encountered in clinical practice will present with the isolated, childhood onset, chronic movement disorder of motor and vocal (phonic) tics. In fact, most patients will have a range of additional neuropsychiatric features, the recognition of which is paramount for the introduction of efficient treatment strategies to promote healthy development and good quality of life. These neuropsychiatric features include GTS-related comorbidities (attention-deficit/hyperactivity disorder, ADHD; obsessive compulsive disorder, OCD; autism spectrum disorder, ASD), coexistent psychopathologies such as anxiety and personality disorders and/or depression, and features considered integral to GTS as self-injurious behaviors and nonobscene socially inappropriate symptoms/behaviors.[4,17] In fact, only approximately 10% of patients will present with the pure movement disorder of GTS (also termed "pure" or "uncomplicated" GTS), whereas the rest (90%) of patients will exhibit comorbid symptoms of ADHD, OCD, and/or ASD.[4,17,18]

Despite divergent prevalence estimates, which largely depend on studied patient cohorts of different ages and the applied screening tools for aforementioned psychopathologies, it appears that ADHD is the most common comorbidity that affects up to 60% of GTS patients, particularly boys.[19] Although the manifestation of ADHD symptoms precedes the onset of tics, its presence has been associated with earlier tic onset (5.8 vs 6.2 years) compared with GTS patients without ADHD.[19] Also, the presence of ADHD in GTS children and adolescents has been associated with further profiles of psychopathology to include OCD, anxiety disorder, anger control, sleep problems, poor social skills, conduct disorder/oppositional defiant disorder, and mood disorders.[18,19]

Prevalence rates of comorbid OCD in GTS vary largely with estimations between 19.3% and 66%, particularly if obsessive-compulsive symptoms or behavior (OCS/OCB) that are below diagnostic threshold are taken into account.[18,20] From a clinical point of view, the presence of OCS/OCB/OCD may pose diagnostic difficulties in certain motor behaviors encountered in GTS patients that seem to fall between the phenomenological spectra of tics and obsessions/compulsions.[4,21,22] However, characteristic clinical features aid the diagnostic distinction and classification between different phenomena. For example, in pure OCD, obsessions that lead to compulsions are sources of major anxiety and discomfort, are intrusive and disruptive (or "ego-dystonic"), and are commonly related to fears of contamination and/or causing harm.[4] In contrast, in GTS, they are largely a result of an inner urge and are most often associated with symmetry behaviors, "just right" experiences, and repetitive touching.[4,21,22] However, in certain cases, these behaviors overlap and may also change with development, in support of the pathophysiologic commonalities between OCD and GTS suggested also by genetic and imaging findings.[23,24] Of note, comorbid OCD in a large sample of children and adolescents with GTS (n = 5060) was found to be associated with ADHD, mood and anxiety disorders, conduct disorder/oppositional defiant disorder, and ASD.[20]

The association of ASD as a comorbid condition to GTS has only been made in the last 15 years with a prevalence of ASD in GTS up to 12.9%.[18,25,26] Patients with GTS and comorbid ASD usually exhibit mild tics[26,27] but have higher rates for other common comorbidities, such as ADHD, oppositional defiant disorder, as well as rage attacks.[26] Of note, rage attacks/explosive outbursts are a common phenomenon in patients with GTS,[28] the presence of which merits clinical attention and further exploration, because they might lead to physical harm with often medicolegal implications.

Finally, as mentioned in the beginning of this section, the clinician should be aware and enquire of the presence of further psychopathological behaviors, including self-injurious behavior (encountered up to 60% in GTS patients[29]), anxiety,[4] personality disorders,[30] and depression (lifetime risk 10%).[31] These symptoms/behaviors are often a greater cause of distress than tics and, together with the aforementioned comorbidities, have a negative impact on GTS patients' quality of life.[32–34]

THE SPECTRUM OF GILLES DE LA TOURETTE SYNDROME THROUGHOUT DEVELOPMENT

The diversity of phenotypic presentations in GTS with tics, echophenomena, paliphenomena, and coprophenomena and the variable expressions of associated psychopathological behaviors during different developmental stages strongly indicate that it is a heterogeneous condition.[35] In fact, results from hierarchical cluster, principal component factor, latent class, and cluster analyses further support this (reviewed in[36]). The only clinical subtype that could be replicated across studies was that of "pure" GTS.

Complicating matters further, even the profile of an individual patient with regard to tics and neuropsychiatric behaviors may change throughout development.[37] However, it is important to point out that in most cases tics will largely remit.[38,39] Of note, GTS patients with comorbidities have less satisfactory symptom control with pharmacologic treatment compared with pure GTS patients.[37]

A Functional Neuroanatomical Approach to Tic Pathophysiology

The mainstay of research in GTS has been the elucidation of tic generation. The fact that tics resemble voluntary actions and can be inhibited on demand but appear purposelessly and in excess has the following pathophysiologic implications. On one hand, it suggests that the same pathways involved in the generation of voluntary actions are also involved in the generation of tics. It also implies that some basic neural structures involved in motor inhibitory control fail to suppress the generation of abnormal motor programs (ie, tics), while others that exert top-down inhibitory control on the execution of these not yet performed motor programs function within normal limits (for review on the functional anatomy of GTS, please see[40]).

Indeed, structural and functional abnormalities were demonstrated in patients with GTS at numerous levels of the corticostriatothalamocortical loops (CSTC), a series of circuits that are fundamental in formation and implementation of voluntary actions, suggesting a relationship between found changes in these structures and tic generation.[40] With a view to subcortical structures and on a microscopic level, 2 neuropathological studies on a limited sample of previously medicated GTS adults have provided evidence of structural alterations in the composition of inhibitory interneuronal GABAergic and cholinergic populations, particularly in sensorimotor parts of the striatum[41] and internal segment of globus pallidus,[42] boosting the hypothesis of a functional imbalance between inhibition/excitation in these structures.[42] Furthermore, functional studies in rodents and monkeys have shown that the injection of the $GABA_A$-antagonist bicuculline in motor parts of the striatum, but also pallidum, leads to disinhibition of the CSTC-loops and to generation of ticlike jerks.[43] Ticlike generation in one of these models was not random, but in fact, followed the somatotopical distribution of respective disinhibited striatal motor areas.[44] In addition, structural neuroimaging studies in GTS patients have provided further evidence of abnormalities in CSTC loops. Smaller caudate volumes were found in a large sample of GTS children and adults with comorbid symptoms of ADHD and/or OCD ($n = 154$, age range: 6–63 years).[45] Interestingly, caudate volumes at that time point of the study predicted future tic severity in a pediatric subsample of patients ($n = 43$) who were re-evaluated at a mean time of 7.5 years later.[46] Also, in the same original study sample, age-dependent hippocampal and amygdala volume changes correlating with tic severity, as well as age-independent and tic-independent thalamic volume enlargements, were demonstrated.[47,48] However, it is noteworthy that these results were not replicated in 2 subsequent studies using different methodologies in treatment-naïve and comorbidity-free GTS adolescent boys.[49,50] On the other hand, the exploration of structural properties of the white matter in the CSTC circuitry has documented further alterations in GTS patients.[24]

Within the primary sensorimotor cortex, structural and functional data also suggest direct involvement in the pathophysiology of tics. Despite clinical and methodological heterogeneity across studies, thinning of sensorimotor cortices has been identified in children and adults with GTS, with correlation between the degree of cortical thinning and tic severity.[51–53] On a functional level, the primary somatosensory cortex was active in 4 studies examining tic-related neural activations as studied by blood oxygenation level–dependent imaging.[54–57] Interestingly, one of these studies compared the patterns of neural activation during the performance of tics and voluntary actions and demonstrated overt similarities between the two.[55] Hence, the dearth of presented evidence supports the clinical hypothesis that tics and voluntary actions share the same sensorimotor pathways (a representative illustration of the affected structures/systems is shown in **Fig. 1**), with data suggesting that striatal disinhibition is central to tic generation.

Interestingly, the disinhibition or hyperexcitability of the striatum and CSTC loops underlying tics might be related to a broader deficit in motor control, reflecting GTS patients' inability to continuously control tic behaviors and possibly predicting wider deficits in other aspects of motor inhibition. Structural neuroimaging data showing alterations of prefrontal cortical areas,[58–60] classically involved in action inhibition, have

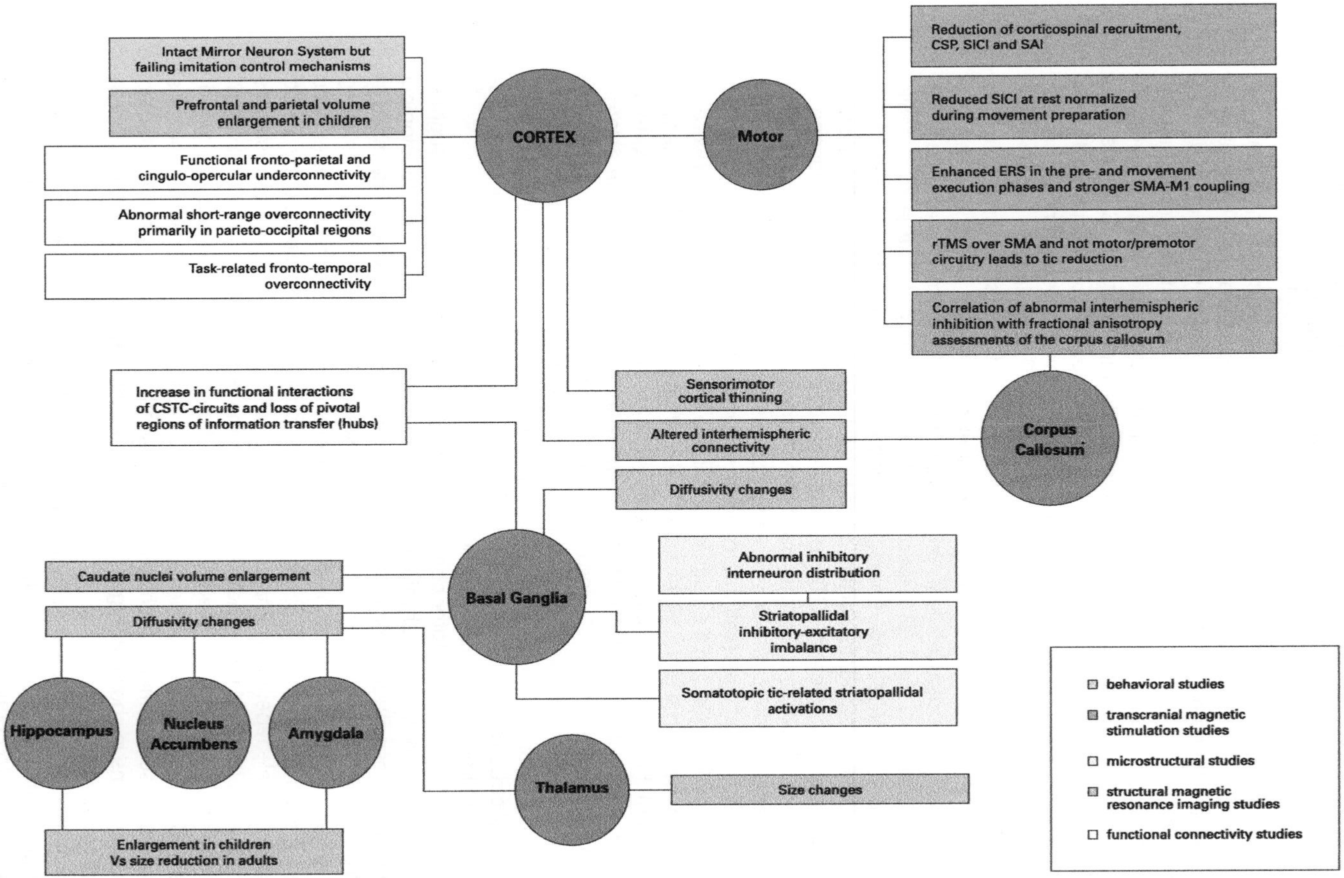

Fig. 1. Illustration of predominantly affected structures/systems in GTS. CSP; ERS; rTMS; SAI; SICI; SMA-M1. CSP, cortical silent period; ERS, event-related synchronization; rTMS, repetitive transcranial magnetic stimulation; SAI, short latency afferent inhibition; SICI, short latency intracortical inhibition; SMA-M1, supplementary motor area — primary motor area. (*Adapted from* Ganos C, Roessner V, Munchau A. The functional anatomy of Gilles de la Tourette syndrome. Neurosci Biobehav Rev 2013;37:1059; with permission.)

been used to support this hypothesis. However, a critical view on behavioral as well as functional neuroimaging studies argues against this hypothesis. In fact, action (response) inhibition has been shown to be normal in GTS children and adults,[61–63] but the neural mechanism underlying this functional domain seems to differ between GTS patients and healthy controls.[61] Furthermore, although tic severity may interfere with different aspects of cognitive control,[64–66] the capacity of tic inhibition *on demand* and behavioral correlates of action inhibition are functionally dissociated.[61] Hence, better voluntary control of tics does not imply better control of actions. Of note, some evidence has also argued in favor of enhanced control of motor responses as an adaptation to the constant need to monitor and inhibit tics.[67–69] Thus, the notion of a presumed deficit in motor inhibition leading to the generation of tics that also disrupts control of voluntary actions is not supported by more recent evidence.

DIFFERENTIAL DIAGNOSIS OF TIC DISORDERS

The clinical diagnosis of tics is in most cases straightforward. However, on rare occasions diagnostic errors may occur. On one hand, tics may be overlooked or labeled as secondary to psychological factors. Such misconception might lead to additional burden in patients and relatives, because the continuous and fruitless search of psychological causes produces feelings of guilt and anxiety. On the other hand, patients with GTS might also have additional abnormal movements, such as dystonia, paroxysmal dyskinesia, or movement disorders secondary to neuroleptic treatments, which may be missed or in fact mislabeled as tics.[70,71] Also, the overlapping phenomenological features of tics with other movement disorders may cause diagnostic confusion, and meticulous history taking paralleled by careful clinical examination is necessary to avoid misdiagnoses. Examples of other movement disorders that can be misdiagnosed as tics include stereotypies, myoclonus or chorea, faciobrachial dystonic seizures due to LGI1 antibodies, but also functional ("psychogenic") ticlike jerks (differential diagnosis of tics is presented in **Fig. 2**). Tic-specific characteristics in GTS such as an anatomic rostrocaudal gradient in tic distribution, awareness of premonitory urges, tic suggestibility, the presence of echophenomena, paliphenomena, and in some instances coprophenomena, the capacity to inhibit tics on demand and personal or family history of aforementioned neuropsychiatric comorbidities are helpful diagnostic clues.[72] Finally, a long list of conditions may present with secondary tics, including neurodevelopmental disorders, acute brain lesions, neurodegenerative illnesses, immune-mediated conditions, and drugs or toxins. A later age at onset (eg, late adolescence or adulthood), abrupt onset, and association with other neurologic manifestations represent red flags that should prompt the exclusion of secondary causes of tics (**Boxes 1** and **2** provide a comprehensive list of secondary causes of tics).

MANAGEMENT

General Considerations

The management of tic disorders differs significantly across patients, as a result of interindividual variability in symptom severity, comorbidity profile, and degree of functional impairment. It is a priority to collect a comprehensive history of the patient's ailments, ideally with a suitable informant, and administer a general set of assessment tools to measure the current severity of tics and related features, primarily OCS, features of ADHD, as well as anxiety and depressive symptoms (**Fig. 3**). Evaluating tic severity in clinic may be challenging, given the high dependency of tics on the environmental context; if patients perceive the consultation as a safe environment, their tic

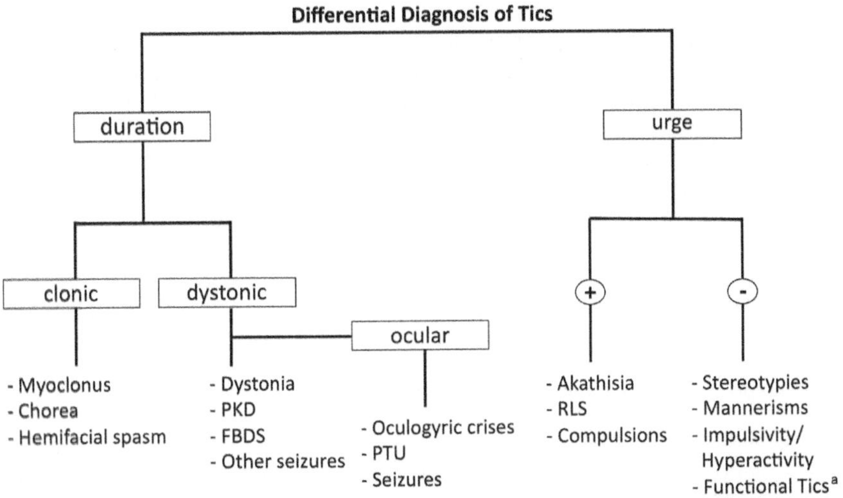

Fig. 2. List of differential diagnoses of tics on the grounds of phenomenology. FBDS, faciobrachial dystonic seizures; PKD, paroxysmal kinesigenic dyskinesia; PTU, paroxysmal tonic upgaze; RLS, restless legs syndrome. [a] A nonlocalized premonitory sensation may be reported. (*Adapted from* Ganos C, Münchau A, Bhatia K. The semiology of tics, Tourette's and their associations. Mov Disord Clin Pract 2014;1:149; with permission.)

severity might temporarily diminish and become underrated by the specialist, hence the crucial role of an adequate informant.

The first step of tic management is psychoeducation, in which patients and families are informed of the natural history of the condition, on the relevance of contextual factors, and on the complexity of the psychopathological spectrum. Scope of this intervention is to maximize acceptance of symptoms and coping strategies with the disorder to assess the actual requirements of more "invasive" interventions. Even when the lifetime history suggests that additional intervention may be needed, this may be postponed if symptom severity is not significant in that moment.

Under what circumstances do tics need prompt intervention? In a minority of cases, tics can be violent (for example, tics consisting of violent head, trunk, or limb movements), or even harmful (eg, spinal damage secondary to violent head thrusts). Moreover, tic-related pain (particularly headache) is an underestimated feature of these disorders. If the social environment is poorly informed, particularly within the school, tics may be stigmatizing, causing isolation and favoring bullying behaviors, with subsequent increase of anxiety levels, worsening of depression and self-esteem, and deterioration of school performance.[73]

Specialists should decide whether treatment should address tics, comorbid symptoms, or both. Any additional treatment of GTS beyond the mere psychoeducation should be tailored to each individual patient, based on the prominent and most disabling symptoms, the social context, patient and family compliance, and local availability of treatment options. **Fig. 4** proposes a therapeutic algorithm adapted from recently published guidelines.[73–75]

Pharmacologic Treatment

The choice of pharmacologic treatment of tics is still based, in most cases, on personal experience. Overall, randomized placebo-controlled trials recruited relatively small samples and had brief duration, and active comparator trials between different

Box 1
Secondary causes of tics

- Neurodevelopmental disorders
  - Mental retardation
  - Autistic spectrum disorders (including Asperger syndrome)
  - Rett syndrome
  - Genetic and chromosomal abnormalities
  - X-linked mental retardation (*MRX23*)
  - Albright hereditary osteodystrophy
  - Duchenne muscular dystrophy
  - Factor VIII hemophilia
  - Fragile X syndrome
  - Lesch-Nyhan syndrome
  - Triple X and 9p mosaicism
  - 47 XXY karyotype
  - Partial trisomy 16
  - 9p monosomy
  - Beckwith-Wiedemann syndrome
  - Tuberous sclerosis
  - Congenital adrenal hyperplasia due to 21-hydroxylase deficiency
  - Phenylketonuria
  - Corpus callosum dysgenesis
  - Craniosynostosis
  - Klinefelter syndrome
  - Neurofibromatosis
  - Developmental stuttering
- Acute brain lesions
  - Posttraumatic
  - Vascular
  - Infectious
  - Varicella-zoster virus
  - Herpes simplex encephalitis
  - *Mycoplasma pneumoniae*
  - Lyme disease
- Postinfectious
  - Sydenham chorea
  - Pediatric autoimmune neuropsychiatric disorder associated with streptococcal infections
- Neurodegenerative diseases
  - Huntington disease
  - Neuroacanthocytosis syndromes

Neurodegeneration with brain iron accumulation

- Other systemic diseases
    - Behçet syndrome
    - Antiphospholipid syndrome
- Peripheral trauma
- Medications and toxins (see **Box 2**)
- Functional ticlike jerks

medications and between pharmacologic and nonpharmacological treatments are scanty (**Table 1** shows an overview of medications used to treat tics). An additional limitation of evaluating the response to drugs for tics is the natural "waxing and waning" characteristic of tics, which is highly influenced by psychosocial stress or other contextual factors. This inevitably confounds the clinician's judgment as to whether a given treatment is effective or not and requires a sufficiently prolonged baseline observation of patients off treatment before a medication is introduced. Tic severity is influenced also by the coexistence of comorbid disorders, such as ADHD or OCD, which, apart from some exceptions, are not targeted by antitic medications. Even less is known on the medium-term and long-term tolerability of medications in GTS patients, and more work is needed to introduce this crucial aspect in the treatment decisional process.

Antipsychotic medications have been reported to be effective in reducing tics since the first open-label studies in the 1970s and 1980s, which documented a good response to D2 dopamine receptor blockers in up to 70% of patients. The efficacy

Box 2
Tic-inducing or tic-exacerbating agents

- Amphetamines
- Cocaine
- Heroin
- Methylphenidate
- Pemoline
- Antipsychotics (D2 blockers)
    - Fluphenazine
    - Perphenazine
    - Thiothixene
- Antidepressants
- Antiepileptics
    - Carbamazepine
    - Phenytoin
    - Phenobarbital
    - Lamotrigine
- L-Dopa

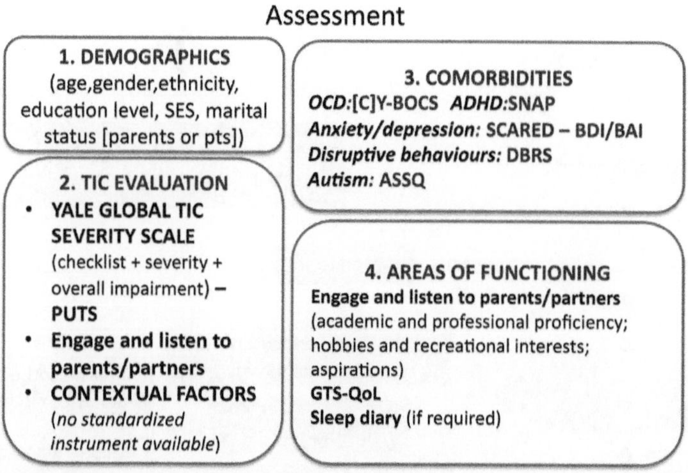

Assessment
1. DEMOGRAPHICS
(age,gender,ethnicity, education level, SES, marital status [parents or pts])
2. TIC EVALUATION
• YALE GLOBAL TIC SEVERITY SCALE (checklist + severity + overall impairment) – PUTS
• Engage and listen to parents/partners
• CONTEXTUAL FACTORS (no standardized instrument available)
3. COMORBIDITIES
OCD:[C]Y-BOCS ADHD:SNAP
Anxiety/depression: SCARED – BDI/BAI
Disruptive behaviours: DBRS
Autism: ASSQ
4. AREAS OF FUNCTIONING
Engage and listen to parents/partners
(academic and professional proficiency; hobbies and recreational interests; aspirations)
GTS-QoL
Sleep diary (if required)

Fig. 3. A comprehensive assessment is key to good management in GTS. The authors propose an assessment strategy divided into 4 main sections: (1) Collection of demographic data to understand the cultural background of the patient and family and choose the right idiom to discuss symptoms, according to patients', parents', or partners' sensibility. (2) Evaluation of tics, comprising in full the Yale Global Tic Severity Scale (YGTSS: checklist of tics, severity, overall impairment). The Premonitory Urges for Tics Scale (PUTS) might help particularly with older children, teens, or adults capturing the actual baseline awareness of their urges. Parents ideally should have the possibility to discuss without the child present at some point during the assessment. Understanding triggers, exacerbants, and alleviators of tics is very important to understand the patient's tic disorder and to foster the ability of patients to master their tics effectively. (3) For many patients, comorbidities are more impairing and should be prioritized in management. Comorbidities require specific behavioral and pharmacologic interventions; it is crucial to assess the severity of these comorbidities and establish treatment priorities between them. The figure suggests a nonexhaustive series of widely used rating scales for the main comorbidities. ASSQ, Autism Spectrum Screening Questionnaire; BAI, Beck Anxiety Inventory; BDI, Beck Depression Inventory; [C]Y-BOCS, Children's Yale-Brown Obsessive-Compulsive Scale; DBRS, Disruptive Behaviors Rating Scale; SCARED, Screen for Child Anxiety-Related Disorders; SNAP, Swanson, Nolan, and Pelham Questionnaire. (4) Focus on areas of functioning to evaluate what aspect of symptoms should be prioritized for treatment. GTS-QoL, Gilles de la Tourette Syndrome Quality-of-Life scale.

of pimozide and haloperidol in treating tics compared with placebo has been documented by 6 and 3 randomized controlled trials (RCTs) of fair quality, respectively.[75–77] Direct comparison between the 2 agents did not show any significant difference in total tic scores, with a worse tolerability profile for haloperidol due to higher rates of sedation, lethargy, and, in particular, extrapyramidal symptoms. The use of fluphenazine is supported by open-label studies,[78] retrospective case series,[79] and one single-blind, placebo-controlled crossover study[75]; there is moderate evidence that fluphenazine has fewer adverse effects than haloperidol. The use of first-generation antipsychotics is limited by their tolerability profile; these drugs can cause increased anxiety and dysphoria (also after withdrawal), hyperprolactinemia (leading to gynecomastia, galactorrhea, irregular menses, and sexual dysfunction), hypotension, electrocardiographic changes, and weight gain. Pimozide was also recently shown to be associated with significant increases in glycemia in pediatric patients.[80] Benzamides like tiapride and sulpiride are more frequently prescribed in Europe, and their efficacy

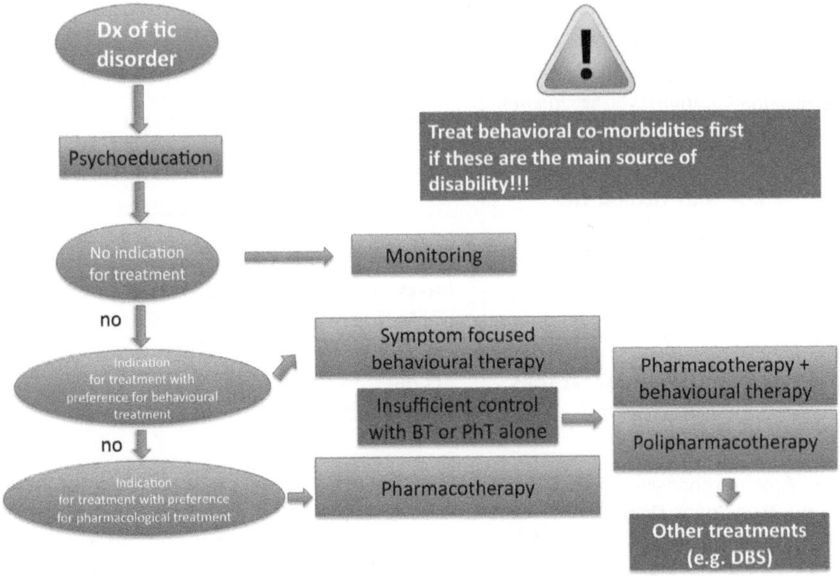

Fig. 4. Flowchart of treatment options in TS. (*Adapted from* Roessner V, Plessen KJ, Rothenberger A, et al. European clinical guidelines for Tourette syndrome and other tic disorders. Part II: pharmacological treatment. Eur Child Adolesc Psychiatry 2011;20:173–96.)

is supported by small controlled studies[73]; sedation remains a common issue when using sulpiride.

Among second-generation antipsychotics, risperidone is the agent for which the highest quality of evidence in favor of efficacy in treating tics has been acquired. Five RCTs have confirmed the superiority to placebo of risperidone, and similar efficacy to pimozide and clonidine in active comparator trials. A recent meta-analysis found no significant difference in the efficacy of risperidone (daily dose range 1–6 mg), haloperidol, pimozide, and ziprasidone, confirming significant superiority to placebo for all 4 agents.[81] Preliminary evidence suggests a potential added value of risperidone in GTS patients with comorbid OCS and impulse control disorder. Importantly, risperidone treatment requires monitoring for motor and metabolic side effects. There is limited and mixed evidence for olanzapine and quetiapine, both of which are associated with metabolic side effects (body mass index increases and alteration in lipid profile). Aripiprazole is a promising molecule that has D2 antagonistic properties in hyperdopaminergic conditions, and agonist effects in hypodopaminergic states. One fair-quality RCT showed superiority to placebo[82] and 5 prospective open-label studies on relatively large clinical samples reported significant reduction in tic severity in approximately 60% of children and adults with GTS treated with aripiprazole, with effects lasting more than 1 year in up to 50% of responders.[75,83] The tolerability profile of this drug in GTS patients seems slightly more favorable than that of other second-generation antipsychotics, particularly with respect to electrocardiographic (QT interval prolongation), whereas its use has been associated with movement disorders and raised serum cholesterol levels in children with GTS.[80] There is no convincing evidence that the use of very low doses of dopamine agonists like ropinirole and pramipexole is efficacious, despite the observation of a moderate effect on comorbid ADHD.[84]

Table 1
Medications for the treatment of tics

Medication	Daily Dose (mg)	Adverse Effects	Level of Evidence
Clonidine	0.05–3	Sedation, dry mouth, headache, irritability, mid-sleep awakenings, rebound hypertension, tics and anxiety following abrupt discontinuation	CG: moderate quality, strong recommendation ESSTS: level A evidence
Guanfacine	0.5–4	Orthostatic hypotension, bradycardia, sedation, headache	CG: moderate quality, strong recommendation ESSTS: level A evidence
Haloperidol	0.5–10	Rigidity, parkinsonism, tardive involuntary movements and akathisia, appetite changes, weight gain, salivary changes, constipation, depression, anxiety, fatigue, sedation, hyperprolactinemia (galactorrhea, gynecomastia, irregular menses, sexual dysfunction)	CG: high quality, weak recommendation ESSTS: level A evidence
Pimozide	0.5–6	Similar to haloperidol but with less movement disorders; QTc interval prolongation	CG: high quality, weak recommendation ESSTS: level A evidence
Risperidone	0.5–16	Sedation, fatigue, depression, acute phobic reactions, weight gain	CG: high quality, weak recommendation ESSTS: level A evidence
Aripiprazole	5–30	Weight gain, increase in BMI and waist circumference, nausea, fatigue, sedation, akathisia, movement disorders, sleep problems, probably lower risk of QT prolongation than with other antipsychotics	CG: moderate quality, weak recommendation ESSTS: level B evidence
Ziprasidone	5–40	Sedation, anxiety, akathisia, movement disorders	CG: low quality, weak recommendation ESSTS: level B evidence
Olanzapine	2.5–20	Sedation, weight gain and increased appetite, dry mouth, transient hypoglycemia	CG: low quality, weak recommendation ESSTS: level B evidence
Fluphenazine	0.5–20	Similar to haloperidol, but less frequent	CG: low quality, weak recommendation ESSTS: not evaluated
Sulpiride Tiapride	50–200	Sedation; less commonly, paradoxic depression, restlessness, sleep problems, weight gain, hyperprolactinemia	CG: not evaluated ESSTS: level B evidence

(*continued on next page*)

Table 1
(*continued*)

Medication	Daily Dose (mg)	Adverse Effects	Level of Evidence
Topiramate	50–150	Weight loss, paraesthesia	CG: low quality, weak recommendation ESSTS: not evaluated
Botulinum toxin		Focal weakness, hypophonia	CG: low quality, weak recommendation
δ-9-THC	10	Anxiety, dizziness, fatigue, dry mouth, mood changes, memory loss, psychosis, blurred vision	CG: low quality, weak recommendation
Quetiapine	50–250	Sedation	CG: very low quality, weak recommendation ESSTS: level C evidence
Tetrabenazine	25–150	Sedation, fatigue, nausea, insomnia, akathisia, parkinsonism, depression	CG: very low quality, weak recommendation

Abbreviations: BMI, body mass index; CG, Canadian guidelines; ESSTS, European Society for the Study of Tourette Syndrome guidelines.
Adapted from Refs.[73,75,110]

α-2-Agonists have been known to be effective as treatment for tics for more than 30 years. Clonidine has been tested in 6 RCTs of heterogeneous quality, overall providing a moderate degree of evidence quality in favor of superiority to placebo for both the oral and the transdermal formulations.[75] Two RCTs and 2 open-label studies assessed the efficacy of guanfacine in children with GTS; this drug has a longer half-life than clonidine and might be administered in a single daily dose. These 2 medications are considered first-line therapy in the United States and Canada, primarily because of their preferable side-effect profile, compared with antipsychotics, whereas in Europe they are definitely less commonly used than antipsychotics.[73,75] A recent meta-analysis confirmed superiority to placebo for both α-2-agonists; however, this benefit was significant only for GTS children/adolescents with comorbid ADHD, and minimal in GTS patients without ADHD.[81] Patients on clonidine should be monitored for reduced blood pressure, sedation, headache, irritability, dysphoria, and interrupted night sleep; moreover, clonidine should be titrated gradually to minimize side effects and discontinued gradually to avoid rebound hypertension.

Baclofen and topiramate showed moderate efficacy in 2 relatively small, double-blind RCTs involving patients of different age groups. Topiramate showed moderate improvement of tic severity from baseline, but the study duration was only 70 days and the sample size was relatively small (n = 29). Nevertheless, this result should encourage further study of this agent in GTS, also with a better monitoring of its tolerability profile.[85] The RCT exploring baclofen was smaller and included only children.[86] Tetrabenazine blocks the vesicular VMAT2 protein leading to presynaptic dopamine depletion with relatively minor postsynaptic D2 blockage. Data on its efficacy over tics are limited to one small open-label trial and to retrospective cohort studies, which showed long-lasting (18–24 months) improvement of tic severity in more than 80% of treated patients.[87,88] Although tetrabenazine does not lead to weight gain, drowsiness, fatigue, nausea, and depression may present a problem in some patients. Botulinum toxin injections may treat persistent and localized simple motor and vocal tics, including coprolalia and upper face or neck tics, with potential reduction also of premonitory urges. This finding is supported by several case reports or small series, 3 retrospective cohort studies, and 1 RCT.[89] Hypophonia is a very common side effect of botulinum toxin injections for vocal tics. Two small RCTs tested δ-9-tetrahydrocannabinol, the main active compound of cannabis, in a total of 28 adults with GTS, reporting a modest benefit on some outcome measures and acceptable tolerability.[90] New studies are needed to explore the potential of cannabinoid-modulating agents in GTS. Nicotine has been explored as add-on treatment to haloperidol in several studies. A single controlled trial of nicotine chewing gum and 3 controlled studies of transdermal nicotine patches showed mild reduction of tic frequency, although at the expense of intolerable gastrointestinal side effects.[91] Several other agents (naloxone, naltrexone, calcium channel blockers, flutamide, lecithin, metoclopramide, ondansetron, physostigmine, citalopram, fluvoxamine, propranolol) have been tried for the treatment of tics, but evidence is mainly anecdotal or limited to poor quality trials.

Complementary and alternative medicine approaches in GTS have recently attracted growing interest. The most promising, based on current available evidence, include ω-3 fatty acids, and Chinese Traditional Medicine (Ningdong granule). A recent, double-blind, placebo-controlled trial of ω-3 fatty acids showed reduced tic-related impairment in children and adolescents with GTS, although there was no direct benefit over tics.[92] The beneficial effect of Ningdong granules is only supported by open-label studies.

Behavioral Treatment

There has been a significant development of behavioral therapies targeting tics during the last 10 years, demonstrating a reduction in the severity of motor and vocal tics. The most effective treatment approaches of this kind are habit reversal training (HRT), a related and expanded version of the HRT package called Comprehensive Behavioral Intervention for Tics (CBIT), and Exposure and Response Prevention (ERP) for tics. The main scope of HRT is to train patients to gain control over their tics in real time. It consists of 3 main components: (1) awareness training, whereby patients learn to recognize their premonitory urges and tics when these occur in real-time; (2) competing response training, whereby patients select and implement a motor behavior through which they may counteract the occurrence of tics; (3) social support, whereby a designed support person promotes the use of HRT strategies outside of therapy.[93] There is a large body of evidence that supports the efficacy of HRT. Six RCTs and several smaller observational studies showed that HRT reduces tic severity effectively. Moreover, meta-analyses detected a large treatment effect size, similar to that observed in other widely used behavioral interventions for conditions like OCD or anxiety disorders.[94,95] There have been different attempts to potentiate HRT using additional components. One of these is Cognitive Behavioral Tension Reduction Therapy (CBTRT), which focuses on addressing tension reduction as a means to reduce tic severity. In addition to the first 2 core components of HRT, CBTRT involves also self-monitoring techniques to identify relevant antecedent cues that facilitate the occurrence of tics as well as relaxation training and cognitive restructuring aiming at influencing patterns of thinking about tension and tics. There is also evidence of the efficacy of CBTRT in reducing tics, which, however, seems primarily dependent on the implementation of the core components of HRT rather than of the additional components. HRT has also been combined to Acceptance and Commitment Therapy (ACT), which consists of exercises that help patients to gain distance from distressing cognitions, emotions, and urges. However, convincing evidence that ACT addition increases HRT efficacy is still lacking. CBIT is the most effective extension of HRT. The components added to HRT in the CBIT package are (1) function-based assessment, which targets contextual factors predictably worsening tics and allows working with support persons and patients to identify strategies to counteract tic-prone situations; (2) relaxation training, which per se is not sufficiently effective to improve tics in monotherapy, but works as a stress management tool; (3) psychoeducational interventions.[93] CBIT is delivered in eleven 1-hour long sessions, 6 of which are weekly, 2 are scheduled every 2 weeks, followed by 3 booster monthly sessions, with a fixed protocol of homework assignments. Overall, HRT and CBIT showed a degree of effect in reducing tics that is not inferior to that provided by some pharmacologic interventions. HRT showed efficacy in children, adolescents, and adults aged 8 to 65 years with GTS, regardless of comorbid psychological conditions, use of antitic medications, and type of tics produced. Two multisite RCTs, one with children and one with adults, involved 8 weekly sessions of CBIT followed by booster sessions every 3 months, and demonstrated its superiority to supportive therapy plus psychoeducation by a 3-fold factor.[96,97] Importantly, there were no adverse effects caused by CBIT; attrition was comparable to that of the control active intervention, and improvements were sustained beyond 6 months after treatment, with a positive spinoff also on psychopathological comorbidities. Preliminary evidence has also suggested noninferiority of HRT administration via a telehealth approach compared with face-to-face administration.[98]

Finally, ERP has been originally validated and is very widely used for OCD. With respect to its application in tic disorders, ERP consists of prolonged exposure to premonitory urges through prolonged suppression of tics[99]; this should lead to habituation to the urge and gradual reduction of the motivation of the patient to tic (a counterconditioning type of approach). Only one RCT has shown noninferiority of ERP to HRT, although ERP is generally longer and less cost-effective than HRT or some of its extensions, such as CBIT.[100]

There are obvious limitations to behavioral treatment in GTS (eg, the still relatively restricted number of well-trained teams of therapists and its length of application, 2–3 months on average) associated with costly resources.[101] More research is also needed to increase knowledge of predictors of good response to CBT and patient selection criteria, which might help tailor the therapeutic intervention (ie, deciding whether to treat with CBT, and which CBT approach to use in the individual patient).

Deep Brain Stimulation Surgery

Over the last decade, there has been increasing experience and experimental evidence of the efficacy and tolerability of functional neurosurgery, in particular of deep brain stimulation (DBS), for GTS. DBS is the only active intervention that is extensively being investigated for adult GTS patients who are deemed refractory to pharmacologic and behavioral interventions. Recommendation documents have been issued by North American and European study groups, aimed at guiding clinicians in patient selection and assessment.[102–104] The main patient selection criteria for DBS in GTS discussed in these recommendations can be summarized as follows:

- Diagnosis of GTS or other chronic tic disorder
- Age 18 or above (according to some authors 25 or above)
- Tics as prominent feature of the clinical presentation
- High tic severity (proposed as $\geq$35 on the Yale Global Tic Severity Subscore for a stable period of time, suggested by some authors of at least 12 months) and/or

presence of potentially highly disabling or harmful tics (eg, tics associated with a clear self-injurious component)

- Tics are considered refractory to pharmacologic and behavioral interventions. Failure of pharmacologic treatment implies having tried a course with medications from at least 3 different pharmacologic classes (eg, antipsychotics, α_2-agonists, benzodiazepines), lasting at least 12 weeks (according to other authors, 6 months) for each drug, at adequate dosage and proven compliance. Failure of behavioral therapy implies having tried at least 10 sessions of behavioral treatment (either HRT-based or ERP-based)
- Stable and optimized treatment of medical, cognitive, and behavioral comorbidities
- Expected compliance during monitoring (stable psychosocial environment)

Overall, these criteria are considered merely proposals, and more work is needed to increase consensus on their routine clinical application. In addition to this, consensus on the ideal anatomic target has not yet been reached to date, the main reason being the paucity of RCTs and lack of adequately powered active comparator trials. At present, the most promising targets are the centromedian/parafascicular-substantia periventricularis-nucleus ventralis oralis internus cross-point of the thalamus, the only target for which a small RCT of fair quality is available,[105] and the globus pallidus pars interna (with higher efficacy when the anteromedial, or limbic, portion is targeted).[106,107] DBS has general potential complications that apply to all anatomic targets and indications (eg, hemorrhage and infection of the electrode implant site). More specific adverse events associated with thalamic DBS in GTS include sedation, abulia, fatigue, apathy, sexual dysfunction, and visual disturbances. Importantly, it has been shown by longitudinal observational studies that thalamic DBS does not lead to long-term adverse cognitive sequelae.[108] The opportunity to apply a "tailored" approach, based on the clinical manifestations exhibited by each patients within the Tourette spectrum, as well as a scheduled, rather than continuous, DBS paradigm,[109] have recently been discussed.

SUPPLEMENTARY DATA

Supplementary data related to this article can be found online at http://dx.doi.org/10.1016/j.ncl.2014.09.008.

REFERENCES

1. American Psychiatric Association. Diagnostic and statistical manual of mental disorders. 5th edition. Arlington (VA): American Psychiatric Publishing; 2013.
2. Knight T, Steeves T, Day L, et al. Prevalence of tic disorders: a systematic review and meta-analysis. Pediatr Neurol 2012;47:77–90.
3. Cavanna AE, Rickards H. The psychopathological spectrum of Gilles de la Tourette syndrome. Neurosci Biobehav Rev 2013;37:1008–15.
4. Robertson MM. Tourette syndrome, associated conditions and the complexities of treatment. Brain 2000;123(Pt 3):425–62.
5. Hallett M. Neurophysiology of tics. Adv Neurol 2001;85:237–44.
6. van der Salm SM, Tijssen MA, Koelman JH, et al. The bereitschaftspotential in jerky movement disorders. J Neurol Neurosurg Psychiatry 2012;83:1162–7.
7. Jankovic J. Tourette syndrome. Phenomenology and classification of tics. Neurol Clin 1997;15:267–75.

8. Leckman JF, Walker DE, Cohen DJ. Premonitory urges in Tourette's syndrome. Am J Psychiatry 1993;150:98–102.
9. Kwak C, Dat Vuong K, Jankovic J. Premonitory sensory phenomenon in Tourette's syndrome. Mov Disord 2003;18:1530–3.
10. Banaschewski T, Woerner W, Rothenberger A. Premonitory sensory phenomena and suppressibility of tics in Tourette syndrome: developmental aspects in children and adolescents. Dev Med Child Neurol 2003;45:700–3.
11. Peterson BS, Leckman JF. The temporal dynamics of tics in Gilles de la Tourette syndrome. Biol Psychiatry 1998;44:1337–48.
12. Ganos C, Kahl U, Schunke O, et al. Are premonitory urges a prerequisite of tic inhibition in Gilles de la Tourette syndrome? J Neurol Neurosurg Psychiatry 2012;83:975–8.
13. Woods DW, Himle MB. Creating tic suppression: comparing the effects of verbal instruction to differential reinforcement. J Appl Behav Anal 2004;37: 417–20.
14. Verdellen C, van de Griendt J, Hartmann A, et al. European clinical guidelines for Tourette syndrome and other tic disorders. Part III: behavioural and psychosocial interventions. Eur Child Adolesc Psychiatry 2011;20:197–207.
15. Ganos C, Ogrzal T, Schnitzler A, et al. The pathophysiology of echopraxia/ echolalia: relevance to Gilles De La Tourette syndrome. Mov Disord 2012;27: 1222–9.
16. Freeman RD, Zinner SH, Muller-Vahl KR, et al. Coprophenomena in Tourette syndrome. Dev Med Child Neurol 2009;51:218–27.
17. Cavanna AE, Servo S, Monaco F, et al. The behavioral spectrum of Gilles de la Tourette syndrome. J Neuropsychiatry Clin Neurosci 2009;21:13–23.
18. Freeman RD, Fast DK, Burd L, et al. An international perspective on Tourette syndrome: selected findings from 3,500 individuals in 22 countries. Dev Med Child Neurol 2000;42:436–47.
19. Roessner V, Becker A, Banaschewski T, et al. Psychopathological profile in children with chronic tic disorder and co-existing ADHD: additive effects. J Abnorm Child Psychol 2007;35:79–85.
20. Wanderer S, Roessner V, Freeman R, et al. Relationship of obsessive-compulsive disorder to age-related comorbidity in children and adolescents with Tourette syndrome. J Dev Behav Pediatr 2012;33:124–33.
21. Cath DC, Spinhoven P, Hoogduin CA, et al. Repetitive behaviors in Tourette's syndrome and OCD with and without tics: what are the differences? Psychiatry Res 2001;101:171–85.
22. Worbe Y, Mallet L, Golmard JL, et al. Repetitive behaviours in patients with Gilles de la Tourette syndrome: tics, compulsions, or both? PLoS One 2010;5:e12959.
23. Mathews CA, Grados MA. Familiality of Tourette syndrome, obsessive-compulsive disorder, and attention-deficit/hyperactivity disorder: heritability analysis in a large sib-pair sample. J Am Acad Child Adolesc Psychiatry 2011;50:46–54.
24. Cheng B, Braass H, Ganos C, et al. Altered intrahemispheric structural connectivity in Gilles de la Tourette syndrome. Neuroimage Clin 2013;4:174–81.
25. Burd L, Li Q, Kerbeshian J, et al. Tourette syndrome and comorbid pervasive developmental disorders. J Child Neurol 2009;24:170–5.
26. Pringsheim T, Hammer T. Social behavior and comorbidity in children with tics. Pediatr Neurol 2013;49:406–10.
27. Canitano R, Vivanti G. Tics and Tourette syndrome in autism spectrum disorders. Autism 2007;11:19–28.

28. Chen K, Budman CL, Diego Herrera L, et al. Prevalence and clinical correlates of explosive outbursts in Tourette syndrome. Psychiatry Res 2013;205:269–75.
29. Mathews CA, Waller J, Glidden D, et al. Self injurious behaviour in Tourette syndrome: correlates with impulsivity and impulse control. J Neurol Neurosurg Psychiatry 2004;75:1149–55.
30. Robertson MM, Banerjee S, Hiley PJ, et al. Personality disorder and psychopathology in Tourette's syndrome: a controlled study. Br J Psychiatry 1997;171:283–6.
31. Robertson MM. Mood disorders and Gilles de la Tourette's syndrome: an update on prevalence, etiology, comorbidity, clinical associations, and implications. J Psychosom Res 2006;61:349–58.
32. Eddy CM, Cavanna AE. On being your own worst enemy: an investigation of socially inappropriate symptoms in Tourette syndrome. J Psychiatr Res 2013;47:1259–63.
33. Eddy CM, Cavanna AE, Gulisano M, et al. Clinical correlates of quality of life in Tourette syndrome. Mov Disord 2011;26:735–8.
34. Eddy CM, Cavanna AE, Gulisano M, et al. The effects of comorbid obsessive-compulsive disorder and attention-deficit hyperactivity disorder on quality of life in Tourette syndrome. J Neuropsychiatry Clin Neurosci 2012;24:458–62.
35. Cavanna AE, Critchley HD, Orth M, et al. Dissecting the Gilles de la Tourette spectrum: a factor analytic study on 639 patients. J Neurol Neurosurg Psychiatry 2011;82:1320–3.
36. Robertson MM. Movement disorders: Tourette syndrome–beyond swearing and sex? Nat Rev Neurol 2014;10:6–8.
37. Rizzo R, Gulisano M, Cali PV, et al. Long term clinical course of Tourette syndrome. Brain Dev 2012;34(8):667–73.
38. Bloch MH, Leckman JF. Clinical course of Tourette syndrome. J Psychosom Res 2009;67:497–501.
39. Pappert EJ, Goetz CG, Louis ED, et al. Objective assessments of longitudinal outcome in Gilles de la Tourette's syndrome. Neurology 2003;61:936–40.
40. Ganos C, Roessner V, Munchau A. The functional anatomy of Gilles de la Tourette syndrome. Neurosci Biobehav Rev 2013;37:1050–62.
41. Kataoka Y, Kalanithi PS, Grantz H, et al. Decreased number of parvalbumin and cholinergic interneurons in the striatum of individuals with Tourette syndrome. J Comp Neurol 2010;518:277–91.
42. Kalanithi PS, Zheng W, Kataoka Y, et al. Altered parvalbumin-positive neuron distribution in basal ganglia of individuals with Tourette syndrome. Proc Natl Acad Sci U S A 2005;102:13307–12.
43. Bronfeld M, Bar-Gad I. Tic disorders: what happens in the basal ganglia? Neuroscientist 2013;19:101–8.
44. Bronfeld M, Belelovsky K, Bar-Gad I. Spatial and temporal properties of tic-related neuronal activity in the cortico-basal ganglia loop. J Neurosci 2011;31:8713–21.
45. Peterson BS, Thomas P, Kane MJ, et al. Basal ganglia volumes in patients with Gilles de la Tourette syndrome. Arch Gen Psychiatry 2003;60:415–24.
46. Bloch MH, Leckman JF, Zhu H, et al. Caudate volumes in childhood predict symptom severity in adults with Tourette syndrome. Neurology 2005;65:1253–8.
47. Miller AM, Bansal R, Hao X, et al. Enlargement of thalamic nuclei in Tourette syndrome. Arch Gen Psychiatry 2010;67:955–64.
48. Peterson BS, Choi HA, Hao X, et al. Morphologic features of the amygdala and hippocampus in children and adults with Tourette syndrome. Arch Gen Psychiatry 2007;64:1281–91.

49. Roessner V, Overlack S, Baudewig J, et al. No brain structure abnormalities in boys with Tourette's syndrome: a voxel-based morphometry study. Mov Disord 2009;24:2398–403.
50. Roessner V, Overlack S, Schmidt-Samoa C, et al. Increased putamen and callosal motor subregion in treatment-naive boys with Tourette syndrome indicates changes in the bihemispheric motor network. J Child Psychol Psychiatry 2011; 52:306–14.
51. Fahim C, Yoon U, Das S, et al. Somatosensory-motor bodily representation cortical thinning in Tourette: effects of tic severity, age and gender. Cortex 2010;46:750–60.
52. Sowell ER, Kan E, Yoshii J, et al. Thinning of sensorimotor cortices in children with Tourette syndrome. Nat Neurosci 2008;11:637–9.
53. Worbe Y, Gerardin E, Hartmann A, et al. Distinct structural changes underpin clinical phenotypes in patients with Gilles de la Tourette syndrome. Brain 2010;133:3649–60.
54. Bohlhalter S, Goldfine A, Matteson S, et al. Neural correlates of tic generation in Tourette syndrome: an event-related functional MRI study. Brain 2006;129: 2029–37.
55. Hampson M, Tokoglu F, King RA, et al. Brain areas coactivating with motor cortex during chronic motor tics and intentional movements. Biol Psychiatry 2009; 65:594–9.
56. Neuner I, Schneider F, Shah NJ. Functional neuroanatomy of tics. Int Rev Neurobiol 2013;112:35–71.
57. Wang Z, Maia TV, Marsh R, et al. The neural circuits that generate tics in Tourette's syndrome. Am J Psychiatry 2011;168:1326–37.
58. Ganos C, Kuhn S, Kahl U, et al. Prefrontal cortex volume reductions and tic inhibition are unrelated in uncomplicated GTS adults. J Psychosom Res 2014;76:84–7.
59. Muller-Vahl KR, Kaufmann J, Grosskreutz J, et al. Prefrontal and anterior cingulate cortex abnormalities in Tourette Syndrome: evidence from voxel-based morphometry and magnetization transfer imaging. BMC Neurosci 2009;10:47.
60. Peterson BS, Staib L, Scahill L, et al. Regional brain and ventricular volumes in Tourette syndrome. Arch Gen Psychiatry 2001;58:427–40.
61. Ganos C, Kuhn S, Kahl U, et al. Action inhibition in tourette syndrome. Mov Disord 2014;29(12):1532–8.
62. Ray Li CS, Chang HL, Hsu YP, et al. Motor response inhibition in children with Tourette's disorder. J Neuropsychiatry Clin Neurosci 2006;18:417–9.
63. Watkins LH, Sahakian BJ, Robertson MM, et al. Executive function in Tourette's syndrome and obsessive-compulsive disorder. Psychol Med 2005;35:571–82.
64. Baym CL, Corbett BA, Wright SB, et al. Neural correlates of tic severity and cognitive control in children with Tourette syndrome. Brain 2008;131:165–79.
65. Jackson SR, Parkinson A, Jung J, et al. Compensatory neural reorganization in Tourette syndrome. Curr Biol 2011;21:580–5.
66. Jung J, Jackson SR, Parkinson A, et al. Cognitive control over motor output in Tourette syndrome. Neurosci Biobehav Rev 2012;37:1016–25.
67. Jackson GM, Mueller SC, Hambleton K, et al. Enhanced cognitive control in Tourette Syndrome during task uncertainty. Exp Brain Res 2007;182:357–64.
68. Jung J, Jackson SR, Nam K, et al. Enhanced saccadic control in young people with Tourette syndrome despite slowed pro-saccades. J Neuropsychol 2014. [Epub ahead of print].
69. Mueller SC, Jackson GM, Dhalla R, et al. Enhanced cognitive control in young people with Tourette's syndrome. Curr Biol 2006;16:570–3.

70. Ganos C, Mencacci N, Gardiner A, et al. Paroxysmal kinesigenic dyskinesia may be misdiagnosed in co-occurring Gilles de la Tourette syndrome. Mov Disord Clin Pract 2014;1:84–6.
71. Kompoliti K, Goetz CG. Hyperkinetic movement disorders misdiagnosed as tics in Gilles de la Tourette syndrome. Mov Disord 1998;13:477–80.
72. Ganos C, Münchau A, Bhatia K. The semiology of tics, Tourette's and their associations. Mov Disord Clin Pract 2014;1:145–53.
73. Roessner V, Plessen KJ, Rothenberger A, et al. European clinical guidelines for Tourette syndrome and other tic disorders. Part II: pharmacological treatment. Eur Child Adolesc Psychiatry 2011;20:173–96.
74. Jankovic J, Kurlan R. Tourette syndrome: evolving concepts. Mov Disord 2011; 26:1149–56.
75. Pringsheim T, Doja A, Gorman D, et al. Canadian guidelines for the evidence-based treatment of tic disorders: pharmacotherapy. Can J Psychiatry 2012; 57:133–43.
76. Mogwitz S, Buse J, Ehrlich S, et al. Clinical pharmacology of dopamine-modulating agents in Tourette's syndrome. Int Rev Neurobiol 2013;112:281–349.
77. Pringsheim T, Marras C. Pimozide for tics in Tourette's syndrome. Cochrane Database Syst Rev 2009;(2):CD006996.
78. Goetz CG, Tanner CM, Klawans HL. Fluphenazine and multifocal tic disorders. Arch Neurol 1984;41:271–2.
79. Wijemanne S, Wu LJ, Jankovic J. Long-term efficacy and safety of fluphenazine in patients with Tourette syndrome. Mov Disord 2014;29:126–30.
80. Rizzo R, Eddy CM, Cali P, et al. Metabolic effects of aripiprazole and pimozide in children with Tourette syndrome. Pediatr Neurol 2012;47:419–22.
81. Weisman H, Qureshi IA, Leckman JF, et al. Systematic review: pharmacological treatment of tic disorders–efficacy of antipsychotic and alpha-2 adrenergic agonist agents. Neurosci Biobehav Rev 2013;37:1162–71.
82. Yoo HK, Joung YS, Lee JS, et al. A multicenter, randomized, double-blind, placebo-controlled study of aripiprazole in children and adolescents with Tourette's disorder. J Clin Psychiatry 2013;74:e772–80.
83. Wenzel C, Kleimann A, Bokemeyer S, et al. Aripiprazole for the treatment of Tourette syndrome: a case series of 100 patients. J Clin Psychopharmacol 2012;32:548–50.
84. Kurlan R, Crespi G, Coffey B, et al. A multicenter randomized placebo-controlled clinical trial of pramipexole for Tourette's syndrome. Mov Disord 2012;27:775–8.
85. Jankovic J, Jimenez-Shahed J, Brown LW. A randomised, double-blind, placebo-controlled study of topiramate in the treatment of Tourette syndrome. J Neurol Neurosurg Psychiatry 2010;81:70–3.
86. Singer HS, Wendlandt J, Krieger M, et al. Baclofen treatment in Tourette syndrome: a double-blind, placebo-controlled, crossover trial. Neurology 2001;56:599–604.
87. Chen JJ, Ondo WG, Dashtipour K, et al. Tetrabenazine for the treatment of hyperkinetic movement disorders: a review of the literature. Clin Ther 2012;34: 1487–504.
88. Porta M, Sassi M, Cavallazzi M, et al. Tourette's syndrome and role of tetrabenazine: review and personal experience. Clin Drug Investig 2008;28:443–59.
89. Marras C, Andrews D, Sime E, et al. Botulinum toxin for simple motor tics: a randomized, double-blind, controlled clinical trial. Neurology 2001;56:605–10.
90. Muller-Vahl KR. Treatment of Tourette syndrome with cannabinoids. Behav Neurol 2013;27:119–24.

91. Silver AA, Shytle RD, Philipp MK, et al. Transdermal nicotine and haloperidol in Tourette's disorder: a double-blind placebo-controlled study. J Clin Psychiatry 2001;62:707–14.
92. Gabbay V, Babb JS, Klein RG, et al. A double-blind, placebo-controlled trial of omega-3 fatty acids in Tourette's disorder. Pediatrics 2012;129:e1493–500.
93. Capriotti M, Woods D. Cognitive-behavioral treatment for tics. In: Martino D, Leckman JF, editors. Tourette syndrome. New York: Oxford University Press; 2013. p. 503–23.
94. McGuire JF, Piacentini J, Brennan EA, et al. A meta-analysis of behavior therapy for Tourette Syndrome. J Psychiatr Res 2014;50:106–12.
95. Wile DJ, Pringsheim TM. Behavior therapy for tourette syndrome: a systematic review and meta-analysis. Curr Treat Options Neurol 2013;15:385–95.
96. Piacentini J, Woods DW, Scahill L, et al. Behavior therapy for children with Tourette disorder: a randomized controlled trial. JAMA 2010;303:1929–37.
97. Wilhelm S, Peterson AL, Piacentini J, et al. Randomized trial of behavior therapy for adults with Tourette syndrome. Arch Gen Psychiatry 2012;69:795–803.
98. Himle MB, Freitag M, Walther M, et al. A randomized pilot trial comparing videoconference versus face-to-face delivery of behavior therapy for childhood tic disorders. Behav Res Ther 2012;50:565–70.
99. van de Griendt JM, Verdellen CW, van Dijk MK, et al. Behavioural treatment of tics: habit reversal and exposure with response prevention. Neurosci Biobehav Rev 2013;37:1172–7.
100. Verdellen CW, Keijsers GP, Cath DC, et al. Exposure with response prevention versus habit reversal in Tourettes's syndrome: a controlled study. Behav Res Ther 2004;42:501–11.
101. Scahill L, Woods DW, Himle MB, et al. Current controversies on the role of behavior therapy in Tourette syndrome. Mov Disord 2013;28:1179–83.
102. Ackermans L, Kuhn J, Neuner I, et al. Surgery for Tourette syndrome. World Neurosurg 2013;80:S29.e15–22.
103. Mink JW, Walkup J, Frey KA, et al. Patient selection and assessment recommendations for deep brain stimulation in Tourette syndrome. Mov Disord 2006;21:1831–8.
104. Piedad JC, Rickards HE, Cavanna AE. What patients with gilles de la tourette syndrome should be treated with deep brain stimulation and what is the best target? Neurosurgery 2012;71:173–92.
105. Ackermans L, Duits A, van der Linden C, et al. Double-blind clinical trial of thalamic stimulation in patients with Tourette syndrome. Brain 2011;134:832–44.
106. Cannon E, Silburn P, Coyne T, et al. Deep brain stimulation of anteromedial globus pallidus interna for severe Tourette's syndrome. Am J Psychiatry 2012;169:860–6.
107. Martinez-Fernandez R, Zrinzo L, Aviles-Olmos I, et al. Deep brain stimulation for Gilles de la Tourette syndrome: a case series targeting subregions of the globus pallidus internus. Mov Disord 2011;26:1922–30.
108. Porta M, Brambilla A, Cavanna AE, et al. Thalamic deep brain stimulation for treatment-refractory Tourette syndrome: two-year outcome. Neurology 2009;73:1375–80.
109. Okun MS, Foote KD, Wu SS, et al. A trial of scheduled deep brain stimulation for Tourette syndrome: moving away from continuous deep brain stimulation paradigms. JAMA Neurol 2013;70:85–94.
110. Martino D, Mink JW. Tic disorders. Continuum (Minneap Minn) 2013;19:1287–311.

Paroxysmal Movement Disorders

Olga Waln, MD[a], Joseph Jankovic, MD[b,*]

KEYWORDS

- Paroxysmal dyskinesia • Paroxysmal choreoathetosis • Paroxysmal dystonia
- Episodic ataxia

KEY POINTS

- Paroxysmal dyskinesias represent a group of episodic abnormal involuntary movements manifested by recurrent attacks of dystonia, chorea, athetosis, or a combination of these hyperkinetic movement disorders.
- Paroxysmal kinesigenic dyskinesia, paroxysmal nonkinesigenic dyskinesia, paroxysmal exertion-induced dyskinesia, and paroxysmal hypnogenic dyskinesia can be distinguished clinically by precipitating factors, duration and frequency of the attacks, and the response to medications.
- Primary paroxysmal dyskinesias are usually autosomal dominant genetic conditions.
- Secondary paroxysmal dyskinesias can be the symptoms of different neurologic and medical disorders.

Videos of paroxysmal dyskinesias accompany this article at http://www.neurologic.theclinics.com/

INTRODUCTION

Paroxysmal dyskinesias are a group of rare movement disorders characterized by the recurrent episodes of dystonia, chorea, athetosis, ballism, or a combination of these abnormal movements, with normal neurologic examination between the episodes.

Mount and Reback[1] first defined paroxysmal dyskinesia as a movement disorder and not epilepsy in 1940, when they described a patient with a personal and family history of the attacks of dystonia and chorea precipitated by caffeine, alcohol, or fatigue. Paroxysms of choreoathetosis triggered by sudden movement were described in 1967 by Kertesz[2] and named "paroxysmal kinesigenic choreoathetosis". A decade

---

Disclosures: The authors have nothing to disclose.
[a] Department of Neurology, Houston Methodist Neurological Institute, 6560 Fannin, Suite 802, Houston, TX 77030, USA; [b] Department of Neurology, Parkinson's Disease Center and Movement Disorders Clinic, Baylor College of Medicine, 6550 Fannin, Suite 1801, Houston, TX 77030, USA
* Corresponding author.
E-mail address: josephj@bcm.edu

later, another type of episodic chorea induced by prolonged exercise was described by Lance.[3] Finally, paroxysms of abnormal movements in sleep were reported in some patients by Lugaresi and Cirignotta.[4]

CLASSIFICATION

The classification of paroxysmal dyskinesias was first proposed by Lance[3] in 1977, was based on the duration of the paroxysms, precipitating factors, and phenomenology of abnormal movements:

1. Paroxysmal kinesigenic choreoathetosis with movement-induced short attacks
2. Paroxysmal dystonic choreoathetosis with long attacks not induced by movements
3. Paroxysmal exercise-induced dyskinesia with intermediate duration of the attacks

Later, this classification was replaced with the one proposed by Demirkiran and Jankovic,[5] based solely on precipitating factors of the attacks and not on phenomenology, because each type of paroxysmal dyskinesia can manifest as dystonia, chorea, athetosis, or a combination of abnormal movements. This new classification includes paroxysmal kinesigenic dyskinesia (PKD), paroxysmal nonkinesigenic dyskinesia (PNKD), paroxysmal exertion-induced dyskinesia (PED), and paroxysmal hypnogenic dyskinesia (PHD).[5]

Depending on etiology, paroxysmal dyskinesias can be primary or idiopathic (including familial and sporadic disorders), and secondary (**Box 1**).

CLINICAL PRESENTATION AND CAUSES OF PAROXYSMAL DYSKINESIAS

Primary paroxysmal dyskinesias are idiopathic or genetic disorders inherited predominantly in autosomal dominant fashion, with normal neurologic examination between the paroxysms.

Paroxysmal Kinesigenic Dyskinesia

The paroxysms in PKD are usually precipitated by a sudden movement, sudden acceleration or change in direction of movement, or startle (Videos 1 and 2). Most commonly, PKD manifests as brief attacks of dystonia in 1 or more extremities not associated with altered consciousness, lasting seconds to a few minutes, recurring up to 100 times per day. Paroxysmal chorea, athetosis, and ballism with or without

Box 1
Classification of paroxysmal dyskinesias

Precipitating factor:

1. Paroxysmal kinesigenic dyskinesia
2. Paroxysmal nonkinesigenic dyskinesia
3. Paroxysmal exertion-induced dyskinesia
4. Paroxysmal hypnogenic dyskinesia

Etiology:

1. Primary (idiopathic):
   I. Familial
   II. Sporadic
2. Secondary

dystonia are less common presentations.[5,6] Most patients describe sensory aura before the attacks, such as limb paresthesia or vague premonitory sensation in the head or abdomen.[6,7] Thus PKD is an example of a movement disorder associated with a sensory phenomenon.[8]

The onset of PKD is between 1 and 20 years in familial disorders and more variable in sporadic cases. Frequency of the attacks commonly decreases in adulthood, with about one-fourth of the patients having complete remission in their 20s or 30s and another one-fourth marked reduction in frequency of the attacks.[6] Forty-two percent of patients with PKD might have a history of nonfebrile infantile seizures,[9] or a family history of infantile convulsions without PKD representing infantile convulsions and choreoathetosis syndrome.[10–12] Other seizure syndromes, common and hemiplegic migraine, and episodic ataxia, are also more prevalent in PKD families than in the general population.[6,7,13–19]

Mutations in the *PRRT2* gene on chromosome 16 were recently identified in multiple families of different ethnicities affected by PKD with or without infantile convulsions.[11,15,16,20–26] *PRRT2* gene is located within locus 16p11.2-q12.1, previously associated with episodic kinesigenic dyskinesia type 1 (EKD1) and categorized as a form of dystonia with a designation of DYT10.[27] PRRT2 (proline-rich transmembrane protein 2) is highly expressed in the basal ganglia and is thought to play an important role in calcium-induced neuronal exocytosis by interacting with synaptosome-associated protein of 25 kDa (SNAP25), a presynaptic membrane protein involved in synaptic vesicle fusion. PKD associated with *PRRT2* mutation is usually an autosomal dominant disorder; however, variable penetrance and de novo mutations in the *PRRT2* gene have been reported.[28–31] Other *PRTT2*-negative families with PKD were found to have a gene mutation linked to chromosome 16q13-q22.1 (EKD2, or DYT19), or no mutation on chromosome 16 (EKD3).[9,32,33] PKD patients with PRRT2 mutations were found to have younger age of onset, higher frequency of attacks, presence of premonitory sensation, and better response to low-dose anticonvulsants than PRRT2-negative patients.[7,34]

Paroxysmal Nonkinesigenic Dyskinesia

The attacks in PNKD are precipitated by caffeine, alcohol, fatigue, or emotional stress, and manifest as episodes of dystonia, chorea, or athetosis involving 1 limb and gradually spreading to other limbs and face. The paroxysms last for minutes to hours, sometimes up to a day, and occur a few times per week or just a few times in a lifetime. Consciousness is always preserved, although some patients with facial involvement might have difficulty talking during the episodes. An aura in the form of limb numbness or stiffness, or an internal feeling of restlessness, can be experienced by about half of the patients with PNKD.[35]

Familial forms of PNKD typically have onset in early childhood up to the early 20s. PNKD can be associated with spastic paraparesis or have a higher prevalence of migraine.[35–37]

Up to now 3 distinct mutations in the *PNKD* gene, previously referred to as the myofibrillogenesis regulator gene (MR-1), on chromosome 2q35 have been identified.[38,39] The gene product, proline-rich transmembrane protein of unknown function, which has been reported to interact with the t-SNARE, SNAP25, localizes to axons but not to dendritic processes, and participates in metabolic detoxification of methylglyoxal, a by-product of oxidative stress and a substance found in coffee and alcohol.[38] The protein also seems to play an important role in protection against neurotoxicity, possibly by participating in glutathione regeneration and maintaining cellular redox status.[40] *PNKD*-positive PNKD is also categorized as DYT8.[27] PNKD with spastic paraparesis, also known as DYT9, was linked to a mutation in *SLC2A1* gene on chromosome 1–encoding glucose transporter (GLUT1).[36,37] Mutation in the calcium-sensitive potassium channel (*KCNMA1*) gene mutation on chromosome 10q22 was identified in a family with PNKD and epilepsy.[41] Another gene candidate was mapped on chromosome 2q31 and designated as DYT20.[42]

Paroxysmal Exertion-Induced Dyskinesia

PED attacks are typically precipitated by prolonged exercise, and rarely by muscle vibration, cold, passive movements, or electric nerve stimulation. The paroxysms manifest as leg dystonia lasting for a few minutes and rarely up to 2 hours, and recur daily or just a few times per month. The onset of PED is between 2 and 30 years.

SLC2A1 gene mutations on chromosome 1p35-p31.3 encoding GLUT1 were implicated in PED with or without epilepsy and hemiplegic migraine, also referred to as DYT18.[43] Other symptoms associated with GLUT1 defect can be seen in PED patients with *SLC2A1* mutations, including developmental delay, infantile seizures, alternating hemiplegia, and hypoglycorrhachia.[44,45] Mutations in the GTP-cyclohydrolase 1 gene were also associated with PED along with other movement disorders such as dopa-responsive dystonia, restless legs syndrome, and familial Parkinson disease.[46]

Runner's dystonia is a sporadic variant of PED, described in marathon runners as paroxysms of leg or foot dystonia provoked by prolonged running.[47] This condition has some clinical features of other forms of primary focal dystonia (sensory trick), PKD (good response to anticonvulsants), or peripherally induced dystonia (history of injury to the affected limb before the onset of dystonia). In a series of 7 cases with a mean age of symptom onset of 53.7 ± 6.1 years, various forms of exercise (cycling, hiking, long-distance running, drumming) triggered dystonia in the lower extremities.[48] Various treatments (eg, botulinum toxin injections, benzodiazepines, physical therapy, bracing, body weight supported gait training, and/or functional electrical stimulation of the peroneal nerve) improved gait, and 6 patients were able to return to their exercise routine albeit with some limitations.

Cases of paroxysmal dyskinesias sharing features of PKD and PNKD have also been described, manifesting as very brief and frequent attacks of choreoathetosis, responding well to anticonvulsants (resembling PKD cases) but precipitated by hyperventilation (similarly to PNKD).[49]

Paroxysmal Hypnogenic Dyskinesia

PHD typically manifests as attacks of dystonia, chorea, ballism during non–rapid eye movement (REM) sleep associated with sudden awakening, whistling, uttering guttural sounds, and appearing frightened.[4,50] The paroxysms may last from 30 seconds to 50 minutes, and occur from a few per night to a few per year.[4] The onset is commonly in childhood or early adulthood, with most cases being sporadic. PHD patients might have abnormal, epileptiform, or ictal electroencephalogram (EEG), personal or family history of convulsive seizures or parasomnias, or daytime paroxysmal dyskinesia.[50–52]

Some families with PHD were found to have mutations in genes coding for nicotinic acetylcholine receptor subunits associated with autosomal dominant nocturnal frontal lobe epilepsy: *CHRNA4* gene on chromosome 20q13.2-q13.3, *CHRNB2* gene on chromosome 1q21, and loci on chromosomes 15q24 and 8p21.[52–54]

The most important clinical and genetic data related to primary paroxysmal dyskinesias are presented in **Table 1**.

Secondary Paroxysmal Dyskinesias

A variety of neurologic and medical diseases can produce the symptoms resembling PKD or PNKD (**Box 2**).[55,56] Many patients with secondary paroxysmal dyskinesias

Table 1
Summary of clinical and genetic data of the primary paroxysmal dyskinesias

	PKD	PNKD	PED	PHD
Inheritance	AD	AD	AD	Usually sporadic
Gender M:F	4:1	2:1	2:3	7:3
Age at onset, years	<1–20	<1–20	2–30	4–20
Phenomenology of abnormal movements	Dystonia with or without chorea/ballism, unilateral or bilateral	Dystonia with or without choreoathetosis, unilateral or bilateral, rarely spasticity	Dystonia, sometimes in combination with choreoathetosis, unilateral or bilateral	Dystonia, chorea, ballism
Triggers	Sudden movement, change in direction, acceleration, startle	Alcohol, caffeine, emotions, fatigue	Prolonged exercise, muscle vibration	Sleep
Duration of paroxysms	Seconds up to 5 min	2 min to 4 h	5 min to 2 h	30 min up to 50 min
Frequency of paroxysms	1 per month to 100 per day	Few per week to few in a lifetime	Few per month	Few per year to few per night
Genetics	1. EKD1: 16p11.2-q12.1 (DYT10) with *PRRT2* gene within this region 2. EKD2: 16q13-q22.1 (DYT19) 3. EKD3: no mutation on chromosome 16	1. *PNKD*: 2q35 (DYT8) 2. *SCL2A1*: chromosome 1 (DYT9) 3. *KCNMA1*: 10q22 4. locus on 2q31 (DYT20)	1. *SCL2A1*: 1p35-p31.3 (DYT18)	1. *CHRNA4*: 20q13.2-q13.3 2. *CHRNB2*: chromosome 1q21 3. Locus on chromosome 15q24 4. Locus on chromosome 8p21
Treatment	Anticonvulsants (carbamazepine, phenytoin, others)	Avoiding triggers, benzodiazepines (clonazepam)	Avoiding triggers, ketogenic diet (in GLUT1 deficiency)	Anticonvulsants

Abbreviations: AD, autosomal dominant; PED, paroxysmal exertion-induced dyskinesia; PHD, paroxysmal hypnogenic dyskinesia; PKD, paroxysmal kinesigenic dyskinesia; PNKD, paroxysmal nonkinesigenic dyskinesia.

Box 2
Secondary paroxysmal dyskinesias

Structural central nervous system (CNS) lesions: multiple sclerosis,[57] stroke in basal ganglia or thalamus, traumatic brain injury (onset of dyskinesias is often delayed by several months),[5] primary CNS lymphoma, brain tumors

Neurovascular disorders: transient ischemic attacks, severe carotid stenosis or occlusion,[58] moya-moya disease,[59] arteriovenous malformation

Neurodegenerative disorders: progressive supranuclear palsy,[60] Fahr disease,[61] neuroacanthocytosis,[62] Parkinson disease[63]

CNS infections: human immunodeficiency virus encephalitis,[64] subacute sclerosing panencephalitis,[65] cytomegalovirus encephalitis, meningovascular syphilis

Systemic metabolic disorders: hypoparathyroidism, pseudohypoparathyroidism, hyperglycemia, hypoglycemia, thyrotoxicosis, Wilson disease,[66] kernicterus[55]

CNS and systemic immune disorders: antiphospholipid syndrome,[67,68] poststreptococcal autoimmune neuropsychiatric syndrome,[69] voltage-gated potassium channel antibody encephalitis,[70] celiac disease,[71] Sjögren syndrome,[72] Hashimoto encephalopathy[73]

Other disorders: peripheral nerve injury,[55] perinatal hypoxic encephalopathy, migraine aura,[55] cerebral palsy (often delayed-onset paroxysmal dyskinesia)[74]

might have interictal neurologic symptoms reflecting the underlying disorder, as opposed to primary paroxysmal dyskinesias with normal neurologic examination between the paroxysms.

Other Paroxysmal Movement Disorders

Episodic ataxias (EA) are rare genetic disorders caused by the mutations in the genes encoding membrane ion-channel proteins inherited in autosomal dominant fashion. EA manifest as brief recurrent attacks of ataxia, sometimes associated with other ictal symptoms, and typically normal interictal neurologic examination except for myokymia, nystagmus, or mild ataxia in some types of EA.[75] The onset in most EA types is in childhood or early adulthood. A summary of clinical manifestations and genetics of EA is presented in **Box 3**.

Familial dyskinesia with facial myokymia (FDFM) is a rare autosomal dominant disease characterized by childhood onset of choreiform movements in the limbs associated with perioral and periorbital myokymia.[84,85] The paroxysms are precipitated by anxiety and not by sudden movements, caffeine, or alcohol. A high prevalence of heart disease in adult patients with FDFM has been reported.[85] Mutations in the adenylyl cyclase 5 (*ADCY5*) gene were identified in familial and sporadic cases of FDFM.[86]

Pediatric Paroxysmal Movement Disorders

In addition to the paroxysmal dyskinesias already discussed, many of which begin in childhood, there are many other paroxysmal movement disorders that occur predominantly or solely in childhood.

Paroxysmal torticollis in infancy is a self-limiting disorder in infants characterized by paroxysms of head tilt or turn to alternating sides, lasting for minutes to 2 weeks.[87] The attacks remit by the age of 2 years. Transient paroxysmal dystonia in infancy is another self-limiting disease of children younger than 2 years, manifesting as attacks of dystonia in the neck and limbs, and opisthotonus of a few minutes'duration.[88]

Benign paroxysmal tonic upgaze (a familial disorder with the attacks of tonic upward deviation of the eyes) and spasmus nutans (a slow tremor of the head associated with

Box 3
Types of episodic ataxia (EA)

EA-1 (with interictal myokymia/neuromyotonia):

- Attacks of ataxia last a few seconds up to 2 minutes; precipitated by sudden movement or startle
- Interictal facial myokymia
- Linked to *KCNA1* gene mutations on chromosome 12p13 encoding voltage-gated potassium channel[76]

EA-2 (with nystagmus):

- Attacks of ataxia and dysarthria last a few hours to days; precipitated by exercise, stress, alcohol, fatigue
- Normal interictal examination
- Linked to CACNA1A gene mutations on chromosome 19p13.2 encoding P/Q calcium channel[77]

EA-3 (with tinnitus and headaches):

- Attacks of ataxia, vertigo, tinnitus, headaches; no identified precipitating factors
- Interictal facial myokymia and mild ataxia
- Linked to a gene on 1q42 chromosome[78]

EA-4 (with ocular motility dysfunction):

- Attacks of ataxia, vertigo, tinnitus, diplopia lasting minutes to hours; precipitated by sudden change in head position, fatigue[79]
- Normal interictal examination
- Episodes gradually become more frequent and transform into progressive ataxia
- No gene candidate

EA-5 (with vertigo and juvenile epilepsy):

- Attacks of ataxia and vertigo; unclear precipitating factors
- Interictal nystagmus; associated with juvenile epilepsy
- Linked to CACNB4 gene mutations on chromosome 2q22-23[80]

EA-6 (with episodes of ataxia from birth to 20 years):

- Attacks of ataxia, vertigo, diplopia, dysarthria, migraines with photophobia, phonophobia, nausea, alternating hemiplegia lasting 2 to 3 hours; precipitated by exercise, excitement, fatigue, alcohol, caffeine
- Mild ataxia and nystagmus interictally
- Linked to SLC1A3 gene on chromosome 5p13 encoding glutamate transporter EAAT1[81]

EA-7 (with episodes of ataxia in juveniles):

- Attacks of ataxia, dysarthria, and weakness; precipitated by emotions or exercise
- Linked to chromosome 19q13[82]

Recently described family with EA:

- Attacks of ataxia, generalized weakness, dysarthria; precipitated by fatigue or stress
- Linked to *UBR4* gene[83]

pendular nystagmus) are 2 other paroxysmal, self-limiting conditions of early childhood.[89,90]

Paroxysmal stiffening, upward gaze, and hypotonia were described in infants with sepiapterin reductase deficiency, a dopa-sensitive neurotransmitter disorder linked to chromosome 2p14-p12.[91]

PATHOPHYSIOLOGY OF PAROXYSMAL DYSKINESIAS

For decades there has been controversy regarding whether paroxysmal dyskinesias are epileptic disorders or movement disorders caused by basal ganglia dysfunction. Clinical similarities between paroxysmal dyskinesias and seizures include manifestation of both conditions as brief, unpredictable attacks of involuntary movements with normal interictal examination, presence of aura in many patients, good response to anticonvulsants (particularly in PKD), and personal and family history of convulsive epilepsy.[92] Most clinical studies reported normal EEG in patients with paroxysmal dyskinesia, but a few described ictal or interictal paroxysmal discharges on EEG arising from frontocentral or supplemental sensorimotor cortex, or from subcortical structures including the caudate nuclei.[92,93]

On the other hand, some paroxysmal dyskinesias respond to levodopa, and have perfusion changes in basal ganglia on single-photon emission computed tomography imaging during the attacks or even interictally.[94–97] Decreased inhibition of the thalamic reticular nuclei by medial globus pallidus and substantia nigra was proposed as a possible pathophysiologic mechanism of paroxysmal dyskinesias.[56] Animal models with PNKD also demonstrated dopamine dysregulation in the basal ganglia.[98]

PHD has the strongest evidence of being an epileptic disorder rather than a nonepileptic condition caused by basal ganglia dysfunction. Clinically, the paroxysms of PHD closely resemble nocturnal frontal lobe epilepsy, with abnormal EEG in many patients.[51] Dystonic rather than tonic-clonic paroxysms in PHD can be potentially explained by the spread of epileptic activity from the mesial frontal lobe to the basal ganglia. At present, PHD is classified as a form of frontal lobe epilepsy termed autosomal dominant nocturnal frontal lobe epilepsy (ADNFE).[99]

EA are channelopathies, or a group of disorders caused by abnormal function of the membrane ion channels or transmembrane transporters. The notion that paroxysmal dyskinesias represent channelopathies[100] was not supported by a recent discovery of *PRRT2* mutations, presumably resulting in an abnormal protein that does not seem to mediate channel functions.

DIAGNOSIS AND DIFFERENTIAL DIAGNOSIS

The diagnosis of paroxysmal dyskinesias and other paroxysmal movement disorders may be difficult to make because many patients might not have any paroxysms during their visits with the physician. The diagnosis is often based on a description of the symptoms by the patients, observation of the attacks of abnormal movements in person or on home video, and after exclusion of other neurologic and medical conditions, including seizure disorders. EEG, including continuous video-EEG monitoring, should be considered in cases of suspected paroxysmal dyskinesia to rule out seizure disorder. All patients with a clinical presentation of paroxysmal movement disorders should undergo laboratory workup for metabolic disorders including thyroid disease, hypoglycemia or hyperglycemia, and electrolyte disturbance (hypocalcemia). MRI of the brain and spine should be reserved for the patient with atypical presentation including later age at onset, neurologic deficit observed between the paroxysms, and other symptoms associated with the paroxysms (headaches, visual changes, and sensory deficit). In patients with suspected central nervous system infection, demyelinating disease, or GLUT1 deficiency, lumbar puncture should be performed. The latter is typically associated with hypoglycorrhachia caused by defective glucose transport across the blood-brain barrier.

Although genetic testing is now commercially available for PNKD (*PNKD*), PKD (*PRRT2*), PED (*SLC2A1*), EA-1 (*KCNA1*), and EA-2 (*CACNA1A*), a systematic approach should be taken before pursuing genetic testing. As there is not always a complete phenotypic-genotypic correlation (eg, patients with *PRRT2* mutations may present with PNKD and PED phenotype and patients with *SLC2A1* mutations can have PNKD), an algorithm has been proposed for genetic testing (**Fig. 1**).[15]

The differential diagnosis of paroxysmal movement disorders is summarized in **Box 4**.

Despite the fact that that paroxysmal dyskinesia attacks are stereotypic, precipitated by certain factors, and not accompanied by loss of consciousness, they can be difficult to distinguish from seizure disorder. Both conditions can have abnormal ictal and interictal EEG, or have no EEG changes. Response to anticonvulsants provides further support for the apparent overlap between epilepsy and paroxysmal dyskinesia.

Some dystonias can also be exacerbated by certain motor tasks such as walking, writing, or playing a musical instrument (task-specific dystonia), thus resembling PED or PKD. However, focal dystonia is restricted to a certain body part, often relieved by a sensory trick, and does not respond to antiepileptics. Diurnal fluctuation and precipitation of dystonia (typically in the lower limbs) by physical exercise or walking is a characteristic feature of dopa-responsive dystonia, thus resembling PED or PKD. In clinically uncertain cases, a trial of levodopa should be considered in all patients, and in fact can serve as a diagnostic tool.

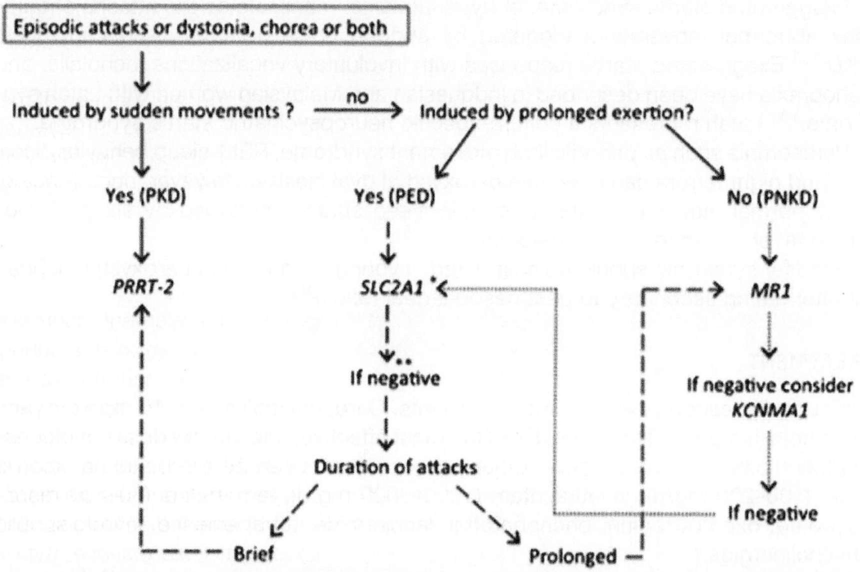

Fig. 1. Suggested algorithm for genetic testing. PED, paroxysmal exertion-induced dyskinesia; PKD, paroxysmal kinesigenic dyskinesia; PNKD, paroxysmal nonkinesigenic dyskinesia. (*From* Erro R, Sheerin UM, Bhatia KP. Paroxysmal dyskinesias revisited: a review of 500 genetically proven cases and a new classification. Mov Disord 2014;29(9):1113; with permission.)

Box 4
Differential diagnosis of paroxysmal movement disorders

Seizures (frontal lobe epilepsy, temporal lobe epilepsy, juvenile myoclonic epilepsy, eating reflex seizures, head-nodding syndrome)[101]

Dystonia (writer's cramp, musician's dystonia, other task-specific focal dystonias, dopa-responsive dystonia)

Tics

Psychogenic movement disorders and nonepileptic pseudoseizures

Hyperekplexia and neuropsychiatric startle syndromes

Parasomnia (periodic limb movement syndrome, rapid eye movement sleep behavior disorder, night terrors)

Sandifer syndrome

Tics are very brief jerks or dystonic posturing that are typically shorter in duration than paroxysmal dyskinesias. Premonitory sensation can be reported by patients with both conditions.

Psychogenic movement disorders and pseudoseizures are often difficult to distinguish from paroxysmal dyskinesias or EA, as both conditions manifest as paroxysms with normal interictal neurologic examination. Distractibility, variability of clinical presentation of different paroxysms, and suggestibility are the features of psychogenic disorders. Other red flags for suspecting psychogenic disorder are adult age at onset, altered level of responsiveness during the attacks, additional psychogenic physical signs, medically unexplained somatic symptoms, and atypical response to medications.[102]

Exaggerated startle syndrome, or hyperekplexia, manifests as the attacks of complex abnormal movements triggered by sudden noise or touch, and can mimic PKD.[103] Exaggerated startle responses with involuntary vocalizations, echolalia, and echopraxia have been described in Indonesian and Malaysian women with Latah syndrome.[104] Latah represents a culture-specific neuropsychiatric startle syndrome.

Parasomnia such as periodic limb movement syndrome, REM-sleep behavior disorder, and night terrors can resemble paroxysmal dyskinesias. However, occurrence of the abnormal movements only in certain sleep stages confirmed by sleep studies would favor a diagnosis of parasomnia.

Sandifer syndrome should be suspected in young children with paroxysms of head tilt after eating secondary to gastroesophageal reflux.[105]

TREATMENT

PKD usually responds well to anticonvulsants. Carbamazepine (1.5–15 mg/kg/d) and phenytoin (5 mg/kg/d) are considered the most effective, often in low doses. If they are contraindicated or not effective, other anticonvulsants can be tried, such as topiramate (100–200 mg/d), levetiracetam (1000–3000 mg/d), lamotrigine (50–400 mg/d), valproate, oxcarbazepine, phenobarbital, lacosamide. tetrabenazine, levodopa, and anticholinergics.[5]

In PNKD, anticonvulsants are unlikely to be effective. Clonazepam (2–4 mg/d) and other benzodiazepines can decrease the frequency and severity of the attacks in some patients. Use of haloperidol, anticholinergics, levetiracetam, acetazolamide, and levodopa has been reported in some cases.[106,107] Recognition and avoidance of precipitating factors is the most important strategy in the management of PNKD. A few patients have been treated successfully with deep brain stimulation of thalamic nuclei or globus pallidus.[108,109]

Avoiding prolonged exercise is paramount in the management of PED because medications are usually ineffective. Anticholinergics, levodopa, and acetazolamide were tried in some cases.[5,106] In patients with PED secondary to GLUT1 mutations, a ketogenic diet has been found to be fairly effective.[110]

Management of secondary paroxysmal dyskinesias includes symptomatic treatment with the same medications used in primary paroxysmal dyskinesia in combination with disease-specific treatment of causative conditions.

EA types 2, 3, 5, and 6 may respond well to acetazolamide. Anticonvulsants can be effective in EA-1. The potassium-channel blocker 4-aminopyridine (15 mg daily in 3 doses) was reported to be effective in some patients with EA.[111]

SUMMARY

Paroxysmal dyskinesia represents a group of episodic, intermittent disorders manifested by transient dystonia, chorea, athetosis, ballism, or a combination of these and other hyperkinesias. The original classification by precipitating or triggering factors[5] has been validated by subsequent studies. However, as a result of the identification of genetic mutations linked to the different forms of paroxysmal dyskinesias, a phenotypic overlap may occur. In addition to a growing number of genetic causes for paroxysmal dyskinesias, secondary etiology is also being increasingly recognized. Correct diagnosis of the paroxysmal dyskinesia often leads to an appropriate and effective treatment.

SUPPLEMENTARY DATA

Supplementary data related to this article can be found online at http://dx.doi.org/10.1016/j.ncl.2014.09.014.

REFERENCES

1. Mount LA, Reback S. Familial paroxysmal choreoathetosis: preliminary report on a hitherto undescribed clinical syndrome. Arch Neurol Psychiatry 1940;44:841–7.
2. Kertesz A. Paroxysmal kinesigenic choreoathetosis: an entity within paroxysmal choreoathetosis syndrome. Description of ten cases including one autopsied. Neurology 1967;17:680–90.
3. Lance JW. Familial paroxysmal dystonic choreoathetosis and its differentiation from related syndromes. Ann Neurol 1977;2:285–93.
4. Lugaresi E, Cirignotta F. Hypnogenic paroxysmal dystonia: epileptic seizure or a new syndrome? Sleep 1981;4:129–38.
5. Demirkiran M, Jankovic J. Paroxysmal dyskinesias: clinical features and classification. Ann Neurol 1995;38:571–9.
6. Bruno MK, Hallett M, Gwinn-Hardy K, et al. Clinical evaluation of idiopathic paroxysmal kinesigenic dyskinesia: new diagnostic criteria. Neurology 2004;63:2280–7.
7. Tan LC, Methawasin K, Teng EW, et al. Clinico-genetic comparisons of paroxysmal kinesigenic dyskinesia patients with and without PRRT2 mutations. Eur J Neurol 2014;21(4):674–8.

8. Patel N, Jankovic J, Hallett M. Sensory aspects of movement disorders. Lancet Neurol 2014;13:100–12.
9. Tomita H, Nagamitsu S, Wakui K, et al. Paroxysmal kinesigenic choreoathetosis locus maps to chromosome 16p11.2-q12.1. Am J Hum Genet 1999;65:1688–97.
10. Torisu H, Watanabe K, Shimojima K, et al. Girl with a PRRT2 mutation and infantile focal epilepsy with bilateral spikes. Brain Dev 2014;36(4):342–5.
11. Lee HY, Huang Y, Bruneau N, et al. Mutations in the novel protein PRRT2 cause paroxysmal kinesigenic dyskinesia with infantile convulsions. Cell Rep 2012; 1(1):2–12.
12. Schmidt A, Kumar KR, Redyk K, et al. Two faces of the same coin: benign familial infantile seizures and paroxysmal kinesigenic dyskinesia caused by PRRT2 mutations. Arch Neurol 2012;69:668–70.
13. Szepetowski P, Rochette J, Berquin P, et al. Familial infantile convulsions and paroxysmal choreoathetosis: a new neurological syndrome linked to the pericentromeric region of human chromosome 16. Am J Hum Genet 1997;61:889–98.
14. Marini C, Conti V, Mei D, et al. PRRT2 mutations in familial infantile seizures, paroxysmal dyskinesia, and hemiplegic migraine. Neurology 2012;79(21): 2109–14.
15. Erro R, Sheerin UM, Bhatia KP. Paroxysmal dyskinesias revisited: a review of 500 genetically proven cases and a new classification. Mov Disord 2014;29(9): 1108–16.
16. Cloarec R, Bruneau N, Rudolf G, et al. PRRT2 links infantile convulsions and paroxysmal dyskinesia with migraine. Neurology 2012;79(21):2097–103.
17. Dale RC, Gardiner A, Antony J, et al. Familial PRRT2 mutation with heterogeneous paroxysmal disorders including paroxysmal torticollis and hemiplegic migraine. Dev Med Child Neurol 2012;54(10):958–60.
18. Castiglioni C, López I, Riant F, et al. PRRT2 mutation causes paroxysmal kinesigenic dyskinesia and hemiplegic migraine in monozygotic twins. Eur J Paediatr Neurol 2013;17(3):254–8.
19. Riant F, Roze E, Barbance C, et al. PRRT2 mutations cause hemiplegic migraine. Neurology 2012;79(21):2122–4.
20. Fabbri M, Marini C, Bisulli F, et al. Clinical and polygraphic study of familial paroxysmal kinesigenic dyskinesia with PRRT2 mutation. Epileptic Disord 2013;15(2):123–7.
21. Wang JL, Cao L, Li XH, et al. Identification of PRRT2 as the causative gene of paroxysmal kinesigenic dyskinesias. Brain 2011;134(Pt 12):3493–501.
22. Meneret A, Grabli D, Depienne C, et al. PRRT2 mutations: a major cause of paroxysmal kinesigenic dyskinesia in the European population. Neurology 2012;79(2):170–4.
23. Liu XR, Wu M, He N, et al. Novel PRRT2 mutations in paroxysmal dyskinesia patients with variant inheritance and phenotypes. Genes Brain Behav 2013;12(2): 234–40.
24. Hedera P, Xiao J, Puschmann A, et al. Novel PRRT2 mutation in an African-American family with paroxysmal kinesigenic dyskinesia. BMC Neurol 2012;12:93.
25. Steinlein OK, Villain M, Korenke C. The PRRT2 mutation c.649dupC is the so far most frequent cause of benign familial infantile convulsions. Seizure 2012;21(9): 740–2.
26. Méneret A, Gaudebout C, Riant F, et al. PRRT2 mutations and paroxysmal disorders. Eur J Neurol 2013;20(6):872–8.
27. Albanese A, Bhatia K, Bressman SB, et al. Phenomenology and classification of dystonia: a consensus update. Mov Disord 2013;28(7):863–73.

28. Friedman J, Olvera J, Silhavy JL, et al. Mild paroxysmal kinesigenic dyskinesia caused by PRRT2 missense mutation with reduced penetrance. Neurology 2012;79(9):946–8.
29. van Vliet R, Breedveld G, de Rijk-van Andel J, et al. PRRT2 phenotypes and penetrance of paroxysmal kinesigenic dyskinesia and infantile convulsions. Neurology 2012;79(8):777–84.
30. Guerrini R, Mink JW. Paroxysmal disorders associated with PRRT2 mutations shake up expectations on ion channel genes. Neurology 2012;79(21):2086–8.
31. Shi CH, Sun SL, Wang JL, et al. PRRT2 gene mutations in familial and sporadic paroxysmal kinesigenic dyskinesia cases. Mov Disord 2013;28(9):1313–4.
32. Valente EM, Spacey SD, Wali GM, et al. A second paroxysmal kinesigenic choreoathetosis locus (EKD2) mapping on 16q13-q22.1 indicates a family of genes which give rise to paroxysmal disorders on human chromosome 16. Brain 2000; 123:2040–5.
33. Spacey SD, Valente EM, Wali GM, et al. Genetic and clinical heterogeneity in paroxysmal kinesigenic dyskinesia: evidence for a third EKD gene. Mov Disord 2002;17:717–25.
34. Mao CY, Shi CH, Song B, et al. Genotype-phenotype correlation in a cohort of paroxysmal kinesigenic dyskinesia cases. J Neurol Sci 2014;340(1–2):91–3.
35. Bruno MK, Lee HY, Auburger GW, et al. Genotype-phenotype correlation of paroxysmal nonkinesigenic dyskinesia. Neurology 2007;68:1782–9.
36. Auburger G, Ratzlaff T, Lunkes A, et al. A gene for autosomal dominant paroxysmal choreoathetosis/spasticity (CSE) maps to the vicinity of potassium channel gene cluster on chromosome 1p, probably within 2 cM between D1S443 and D1S197. Genomics 1996;31(1):90–4.
37. Weber YG, Kamm C, Suls A, et al. Paroxysmal choreoathetosis/spasticity (DYT9) is caused by a GLUT1 defect. Neurology 2011;77(10):959–64.
38. Lee HY, Xu Y, Huang Y, et al. The gene for paroxysmal non-kinesigenic dyskinesia encodes an enzyme in a stress response pathway. Hum Mol Genet 2004;13(24):3161–70.
39. Ghezzi D, Viscomi C, Ferlini A, et al. Paroxysmal non-kinesigenic dyskinesia is caused by mutations of the MR-1 mitochondrial targeting sequence. Hum Mol Genet 2009;18(6):1058–64.
40. Shen Y, Lee HY, Rawson J, et al. Mutations in PNKD causing paroxysmal dyskinesia alters protein cleavage and stability. Hum Mol Genet 2011;20(12):2322–32.
41. Du W, Bautista JF, Yang H, et al. Calcium-sensitive potassium channelopathy in human epilepsy and paroxysmal movement disorder. Nat Genet 2005;37:733–8.
42. Spacey SD, Adams PJ, Lam PC, et al. Genetic heterogeneity in paroxysmal nonkinesigenic dyskinesia. Neurology 2006;66(10):1588–90.
43. Weber YG, Storch A, Wuttke TV, et al. GLUT1 mutations are a cause of paroxysmal exertion-induced dyskinesias and induce hemolytic anemia by a cation leak. J Clin Invest 2008;118(6):2157–68.
44. Yang H, Wang D, Engelstad K, et al. Glut1 deficiency syndrome and erythrocyte glucose uptake assay. Ann Neurol 2011;70:996–1005.
45. Leen WG, Wevers RA, Kamsteeg EJ, et al. Cerebrospinal fluid analysis in the workup of GLUT1 deficiency syndrome: a systematic review. JAMA Neurol 2013;70(11):1440–4.
46. Dale RC, Melchers A, Fung VS, et al. Familial paroxysmal exercise-induced dystonia: atypical presentation of autosomal dominant GTP-cyclohydrolase 1 deficiency. Dev Med Child Neurol 2010;52(6):583–6.
47. Wu LJ, Jankovic J. Runner's dystonia. J Neurol Sci 2006;251:73–6.

48. Katz M, Byl NN, San Luciano M, et al. Focal task-specific lower extremity dystonia associated with intense repetitive exercise: a case series. Parkinsonism Relat Disord 2013;19(11):1033–8 pii:S1353-8020(13) 00267–8.
49. Kinast M, Erenberg G, Rothner AD. Paroxysmal choreoathetosis: report of five cases and review of the literature. Pediatrics 1980;65(1):74–7.
50. Provini F, Plazzi G, Lugaresi E. From nocturnal paroxysmal dystonia to nocturnal frontal lobe epilepsy. Clin Neurophysiol 2000;111(Suppl 2):S2–8.
51. Tinuper P, Cerullo A, Cirignotta F, et al. Nocturnal paroxysmal dystonia with short-lasting attacks: three cases with evidence for an epileptic frontal lobe origin of seizures. Epilepsia 1990;31(5):549–56.
52. Van Rootselaar AF, van Westrum SS, Velis DN, et al. The paroxysmal dyskinesias. Pract Neurol 2009;9:102–9.
53. Steinlein OK, Mulley JC, Propping P, et al. A missense mutation in the neuronal nicotinic acetylcholine receptor alpha 4 subunit is associated with autosomal dominant nocturnal frontal lobe epilepsy. Nat Genet 1995;11(2):201–3.
54. De Fusco M, Becchetti A, Patrignani A, et al. The nicotinic receptor beta 2 subunit is mutant in nocturnal frontal lobe epilepsy. Nat Genet 2000;26(3):275–6.
55. Blakeley J, Jankovic J. Secondary paroxysmal dyskinesias. Mov Disord 2002a;17(4):726–34.
56. Blakeley J, Jankovic J. Secondary causes of paroxysmal dyskinesias. Adv Neurol 2002b;89:401–20.
57. De Seze J, Stojkovic T, Destée M, et al. Paroxysmal kinesigenic choreoathetosis as a presenting symptom of multiple sclerosis. J Neurol 2000;247(6):478–80.
58. Sethi KD, Lee KH, Deuskar V, et al. Orthostatic paroxysmal dystonia. Mov Disord 2002;17(4):841–5.
59. Baik JS, Lee MS. Movement disorders associated with moyamoya disease: a report of 4 new cases and a review of literatures. Mov Disord 2010;25(10):1482–6.
60. Adam AM, Orinda DO. Focal paroxysmal kinesigenic choreoathetosis preceding the development of Steele-Richardson-Olszewski syndrome. J Neurol Neurosurg Psychiatr 1986;49(8):957–9.
61. Micheli F, Fernandez Pardal MM, Casas Parera I, et al. Sporadic paroxysmal dystonic choreoathetosis associated with basal ganglia calcifications. Ann Neurol 1986;20(6):750.
62. Tschopp L, Raina G, Salazar Z, et al. Neuroacanthocytosis and carbamazepine responsive paroxysmal dyskinesias. Parkinsonism Relat Disord 2008;14(5):440–2.
63. Bozi M, Bhatia KP. Paroxysmal exercise-induced dystonia as a presenting feature of young-onset Parkinson's disease. Mov Disord 2003;18(12):1545–7.
64. Mirsattari SM, Berry ME, Holden JK, et al. Paroxysmal dyskinesias in patients with HIV infection. Neurology 1999;52(1):109–14.
65. Ondo WG, Verma A. Physiological assessment of paroxysmal dystonia secondary to subacute sclerosing panencephalitis. Mov Disord 2002;17(1):154–7.
66. Micheli F, Tschopp L, Cersosimo MG. Oxcarbazepine-responsive paroxysmal kinesigenic dyskinesia in Wilson disease. Clin Neuropharmacol 2011;34(6):262–4.
67. Engelen M, Tijssen MA. Paroxysmal non-kinesigenic dyskinesia in antiphospholipid syndrome. Mov Disord 2005;20(1):111–3.
68. Baizabal-Carvallo JF, Jankovic J. Movement disorders in autoimmune diseases. Mov Disord 2012;27(8):935–46.
69. Dale RC, Heyman I, Surtees RA, et al. Dyskinesias and associated psychiatric disorders following streptococcal infections. Arch Dis Child 2004;89(7):604–10.

70. Aradillas E, Schwartzman RJ. Kinesigenic dyskinesia in a case of voltage-gated potassium channel-complex protein antibody encephalitis. Arch Neurol 2011; 68(4):529–32.
71. Hall DA, Parsons J, Benke T. Paroxysmal nonkinesigenic dystonia and celiac disease. Mov Disord 2007;22(5):708–10.
72. Alonso-Navarro H, Arroyo M, Parra A, et al. Paroxysmal dystonia associated to primary Sjögren's syndrome. Mov Disord 2009;24(5):788–90.
73. Liu MY, Zhang SQ, Hao Y, et al. Paroxysmal kinesigenic dyskinesia as the initial symptom of Hashimoto encephalopathy. CNS Neurosci Ther 2012;18:271–3.
74. Rosen JA. Paroxysmal choreoathetosis associated with perinatal hypoxic encephalopathy. Arch Neurol 1964;11:385–7.
75. Fahn S, Jankovic J, Hallett M. The paroxysmal dyskinesias. In: Fahn S, Jankovic J, Hallett M, editors. Principles and practice of movement disorders. 2nd edition. Philadelphia: Elsevier Sanders; 2011. p. 476–95.
76. Browne DL, Gancher ST, Nutt JG, et al. Episodic ataxia/myokymia syndrome is associated with point mutations in the human potassium channel gene, KCNA1. Nat Genet 1994;8(2):136–40.
77. Ophoff RA, Terwindt GM, Vergouwe MN, et al. Familial hemiplegic migraine and episodic ataxia type-2 are caused by mutations in the Ca^{2+} channel gene CACNL1A4. Cell 1996;87(3):543–52.
78. Cader MZ, Steckley JL, Dyment DA, et al. A genome-wide screen and linkage mapping for a large pedigree with episodic ataxia. Neurology 2005;65(1):156–8.
79. Farmer T, Mustian VM. Vestibulo-cerebellar ataxia: a newly defined hereditary syndrome with periodic manifestations. Arch Neurol 1963;8:471–80.
80. Escayg A, De Waard M, Lee DD, et al. Coding and noncoding variation of the human calcium-channel beta4-subunit gene CACNB4 in patients with idiopathic generalized epilepsy and episodic ataxia. Am J Hum Genet 2000;66(5):1531–9.
81. Jen JC, Wan J, Howard BD, et al. Mutation in the glutamate transporter EAAT1 causes episodic ataxia, hemiplegia, and seizures. Neurology 2005;65(4):529–34.
82. Kerber KA, Jen JC, Lee H, et al. A new episodic ataxia syndrome with linkage to chromosome 19q13. Arch Neurol 2007;64(5):749–52.
83. Conroy J, McGettigan P, Murphy R, et al. A novel locus for episodic ataxia: UBR4 the likely candidate. Eur J Hum Genet 2014;22:505–10.
84. Fernandez M, Raskind W, Wolff J, et al. Familial dyskinesia and facial myokymia (FDFM): a novel movement disorder. Ann Neurol 2001;49:486–92.
85. Chen YZ, Matsushita MM, Robertson P, et al. Autosomal dominant familial dyskinesia and facial myokymia: single exome sequencing identifies a mutation in adenylyl cyclase 5. Arch Neurol 2012;69:630–5.
86. Chen YZ, Friedman JR, Chen DH, et al. Gain-of-function ADCY5 mutations in familial dyskinesia with facial myokymia. Ann Neurol 2014;75(4):542–9.
87. Snyder CH. Paroxysmal torticollis in infancy. A possible form of labyrinthitis. Am J Dis Child 1969;117(4):458–60.
88. Angelini L, Rumi V, Lamperti E, et al. Transient paroxysmal dystonia in infancy. Neuropediatrics 1988;19(4):171–4.
89. Verrotti A, Trotta D, Blasetti A, et al. Paroxysmal tonic upgaze of childhood: effect of age-of-onset on prognosis. Acta Paediatr 2001;90:1343–5.
90. Antony JH, Ouvrier RA, Wise G. Spasmus nutans: a mistaken identity. Arch Neurol 1980;37:373–5.
91. Dill P, Wagner M, Somerville A, et al. Child neurology: paroxysmal stiffening, upward gaze, and hypotonia: hallmarks of sepiapterin reductase deficiency. Neurology 2012;78(5):e29–32.

92. van Strien TW, van Rootselaar AF, Hilgevoord AA, et al. Paroxysmal kinesigenic dyskinesia: cortical or non-cortical origin. Parkinsonism Relat Disord 2012;18(5): 645–8.
93. Lombroso CT. Paroxysmal choreoathetosis: an epileptic or non-epileptic disorder? Ital J Neurol Sci 1995;16(5):271–7.
94. Loong SC, Ong YY. Paroxysmal kinesigenic choreoathetosis. Report of a case relieved by L-dopa. J Neurol Neurosurg Psychiatr 1973;31:921–4.
95. Ko CH, Kong CK, Ngai WT, et al. Ictal (99m) Tc ECD SPECT in paroxysmal kinesigenic choreoathetosis. Pediatr Neurol 2001;24:225–7.
96. Joo EY, Hong SB, Tae WS, et al. Perfusion abnormality of the caudate nucleus in patients with paroxysmal kinesigenic choreoathetosis. Eur J Nucl Med Mol Imaging 2005;32:1205–9.
97. Kluge A, Kettner B, Zschenderlein R, et al. Changes in perfusion pattern using ECD-SPECT indicate frontal lobe and cerebellar involvement in exercise-induced paroxysmal dystonia. Mov Disord 1998;13(1):125–34.
98. Lee HY, Nakayama J, Xu Y, et al. Dopamine dysregulation in a mouse model of paroxysmal nonkinesigenic dyskinesia. J Clin Invest 2012;122(2):507–18.
99. Sohn YH, Lee PH. Paroxysmal choreodystonic disorders. Handb Clin Neurol 2011;100:367–73.
100. Margari L, Presicci A, Ventura P, et al. Channelopathy: hypothesis of a common pathophysiologic mechanism in different forms of paroxysmal dyskinesia. Pediatr Neurol 2005;32(4):229–35.
101. Winkler AS, Friedrich K, König R, et al. The head nodding syndrome—clinical classification and possible causes. Epilepsia 2008;49(12):2008–15.
102. Ganos C, Aguirregomozcorta M, Batla A, et al. Psychogenic paroxysmal movement disorders – clinical features and diagnostic clues. Parkinsonism Relat -Disord 2014;20:41–6.
103. Bakker MJ, van Dijk JG, van den Maagdenberg AM, et al. Startle syndromes. Lancet Neurol 2006;5(6):513–24.
104. Bakker MJ, van Dijk JG, Pramono A, et al. Latah: an Indonesian startle syndrome. Mov Disord 2013;28(3):370–9.
105. Kirkham FJ, Haywood P, Kashyape P, et al. Movement disorder emergencies in childhood. Eur J Paediatr Neurol 2011;15(5):390–404.
106. Bhatia KP. Paroxysmal dyskinesias. Mov Disord 2011;26(6):1157–65.
107. Mehta SH, Morgan JC, Sethi KD. Paroxysmal dyskinesias. Curr Treat Options Neurol 2009;11:170–8.
108. Loher TJ, Krauss JK, Burgunder JM, et al. Chronic thalamic stimulation for treatment of dystonic paroxysmal nonkinesigenic dyskinesia. Neurology 2001;56(2): 268–70.
109. Kaufman CB, Mink JW, Schwalb JM. Bilateral deep brain stimulation for treatment of medically refractory paroxysmal nonkinesigenic dyskinesia. J Neurosurg 2010;112(4):847–50.
110. Alter AS, Engelstad K, Hinton VJ, et al. Long-term clinical course of Glut1 deficiency syndrome. J Child Neurol 2014. [Epub ahead of print].
111. Strupp M, Kalla R, Claassen J, et al. A randomized trial of 4-aminopyridine in EA2 and related familial episodic ataxias. Neurology 2011;77(3):269–75.

Drug-induced Movement Disorders

Shyamal H. Mehta, MD, PhD[a], John C. Morgan, MD, PhD[b], Kapil D. Sethi, MD, FRCP (UK)[c,d,*]

KEYWORDS

• Movement disorder • Drugs • Dopamine receptor • Tardive dyskinesia
• Tardive Dystonia

KEY POINTS

- Drug induced movement disorders are most commonly associated with but not restricted to atypical & typical neuroleptics. Other drugs such as antidressants, antihistaminics and anti-arrhythmics, etc can also cause abnormal involuntary movements.
- Tardive dyskinesia (TD) can occur following a minimum of 3 months of neuroleptic expusure or even with a 1 month exposure in individuals over age 60.
- TD has not disappeared with the use of newer, more expensive antipsychotics; at higher doses, some of the newer atypical antipsychotics carry a substantially high risk similar to the older neuroleptics.
- It is important to distinguish classic TD from Tardive Dystonia due to treatment implications.

MOVEMENT DISORDERS CAUSED BY DOPAMINE RECEPTOR–BLOCKING AGENTS

The advent of atypical antipsychotics led to the hope that the incidence of drug-induced movement disorders will decrease significantly over time. However, the hope has not been realized, and the movement disorders caused by dopamine receptor–blocking agents (DBA) continue to be a significant problem. The introduction of chlorpromazine in 1952 was a major event in psychiatry but soon it became clear that this drug was associated with major significant acute side effects, such as akathisia, drug-induced parkinsonism, and acute dystonia.[1] A more persistent (late-appearing) dyskinesia was first recognized in the late 1950s.[2] Since then, extensive clinical experience has accumulated with the use of DBA, and the wide range of movement disorders that can be caused by these drugs (**Box 1**).

[a] Mayo Clinic Arizona, Scottsdale, AZ 85259, USA; [b] Georgia Health Sciences University, Augusta, GA 30912, USA; [c] Movement Disorders Program, Georgia Health Sciences University, Augusta, GA 30912, USA; [d] Merz Pharmaceuticals, 4215 Tudor Lane, Greensboro, NC 27410, USA
* Corresponding author. Movement Disorders Program, Georgia Health Sciences University, Augusta, GA 30912.
E-mail address: ksethi@gru.edu

Neurol Clin 33 (2015) 153–174
http://dx.doi.org/10.1016/j.ncl.2014.09.011 neurologic.theclinics.com

Box 1
Movement disorders induced by dopamine-blocking agents

1. Acute
   - Acute dystonia
   - Acute akathisia
   - Drug-induced parkinsonism
2. Chronic
   - Common:
     - Tardive dyskinesia
     - Tardive dystonia
     - Tardive akathisia
   - Uncommon:
     - Tardive myoclonus
     - Tardive tics
     - Tardive tremor
3. Miscellaneous
   - Neuroleptic malignant syndrome

ACUTE MOVEMENT DISORDERS CAUSED BY DOPAMINE RECEPTOR–BLOCKING AGENTS

Acute Dystonia

Acute dystonia occurs shortly after the introduction of DBA and occasionally after a dose increase or a switch to a more potent antipsychotic drug, particularly an injectable high-potency DBA. Often, there is a delay between the administration of the drug and the appearance of dystonia. About a half of patients experience the first signs of dystonia within 48 hours of drug intake, and in most patients signs appear within 5 days of drug initiation.[3] Acute dystonia is more likely to occur with typical DBA; however, the newer atypical drugs, including clozapine, are not devoid of this side effect.[4]

Dystonic reactions are variable in location and severity and are occasionally painful. The usual manifestations are orofacial dystonia, back arching, and neck extension. Life-threatening laryngospasm may occur.[5] Repeated acute dystonic reactions, in the absence of further exposure, has been observed even with a single dose of DBA. Acute dystonic reactions have rarely been reported with selective serotonin reuptake inhibitors (SSRIs), opioids, methylphenidate, rivastigmine, albendazole, gabapentin, cetirizine, foscarnet, quinine, and general anesthetics.[6] A form of subacute dystonic reaction appearing 3 to 10 days after starting DBA that results in truncal lateroflexion is called the Pisa syndrome (pleurothotonus).[7] However, Pisa syndrome may also be seen as a manifestation of Tardive Dystonia.[8]

An oculogyric crisis (OGC) is characterized by tonic conjugate ocular deviation that may last minutes to hours, and OGCs can occur in both acute and Tardive Dystonia.[9] Recurrent OGCs despite withdrawal of neuroleptic drugs are rare but have also been reported.[10] This finding may relate to the long half-life of these drugs or their metabolites.

Frequency and risk factors

The frequency of acute DBA-induced dystonia has varied widely from 2.3% to 94% in different reports.[11] The risk factors for dystonia include male gender, young age (<30 years), high potency and high dose of neuroleptics used, familial predisposition, the type of underlying psychiatric illness, mental retardation, and a history of electroconvulsive therapy.[11] There is a 2:1 risk of drug-induced dystonia in men compared with women. The same ratio holds true for young adults and children. Cocaine abuse may predispose to acute dystonic reactions.[12] Acquired immunodeficiency syndrome (AIDS) has also been associated with increased risk.[13]

Mechanism

Two opposing hypotheses have been proposed as a mechanism of acute dystonia. One hypothesis is that dopaminergic hypofunction results in a relative overactivity of cholinergic mechanisms.[14] This hypothesis is supported by a consistent amelioration of acute dystonia by anticholinergic drugs.

The other hypothesis proposes that there is paradoxic dopaminergic hyperfunction induced by DBA through blockade of presynaptic dopamine receptors. Moreover, as the level of the DBA decreases, sensitized postsynaptic receptors are exposed to the natural release of dopamine from presynaptic terminals.[15]

The possible contribution of other neurotransmitter systems, such as gamma-aminobutyric acid (GABA), is unknown. The role of sigma receptors has been explored. It has been reported that the unilateral microinjection of sigma ligands into the red nucleus induces torticollis in rats.[16] In this model the anticholinergic drug biperiden ameliorates dystonia induced by 2 sigma ligands.

Management

Evidence exists that acute dystonic reactions may be prevented by the use of anticholinergic drugs and that these drugs should be considered in patients at high risk for acute dystonia (young patients, cocaine abusers, and patients with AIDS).[3]

Injectable anticholinergic drugs are particularly effective in the treatment of acute dystonia[17] and so is the antihistamine drug diphenhydramine.[18] Phencyclidine (PCP)-induced dystonia should be considered if a patient with suspected DBA-induced acute dystonia fails to respond to the drugs mentioned earlier.[19] Diazepam has occasionally been used with success. At times, acute dystonic reactions, such as laryngeal dystonia, are severe enough to warrant lifesaving measures (tracheostomy). The patients should be observed for recurrence of acute dystonia even if they receive no further DBA.

Acute Akathisia

Haskovec and colleagues[20] first used the term akathisia (from the Greek, meaning not to sit) in 1901, long before the development of DBAs. The phenomenon of akathisia is paradoxic given that the same drugs that are supposed to calm patients result in restlessness.

There are 2 aspects of akathisia: (1) a subjective report of restlessness or inner tension, particularly referable to the legs, with a consequent inability to maintain a posture for several minutes, and (2) the objective manifestations of restlessness in the form of movements of the limbs, a tendency to shift body position in the chair while sitting or marching while standing.

The temporal association with drug administration is an important feature in the diagnosis of akathisia. The most recognized form of akathisia usually starts within hours or days after the initiation or increase in DBA dosage or change to a high-potency DBA, and even a single dose of DBA is sufficient for the diagnosis.[21] Acute akathisia usually starts within the first 2 weeks[22,23] and almost always within the first 6 weeks of DBA administration.[24] The term pseudoakathisia applies to patients with the objective features of akathisia without the subjective component, which may be hard to elicit from psychotic patients.[25] The reported rates of akathisia range from 21% to 31% in different reports.[22,23] The use of atypical agents has clearly diminished the risk of akathisia, although it has not disappeared. As an example, a study of quetiapine across a dose range 75 to 750 mg/d found a prevalence of 0% to 2% versus 8% and 15% for patients randomized to placebo and haloperidol respectively.[26] Another disorder that must be distinguished from akathisia is restless legs syndrome (RLS). RLS can be interpreted as a focal akathisia mostly affecting legs but with a clear circadian pattern, being worse in the evening. In addition, unlike RLS, periodic limb movements of sleep are not a characteristic finding in patients with akathisia.

Mechanism

DBA cause akathisia by blocking dopamine receptors, especially D2 receptors. The higher rates of akathisia seen with the use of high-potency D2 blocking agents support this hypothesis. Two studies using PET[27,28] showed an association between D2 occupancy in the striatum and the development of akathisia. It is estimated that a 74% to 82% of D2 receptors have to be occupied for extrapyramidal effects including akathisia to occur. However, the D2 antagonism hypothesis does not explain why cholinergic and β-adrenergic antagonists are effective in some cases of akathisia.

An alternative hypothesis proposes that DBA antagonism of mesocortical and mesolimbic dopaminergic projections leads to akathisia.[15] This hypothesis is supported by the observation that lesions of mesocortical dopaminergic neurons lead to increased locomotor activity in rodents.

Management

Anticholinergic and antiadrenergic are the 2 classes of drugs most commonly used in the treatment of acute akathisia. However, a recent Cochrane Database Review concluded that there was insufficient evidence to support their use.[29,30]

Anticholinergics used have included benztropine (dosage range, 0.5–8 mg/d), trihexyphenidyl (1–15 mg/d), procyclidine (7.5–20 mg/d), biperiden (2–8 mg/d), and orphenadrine (100–400 mg/d). Lowest effective dose should be used and peripheral anticholinergic side effects (eg, constipation, dry mouth) and central anticholinergic side effects (confusion, memory disturbance) should be monitored, especially in the elderly.

Of the antiadrenergic drugs, propranolol (a lipophilic, nonspecific β-blocker) has been used most extensively. It seems that a low dose of propranolol is sufficient, with most investigators recommending doses on the order of 60 mg/d and rarely more than 120 mg/d. Clonidine, an α2-adrenergic agonist that reduces central noradrenergic activity, has been beneficial, but side effects such as sedation limit its practical utility.

$5HT_{2A}$ antagonists are increasingly used in the treatment of acute akathisia. A large trial of low-dose mirtazapine compared with propranolol showed that it was just as effective in treating neuroleptic-induced acute akathisia with a more convenient dosing and fewer side effects.[31] Trazodone is another agent with prominent serotonergic antagonistic properties. A recent placebo-controlled, double-blind, crossover study with trazodone (100 mg/d) showed statistically significant clinical improvement in the symptoms of acute akathisia.[32]

Drug-induced Parkinsonism

Drug-induced parkinsonism (DIP) may be an adverse effect of multiple drugs, with DBAs (neuroleptics and nonneuroleptics such as metoclopramide) being the most common causes.[33] **Boxes 2 and 3** list drugs that are likely to occasionally cause or exacerbate parkinsonism.

Prevalence of drug-induced parkinsonism

DIP is a frequent adverse effect of DBA therapy, occurring in 15% to 60% of treated patients.[24] In one study involving a geriatric population, 51% of 95 patients referred for evaluation of parkinsonism likely had DIP.[34] In a general neurology practice, 56.8% of the 306 cases of parkinsonism were either induced or aggravated by drugs.[35] In a community study, 18% of cases initially diagnosed as PD were subsequently reclassified as DIP.[36] These patients are often labeled as having Parkinson disease (PD) and treated with dopaminergic drugs without benefit.

The dose and the potency of DBA therapy are of obvious importance. Although typical neuroleptics have been associated with a high rate of DIP, the second-generation (atypical) neuroleptics (eg, risperidone, olanzapine, aripiprazole) also have this side effect, but the frequency and severity may be lower.[37] Clinical experience has shown that, in patients with PD, even atypical agents (with the exception of clozapine and possibly low-dose quetiapine) can worsen parkinsonism and should be avoided.

Clinical features

PD and DIP may be hard to differentiate clinically. The prevalent teaching has been that DIP tends to be symmetric; however, asymmetry is common, occurring in 30% of cases.[38,39] In addition, as in PD, subgroups exist within DIP; some have primarily bradykinesia, others have predominant tremor and in some the symptoms are mixed. Postural reflexes may be impaired in patients with more severe disease, and many

Box 2
Medications likely to induce or exacerbate parkinsonism

Neuroleptics

Phenothiazines: chlorpromazine, promethazine, levopromazine, triflupromazine, thioridazine, trifluoperazine, prochlorperazine, perphenazine, fluphenazine, mesoridazine, piperazine, acetophenazine, trimeprazine, thiethylperazine

Butyrophenones: haloperidol, droperidol, triperidol

Diphenylbutylpiperidine: pimozide

Indolines: molindone

Substituted benzamides: metoclopramide, cisapride, sulpiride, clebopride, domperidone, veralipride, alizapride, remoxipride, tiapride, veralipride

Benzoquinolizine: tetrabenazine

Rauwolfia derivate: reserpine

Dibenzazepine: loxapine

Thioxanthenes: flupenthixol, chlorprothixene, thiothixene

Atypicals: risperidone, olanzapine, clozapine, quetiapine, ziprasidone, and aripiprazole.

Calcium channel blockers: flunarizine, cinnarizine

Box 3
Medications that occasionally induce or exacerbate parkinsonism

Amphotericin B

Amiodarone

Calcium channel blockers: verapamil, diltiazem, nifedipine, amlodipine

Cyclophosphamide

Cyclosporine

Cytosine arabinoside

Disulfiram

Lithium

Meperidine

Methyldopa

SSRIs: citalopram, fluoxetine, paroxetine, sertraline

Valproate

patients have an abnormal gait. Festination is uncommon, and sudden transient freezing, which is a symptom of PD, is rare.[39,40] The coexistence of a hyperkinetic movement disorder, such as orobuccolingual dyskinesia in a parkinsonian patient in the absence of levodopa treatment, supports a diagnosis of DIP rather than PD. Evidence is emerging that gait dysfunction and nonmotor features such as constipation, sexual dysfunction, and hyposmia may more strongly suggest of a diagnosis of PD than DIP.[41,42]

DIP typically develops between 2 weeks and 1 month following introduction of a neuroleptic or an increase in dose. In one series, 50% to 70% of cases developed within 1 month and 90% within 3 months.[43]

The clinical features of DIP may resolve despite continuing DBA therapy, suggesting tolerance, but prospective studies to address this issue are lacking. Most cases resolve after discontinuing DBA; however, in some patients, symptoms persist for months.[44] If parkinsonism persists for more than 6 months after discontinuing DBA underlying PD that was unmasked by DBAs should be suspected.

Metoclopramide-induced parkinsonism is common. This nonneuroleptic DBA is still frequently prescribed for the treatment of gastroesophageal reflux and diabetic gastroparesis. Metoclopramide is a frequent cause in elderly diabetic patients with renal insufficiency.[33] Parkinsonism typically develops when these patients are taking the conventional dose of 40 mg/d. Metoclopramide is cleared by the kidneys, and in renal failure the dose should be reduced by 50%.

Pathophysiology

By virtue of their D2 receptor–blocking activity DBAs would be expected to result in parkinsonism.[15] DIP seems to develop in almost everyone given high doses of high-potency DBA, thereby achieving concentrations that would block about 80% of central dopamine receptors.[45] However, the reasons why some individuals develop parkinsonism in the usual therapeutic dose range are unclear. Also unexplained is the delay between the pharmacologic blockade of the D2 receptors and the onset of DIP. Although DBAs block dopamine receptors within minutes to hours, DIP typically appears many days or weeks following drug exposure, which suggests that the sole explanation of D2 receptor blockade is overly simplistic.

There seems to be a complex interplay between the potency and dose of the DBA and individual susceptibility in the pathogenesis of DIP. A high ratio between serotonin ($5HT_2$) and D2 dopamine receptor antagonism seems to be less likely to cause movement disorders, including DIP.[46] Also, imaging studies have shown that a rapid dissociation of the drug from the receptor may reduce the motor side effects of DBA.[47]

Older age, female sex, and the presence of cerebral atrophy are some of the individual risk factors. Genetic susceptibility to DIP has been postulated based on case reports indicating a familial predisposition to DIP and may relate to genetic differences in drug metabolism.[48,49]

In some cases DIP may merely be unmasking subclinical PD. DIP in treated patients is more prevalent than is PD in the general population. However, the frequency of older patients with incidental Lewy bodies at autopsy is approximately 15 times the frequency of patients with clinically apparent PD.[50] The evidence for DBA unmasking PD comes from both clinical[51] and pathologic observations.[52] In some cases of DIP, the condition may persist after discontinuing DBA, and some patients may go on to develop PD. More recently, functional neuroimaging has been used to explore this problem. Dopamine transporter (DAT) imaging is now commercially available to study presynaptic nigrostriatal deficit, which is a hallmark of PD. This imaging is helpful in differentiating true nigrostriatal dysfunction seen in PD from DIP. A normal DAT study supports DIP and may predict recovery on stopping DBA.[53] For a detailed discussion on DAT imaging in movement disorders please see Ref.[54]

Management

Prevention of DIP is the most important goal and so DBA should be administered only when necessary. Atypical antipsychotics should be used when possible because of their lower propensity to cause extrapyramidal syndrome including DIP. The use of anticholinergic drugs in prophylaxis is debatable. High-dose anticholinergics may potentially worsen psychiatric problems and can cause confusion and memory difficulties. A reasonable approach may be to treat patients who are at a higher risk prophylactically (eg, patients with AIDS) with anticholinergics. This approach would be particularly useful if a high-dose, high-potency DBA is used. However, prospective data to support this approach are missing.

The treatment of clinically manifest DIP is difficult. The DBA should be withdrawn gradually if possible. In most cases, the condition is reversible once the offending agent is withdrawn. However, there is a potential for recurrence of the psychosis. In cases in which DBA cannot be withdrawn, substitution with an atypical agent should be attempted. Clozapine, an atypical neuroleptic, has a low propensity to cause movement disorders, but it causes agranulocytosis in approximately 1% of patients. The risk of DIP is also low with quetiapine, especially in moderate dosages, but higher doses of even this drug and others such as olanzapine, risperidone, and aripiprazole may cause DIP.

It may be prudent to leave mild DIP untreated. If necessary, the symptoms can be managed with anticholinergic agents, antihistaminic agents, or amantadine. Amantadine is a useful drug and may be superior to anticholinergics, as shown in 2 studies.[55,56]

There are limited data on the use of levodopa or dopamine agonists in the treatment of DIP. In one study, dopaminergic drugs seemed to worsen psychosis,[57] but this approach has not been systematically studied.

Tardive (late-appearing) movement disorders caused by dopamine receptor–blocking agents

DIP may occur in a delayed fashion, but the problems more frequently encountered in a tardive fashion include classic tardive dyskinesia (TD) and its variants and tardive akathisia.

Classic Tardive Dyskinesia

TD has been defined by the American Psychiatric Association Task Force as an abnormal involuntary movement following a minimum of 3 months of neuroleptic treatment in a patient with no other identifiable cause for movement disorders.[58] However, Diagnostic and Statistical Manual of Mental Disorders, Fourth Edition, criteria specify that the duration of exposure to neuroleptics may be only 1 month in individuals aged 60 years and older.[59]

Epidemiology and risk factors

In a review of 56 studies that spanned from 1959 to 1979, Kane and Smith[60] reported point prevalence of TD ranging from 0.5% to 65%, with an average point prevalence of 20%. In a more recent review from 2008, analysis of 12 studies since 2004 (n = 28,051, followed for 463,925 person-years), revealed that the annualized TD incidence was 3.9% for second-generation antipsychotics and 5.5% for first-generation antipsychotics.[61] The clinical significance of both of these figures is limited because they were derived from studies that differed in assessment criteria, methodology, and population characteristics. However, overall, the incidence of TD seems to have diminished with the advent of modern antipsychotic drugs compared with the older neuroleptics. However, TD has not disappeared with the use of newer, more expensive antipsychotics; at higher doses, some of the newer atypical antipsychotics carry a substantially high risk similar to the older neuroleptics.[54] In addition, in high dosages the atypical antipsychotics are also associated with weight gain, diabetes, and increased cardiovascular risk. The treatment therefore has to be individualized, and clinical awareness and continued vigilance are necessary.

Risk factors for development of TD most consistently defined by various epidemiologic studies include affective disorder, old age, female gender, total cumulative drug exposure, diabetes, alcohol and cocaine abuse, persistence of neuroleptic drug use after the development of TD, and a history of electroconvulsive treatment. Advancing age is the most consistently established risk factor for TD, and there seems to be a linear correlation between age and both the prevalence and severity of TD. Several studies have indicated a higher risk in women.[62] The evidence that diabetes increases the risk of TD comes from a study by Woerner and colleagues[63] who reported a risk ratio of 2.3 for diabetics exposed to neuroleptics compared with similarly treated non-diabetics, with the risk being greater in aged diabetics.

Clinical features

Classic TD manifests as repetitive, coordinated, seemingly purposeful movements affecting mainly the orofacial area. Some clinicians prefer to use the term tardive stereotypy to describe these movements. True chorea may occur but usually in the setting of withdrawal dyskinesia (discussed later).

Many patients with TD show a combination of movement disorders. In general, the presence of multiple movement disorders in a patient should alert the physician to the possibility of a drug-induced movement disorder. Most frequently, stereotypy of classic TD is combined with choreic movements of the hands, fingers, arms, and feet or with dystonia. Respiratory dyskinesias, caused by chest muscles and diaphragmatic involvement resulting in noisy and irregular breathing, often lead to pulmonary investigations. The abdominal and pelvic muscles may also be involved, producing truncal or pelvic movements known as copulatory dyskinesia, which is especially common in elderly women given metoclopramide.

Other causes of orobuccolingual dyskinesia should be considered in the differential diagnosis before diagnosing DBA as the cause (**Box 4**).

Withdrawal and Covert Dyskinesia

The abnormal movements occasionally commence when the DBA is discontinued or the dosage is reduced. This form of dyskinesia has been called withdrawal or covert dyskinesia.[64] By convention, the term withdrawal dyskinesia is used when the dyskinesia disappears within 3 months of drug withdrawal. If dyskinesia persists beyond 3 months it is termed covert dyskinesia. This distinction is arbitrary, because some of the covert dyskinesias disappear after prolonged follow-up.

Tardive Dyskinesia Variants

Tardive tourettism

A 2011 review of the literature only found 41 published cases of tardive tourettism (TT), making it a rare variant.[65] Tourettism has been recognized as a complication associated not only with neuroleptics but with other drugs such as anticonvulsants, antidepressants, and stimulants.[65] Patients may develop abnormal movements and vocalizations following chronic neuroleptic treatment. Further, the symptoms shown by the patients are indistinguishable from those of classic Tourette syndrome. A history of tics during childhood excludes the diagnosis of TT. The neuropharmacology underlying TT likely parallels that of TD and idiopathic Tourette syndrome.[66]

Tardive myoclonus

Tardive myoclonus has been described rarely as a late complication of prolonged neuroleptic therapy.[67] It is usually a postural myoclonus of the upper extremities, and associated movement disorders are common. Clonazepam pharmacotherapy ameliorates tardive myoclonus.

Tardive tremor

Tardive tremor has rarely been reported.[68] It is said to be more of a postural and kinetic tremor, compared with the rest tremor of DIP, and it is not usually associated with other signs of parkinsonism. Also, this tremor seems to respond to tetrabenazine or clozapine, which suggests that it is more related to TD than to DIP. Tardive tremor

Box 4
Differential diagnosis of orobuccolingual dyskinesia

1. Spontaneous dyskinesia of elderly (usually dystonic)
2. Hereditary choreas
3. Basal ganglia strokes
4. Systemic lupus erythematosus
5. Edentulous dyskinesia
6. Other drugs causing dyskinesias: levodopa, amphetamines, cocaine, tricyclic antidepressants, cimetidine, flunarizine, antihistamines

is a rare complication, and more patients must be characterized before the phenomenon can be completely understood.

Tardive Dystonia

Keegan and Rajput[69] coined the term dystonia tarda in 1973 but it was not until Burke and colleagues[70] reported a large series of 42 patients with Tardive Dystonia seen in 3 movement disorder centers in 1982 that this entity became better recognized. This variant of TD is common, and in a study of veterans on chronic neuroleptic therapy we found mild dystonic manifestations in 27 of 125 patients.[71] These manifestations most commonly involved the hands and the jaw. This finding represents a prevalence of nearly 20%; approximately 10 times higher than a previous study on this subject.[72] Other studies have found an intermediate prevalence of about 9% to 13%.[73] Drugs such as duloxetine, cetirizine, and amlodipine have also been reported to cause Tardive Dystonia.[74–76]

The reasons to differentiate classic TD from Tardive Dystonia and are as follows: the abnormal movements are distinct from classic TD. Although TD seems to occur most commonly in elderly women, Tardive Dystonia seems to be more common in younger patients, showing no predilection for either sex. Moreover, anticholinergic drugs tend to worsen classic TD but are beneficial in Tardive Dystonia.[77] Tardive Dystonia is said to be more persistent than classic TD, but remissions may occur on withdrawal of the DBA. There is no safe period and Tardive Dystonia may occur after a limited exposure to neuroleptics, and in one large series at least 25% of patients were given neuroleptics for disorders other than psychosis.[78]

The dystonic movements of patients with Tardive Dystonia are indistinguishable from those of idiopathic torsion dystonia. However, in contrast with idiopathic dystonia, other types of involuntary movements, such as orobuccolingual dyskinesia, may coexist. The dystonia may be focal, segmental, and rarely generalized.[77–79] In most patients, Tardive Dystonia is focal at onset, but, when fully developed, many patients have developed segmental dystonia[77–79] by the time of presentation. When the neck is involved, retrocollis is typical, and, when the trunk is involved, truncal extension is the predominant abnormal posture. Truncal flexion may, rarely, be seen. Lateral flexion of the trunk or the Pisa syndrome (pleurothotonus) can occur in Tardive Dystonia and less commonly in idiopathic dystonia.[8] Tardive Dystonia rarely involves the larynx, resulting in upper airway obstruction. Note that the breathing is normal during sleep in such patients.[80]

Even when Tardive Dystonia appears in the setting of DBA therapy, clinicians should rule out other causes, such as Wilson disease and symptomatic dystonia caused by focal lesions in the basal ganglia. Obtaining a good family history is important to rule out inherited dystonias. It was hypothesized that *DYT1* gene mutations may confer increased susceptibility to Tardive Dystonia. However, DYT1 mutations were not found in patients with Tardive Dystonia.[81]

An earlier mean age of onset (36 years) has been reported for Tardive Dystonia compared with classic TD (mean, 61 years).[82] Children exposed to DBA are more likely to get Tardive Dystonia, and as children age they are less likely to develop generalized dystonia.[71] Male predominance has also been a consistent finding in most studies (male/female ratio about 2:1).

Tardive akathisia

In contrast with acute akathisia, tardive akathisia (TA) occurs in a delayed fashion and does not disappear on discontinuation of the DBA. Persistent akathisia is defined as being present for at least 1 month when the patient is on a constant dose of a

DBA.[83] It occurs in about 20% to 40% of schizophrenics treated with DBA.[84] However, other than RLS and PD, persistent akathisia is uncommon, suggesting the role of DBA in TA.

As in classic TD, several types of TA have been described (ie, covert and withdrawal akathisia).[85,86] In one report, the mean age of patients with TA was 58 years and women outnumbered men by 2 to 1.[83] Almost all classes of DBA have been responsible.

The time of onset of TA after the initiation of DBA varied from 2 weeks to 22 years, with a mean of 4.5 years.[83] TA in this clinic population occurred in the first year of exposure in 15 of 45 patients. In another report,[25] 12 of 23 patients with chronic akathisia had an acute onset, with akathisia persisting for 7 months to 11 years. The remaining patients had onset at withdrawal of the DBA (withdrawal akathisia).

It is stated that the subjective experience of distress may be less in TA, but longitudinal studies to support this are lacking. Behavioral features seen in acute akathisia, such as an exacerbation of psychosis or aggressive/suicidal behavior, have not been described with TA. The motor phenomena of TA also are similar to those of acute akathisia, except that many patients with TA tend to pump their legs up and down or abduct/adduct them in a stereotyped manner while sitting. Patients with TA also commonly show truncal movements (rocking back and forth, or shifting while sitting) and respiratory irregularities (including panting, grunting, moaning, or even shouting). Because many patients with TA also have TD or Tardive Dystonia, it is often difficult to attribute a given movement to one or the other. Barnes and Braude[25] reported a moderate to severe orofacial dyskinesia in 39% of their patients with TA and choreoathetoid limb movements in 56%.

Pathophysiology of tardive dyskinesia TD is hard to explain given that the same DBA that block D2 receptors and cause DIP result in TD. Although the exact pathophysiology of TD is incompletely understood, one of the commonly ascribed theories is that of dopamine receptor (in particular D2 receptor) hypersensitivity. As the activation of indirect pathway results in paucity of movements, excess D2 receptor stimulation/activity inhibits the indirect pathway, resulting in hyperkinesia.[87] Several findings support a dopaminergic supersensitivity. First, reduction of DBA dose may precipitate TD (withdrawal emergent syndrome or covert dyskinesia) or worsen existing TD. Likewise, increasing the DBA dose can temporarily mask TD symptoms. Second, dyskinesias induced by levodopa in patients with PD closely resemble the movements seen in TD. However, the clinical course of such dyskinesia is different in that the abnormal movements disappear when levodopa is withdrawn.

Another hypothesis states that the long-term blockade of the D2 receptor and its subsequent hypersensitization can lead to maladaptive plasticity in striatal-cortical transmission, causing an imbalance between the direct and indirect pathway. It is proposed that this continued miscommunication may be responsible for the persistence of symptoms even after the withdrawal of DBAs.[88] Another hypothesis implicates GABA depletion as a possible mechanism. This hypothesis is based on animal studies that showed decreased GABA turnover and upregulation of receptors in animals with the most significant TD.[89] Even a small human postmortem study showed significantly decreased glutamic acid decarboxylase (GAD) activity (the rate limiting enzyme in GABA synthesis) in patients with TD compared with patients without TD.[80] Thus, although conclusive evidence of a single pathophysiologic mechanism is lacking, it seems that a complex interplay between the different neurotransmitter systems (dopaminergic, GABAergic, cholinergic, and glutaminergic) may be important in the development of TD.

Genetics of tardive dyskinesia Several attempts have been made to study genetic polymorphisms for an association with TD in various ethnic populations. Polymorphisms in the genes coding for D2 and D3 dopamine receptors (DRD2, DRD3), catechol-O-methyl-transferase (COMT), $5HT_{2A}$ receptors (HTR2A), manganese superoxide dismutase (MnSOD), and cytochrome P450 gene (CYP2D6) have been shown to influence the risk for TD. In addition, variation in genes related to the other neurotransmitter systems mentioned earlier have also been found: GABAergic pathways (SLCA11, GABRB2, GABRC3), *N*-methyl-D-aspartate receptor (GRIN2A), and oxidative stress–related genes (GSTM1, GSTP1, NQO1, NOS3).[87,90]

New research is not only focused on genetic variations as risk factors for TD but also in predicting response to treatment of TD. In one study the presence of polymorphism Val66Met in the gene for brain-derived neurotrophic factor predicted a good response to *Ginkgo biloba*.[91]

Management of Tardive Syndromes

Orobuccolingual dyskinesia

By definition, TD is iatrogenic and delayed. Preventing development of TD is one of the most important principles in the use of DBA for psychiatric disease or gastrointestinal problems. The need for DBA therapy should be reviewed periodically, even in patients showing no signs of TD. Some patients with acute psychosis do not require the high levels of DBA that were prescribed initially. Every 3 to 6 months patients should be examined for early signs of TD. If signs are present, switching to clozapine or another atypical neuroleptic may prevent further worsening of TD.

A variety of drugs have been used in the symptomatic treatment of TD, but none is uniformly effective. The most important step is to gradually taper off the DBA, if possible.

Dopamine-depleting agents such as reserpine or tetrabenazine are the most often used. The usual dose of reserpine is 0.25 mg/d, and the dose is increased gradually to 3 to 5 mg/d. Tetrabenazine is initiated at 25 mg/d and gradually increased to 150 mg/d.[92,93] Another useful agent is alpha-methyl-p-tyrosine, which forms a false neurotransmitter. It has been used alone or with reserpine.[94] In general, anticholinergic drugs exacerbate orobuccolingual TD and should be discontinued.[95]

A plethora of other medications have been used for symptomatic treatment of TD. However, these treatments are based on small open-label studies or case reports. These medications include amantadine, benzodiazepines, baclofen, valproic acid, donepezil (acting as a cholinomimetic), lithium, zonisamide, melatonin, and zolpidem.[96] Based on the theory that oxidative stress may be implicated in the pathophysiology of TD, several antioxidants have been tried: vitamin E, vitamin B_6, and *G biloba*. There has been a lot of interest in vitamin E, but several studies have yielded conflicting results ranging from it being ineffective to providing modest improvement.[97] A study with 1200 mg of vitamin B_6 per day found some improvement in symptoms of TS, but the data are insufficient to support or refute their use in TS.[97] In terms of antioxidants, *G biloba* has the strongest recommendation for use in TS. A double-blind placebo-controlled study not only found improvement of tardive symptoms but also a continued benefit for ~6 months after discontinuation of the drug. However, due caution should be exercised because of the antiplatelet effect and hemorrhagic complications associated with its use.[97,98] Although neuroleptics can cause these tardive syndromes, some atypical neuroleptics have also been used to treat TD, especially Tardive Dystonia (discussed later). Surgical treatment with either pallidotomy or pallidal deep brain stimulation is reserved for the most severe cases with debilitating symptoms that are refractory to medications.[99]

Tardive tourettism, myoclonus, and tremor

In general, the strategies to manage these variants closely resemble those for classic TD. Whenever possible, DBA should be withdrawn and dopamine-depleting drugs used.

Tardive Dystonia

In Tardive Dystonia the movement disorder is more severe and often more persistent than the other tardive syndromes. If the dystonia is focal (or segmental) botulinum toxin injections may be the most effective symptomatic treatment, particularly for craniocervical dystonia. Tarsy and colleagues[100] reported moderate to marked improvement in 29 of 38 affected body parts injected with botulinum toxin in 34 patients with Tardive Dystonia, all of whom had an incomplete response to a variety of drugs.

For generalized dystonia, several drugs are available for symptomatic treatment. Drug response is variable, and patients often must be switched between various agents or rational polypharmacy must be used.[11] Anticholinergic drugs worsen classic TD but may help patients with Tardive Dystonia.[77] Other medications commonly used are tetrabenazine, benzodiazepines, and baclofen. Less commonly used drugs are levodopa, amantadine, β-blockers, and anticonvulsants. We try an anticholinergic (such as trihexyphenidyl) first and gradually increase the dose as tolerated. Next, tetrabenazine or reserpine is added to anticholinergic drugs. Oral baclofen in increasing doses can be helpful. Intrathecal baclofen for axial (truncal) dystonia can be useful but may be difficult for long-term use because of pump or delivery problems and risk of infection.[11] Severe resistant Tardive Dystonia may be managed by deep brain stimulation of pallidum.

Atypical Neuroleptics in the Treatment of Tardive Syndrome

There is a growing body of literature with reports of improvement of TD when patients were switched from an older neuroleptic to an atypical neuroleptic or even from one atypical to another.[101] In general, these drugs have a lower affinity for the D2 receptor and have a high affinity for histamine, dopamine, and $5HT_2$receptors.[102] A high ratio between $5HT_2$ and D2 dopamine receptor antagonism produces less in the way of movement disorder, including TD. Risperidone (based on class II and III studies) and olanzapine (based on a class III study) may be effective. There is no evidence to determine the efficacy of ziprasidone, aripiprazole, and sertindole in the treatment of tardive syndromes. Thus, the evidence-based practice guidelines from the American Academy of Neurology (AAN) do not recommend using neuroleptics for the treatment of TD.[97] However, clozapine, a dibenzodiazepine, is an atypical neuroleptic that has a low propensity to cause movement disorders. Several uncontrolled observations have suggested that clozapine benefits about 40% of patients with TD, particularly those with Tardive Dystonia.[103,104] However, the data regarding clozapine are confusing. A recent review evaluated reports of clozapine improving TD versus being implicated in causing TD. The investigators concluded that the evidence of beneficial effects of clozapine in TD was greater than for its role in causation/worsening of TS.[105] Hence, we use this drug in the treatment of TD in appropriate patients.

Tardive Akathisia

TA does not consistently respond to any pharmacologic therapy, and patients with this TD variant express symptoms of distress, violence, and even suicidal ideation. However, Burke and colleagues[83] found that 87% of patients showed some improvement with reserpine and 58% with tetrabenazine. They reported complete resolution of symptoms in one-third of patients. Opioids and β-blockers, which help acute akathisia, usually do not ameliorate TA. Beneficial effects of the sigma-1 agonist fluvoxamine on TD and TA have recently been reported in a small case series of 3 patients[106]

Clinical Course of Tardive Syndromes

TD was thought to be persistent in most cases, but several studies have shown that up to 40% of patients improve on cessation of neuroleptic therapy.[107] This outcome is more likely to occur in young patients and in patients with a shorter history of TD. If typical DBAs are continued, it is unlikely that TD will remit. The subtype of TD may also be important. Tardive Dystonia is a persistent disorder, and remissions are infrequent. The remission rate of Tardive Dystonia was low at 10% (21 of 231 patients) after a mean follow-up period of 6.6 years.[71,77] However, these studies are from tertiary care centers, and it is possible that more cases of Tardive Dystonia remit than is generally realized.

Movement Disorders Caused by Other Drugs

A variety of other drugs produce movement disorders. When movement disorders are caused by drugs that are not commonly perceived as causative agents, the diagnosis may be missed for extended periods of time, resulting in unnecessary diagnostic work-up and inappropriate therapy. The diagnosis depends on a compulsive drug history not only from the patient but also from the patient's family, primary physician, and pharmacist. In general, the non–DBA-induced movement disorders differ in the course from TS and remit on discontinuation of the causal agent. Rechallenge may result in a return of the movement disorder but it is not necessary. Although drug-induced movement disorders can occur in previously healthy patients, patients with abnormal development or brain injury are more disposed to develop movements related to these drugs.

Given space constraints, this article lists the major drugs that can cause or exacerbate akathisia, chorea, myoclonus, tics, and tremor in tabular form in **Boxes 5–9**.

Box 5
Drugs that may cause or exacerbate akathisia

Antiepileptics: carbamazepine, ethosuximide

Buspirone

Calcium channel antagonists: diltiazem

Dopamine antagonists/depletors

Lithium

Methysergide

SSRIs

Tricyclic antidepressants

Vestibular sedatives: flunarizine, cinnarizine

Adapted from Sachdev PS. Acute and tardive drug-induced akathisia. In: Sethi KD, editor. Drug-induced movement disorders. New York: Marcel Dekker; 2004. p. 129–64.

Box 6
Drugs that may cause or exacerbate chorea

Anticholinergics

Antidepressants: SSRIs, tricyclic antidepressants

Antiepileptics: carbamazepine, gabapentin, phenytoin, valproate

Antihistamines

Dopamine antagonists

Dopaminergic drugs: dopamine agonists, levodopa

Hormones: thyroid hormone, estrogen

Lithium

Stimulants: amphetamines, cocaine, methylphenidate

Miscellaneous: aminophylline, baclofen, cimetidine, digoxin

Adapted from Bhidayasiri R, Truong DD. Chorea and related disorders. Postgrad Med J 2004;80:527–34.

Box 7
Drugs that may cause or exacerbate myoclonus

Anesthetics: chloralose, etomidate, enflurane, propofol, spinal anesthetics

Antibiotics/antimalarials: cephalosporins, fluoroquinolones, imipenem, mefloquine, penicillins

Antiepileptics: carbamazepine, gabapentin, lamotrigine, phenytoin, valproate, vigabatrin

Antidepressants: monoamine oxidase inhibitors, SSRIs, tricyclics

Antineoplastic drugs: chlorambucil, ifosfamide

Calcium channel antagonists: diltiazem, nifedipine, verapamil

Contrast agents

Dopaminergics: levodopa, dopamine agonists and antagonists

Drugs of abuse: MDMA (Ecstasy)

Gastrointestinal drugs: bismuth salts

Narcotics: methadone, meperidine, morphine, oxycodone

Other drugs: gamma-hydroxybutyrate, tranexamic acid

Abbreviation: MDMA, 3,4-methylenedioxy-methamphetamine.

Data from Refs.[108–110]

Box 8
Drugs that may exacerbate or cause tics

Antiepileptics: carbamazepine, lamotrigine

Drugs of abuse: amphetamines, cocaine, heroin

Levodopa

SSRIs: fluoxetine, sertraline

Stimulants (controversial): methylphenidate

Data from Refs.[111–114]

Box 9
Nonneuroleptic drugs associated with tremor

Major Category	Typical Examples
Postural Tremor	
Antiarrhythmics	Amiodarone, mexiletine, procainamide
Antidepressants/mood stabilizers	Amitriptyline, lithium, SSRIs
Antiepileptics	Valproate
Bronchodilators	Albuterol, salmeterol
Chemotherapeutics	Tamoxifen, Ara-C, ifosfamide
Drugs of abuse	Cocaine, ethanol, MDMA, nicotine
Gastrointestinal drugs	Metoclopramide, cimetidine
Hormones	Thyroxine, calcitonin, medroxyprogesterone
Immunosuppressants	Tacrolimus, cyclosporine, alfa-interferon
Methylxanthines	Theophylline, caffeine
Kinetic and Terminal Kinetic Tremor	
Antibiotics/antivirals/antifungals	Ara-A
Antidepressants/mood stabilizers	Lithium
Bronchodilators	Albuterol, salmeterol
Chemotherapeutics	Ara-C, ifosfamide
Drugs of abuse	Ethanol
Hormones	Epinephrine
Immunosuppressants	Tacrolimus, cyclosporine
Resting Tremor	
Antibiotics, antivirals, antifungals	Trimethoprim/sulfa, amphotericin B
Antidepressants, mood stabilizers	SSRIs
Antiepileptics	Valproate
Chemotherapeutics	Thalidomide
Drugs of abuse	Cocaine, ethanol, MDMA
Gastrointestinal drugs	Metoclopramide
Hormones	Medroxyprogesterone

Adapted from Morgan JC, Sethi KD. Drug- and toxin-induced tremor. In: Lyons KE, Pahwa R, editors. Handbook of essential tremor and other tremor disorders. London: Taylor & Francis; 2005. p. 347; with permission.

REFERENCES

1. Delay J, Deniker P. Chlorpromazine and neuroleptic treatments in psychiatry. J Clin Exp Psychopathol 1956;17(1):19–24.
2. Uhrbrand L, Faurbye A. Reversible and irreversible dyskinesia after treatment with perphenazine, chlorpromazine, reserpine and electroconvulsive therapy. Psychopharmacologia 1960;1:408–18.
3. Keepers GA, Clappison VJ, Casey DE. Initial anticholinergic prophylaxis for neuroleptic-induced extrapyramidal syndromes. Arch Gen Psychiatry 1983; 40(10):1113–7 [Research Support, Non-US Gov't Research Support, US Gov't, Non-P.H.S. Research Support, US Gov't, P.H.S.].
4. Pierre JM. Extrapyramidal symptoms with atypical antipsychotics: incidence, prevention and management [review]. Drug Saf 2005;28(3):191–208.
5. Flaherty JA, Lahmeyer HW. Laryngeal-pharyngeal dystonia as a possible cause of asphyxia with haloperidol treatment [case reports]. Am J Psychiatry 1978; 135(11):1414–5.
6. Burkhard PR. Acute and subacute drug-induced movement disorders. Parkinsonism Relat Disord 2014;20(Suppl 1):S108–12.

7. Suzuki T, Koizumi J, Moroji T, et al. Clinical characteristics of the Pisa syndrome. Acta Psychiatr Scand 1990;82(6):454–7.
8. Suzuki T, Matsuzaka H. Drug-induced Pisa syndrome (pleurothotonus): epidemiology and management [review]. CNS Drugs 2002;16(3):165–74.
9. Sachdev P. Tardive and chronically recurrent oculogyric crises. Mov Disord 1993;8(1):93–7 [Case Reports Research Support, Non-US Gov't].
10. Schneider SA, Udani V, Sankhla CS, et al. Recurrent acute dystonic reaction and oculogyric crisis despite withdrawal of dopamine receptor blocking drugs. Mov Disord 2009;24(8):1226–9.
11. Bhatt M, Sethi KD, Bhatia K. Acute and tardive dystonia. In: Sethi KD, editor. Drug-induced movement disorders. New York: Marcel Dekker; 2004. p. 111–28.
12. van Harten PN, van Trier JC, Horwitz EH, et al. Cocaine as a risk factor for neuroleptic-induced acute dystonia. J Clin Psychiatry 1998;59(3):128–30 [Research Support, Non-US Gov't].
13. van Der Kleij FG, de Vries PA, Stassen PM, et al. Acute dystonia due to metoclopramide: increased risk in AIDS [case reports]. Arch Intern Med 2002;162(3): 358–9.
14. Neale R, Gerhardt S, Liebman JM. Effects of dopamine agonists, catecholamine depletors, and cholinergic and GABAergic drugs on acute dyskinesias in squirrel monkeys. Psychopharmacology (Berl) 1984;82(1–2):20–6.
15. Marsden CD, Jenner P. The pathophysiology of extrapyramidal side-effects of neuroleptic drugs [review]. Psychol Med 1980;10(1):55–72.
16. Matsumoto RR, Hemstreet MK, Lai NL, et al. Drug specificity of pharmacological dystonia. Pharmacol Biochem Behav 1990;36(1):151–5 [Research Support, Non-US Gov't Research Support, US Gov't, P.H.S.].
17. Keepers GA, Casey DE. Clinical management of acute neuroleptic-induced extrapyramidal syndromes [review]. Curr Psychiatr Ther 1986;23:139–57.
18. Waugh WH, Metts JC Jr. Severe extrapyramidal motor activity induced by prochlorperazine. Its relief by the intravenous injection of diphenhydramine. N Engl J Med 1960;262:353–4.
19. Piecuch S, Thomas U, Shah BR. Acute dystonic reactions that fail to respond to diphenhydramine: think of PCP [case reports letter]. J Emerg Med 1999;17(3):527.
20. Haskovec L. Akathisie. Arch Bohemes Med Clin 1902;17:704–8.
21. Healy D, Farquhar G. Immediate effects of droperidol. Hum Psychopharmacol 1998;13(2):113–20 [Clinical and Experimental].
22. Braude WM, Barnes TR, Gore SM. Clinical characteristics of akathisia. A systematic investigation of acute psychiatric inpatient admissions. Br J Psychiatry 1983;143:139–50 [Research Support, Non-US Gov't].
23. Sachdev P, Kruk J. Clinical characteristics and predisposing factors in acute drug-induced akathisia. Arch Gen Psychiatry 1994;51(12):963–74 [Research Support, Non-US Gov't].
24. Ayd FJ Jr. A survey of drug-induced extrapyramidal reactions. JAMA 1961;175: 1054–60.
25. Barnes TR, Braude WM. Akathisia variants and tardive dyskinesia. Arch Gen Psychiatry 1985;42(9):874–8 [Research Support, Non-US Gov't].
26. Arvanitis LA, Miller BG. Multiple fixed doses of "Seroquel" (quetiapine) in patients with acute exacerbation of schizophrenia: a comparison with haloperidol and placebo. The Seroquel Trial 13 Study Group. Biol Psychiatry 1997;42(4): 233–46.
27. Farde L, Nordstrom AL, Wiesel FA, et al. Positron emission tomographic analysis of central D1 and D2 dopamine receptor occupancy in patients treated with

classical neuroleptics and clozapine. Relation to extrapyramidal side effects. Arch Gen Psychiatry 1992;49(7):538–44 [Research Support, Non-US Gov't Research Support, US Gov't, P.H.S.].
28. Nordstrom AL, Farde L, Halldin C. Time course of D2-dopamine receptor occupancy examined by PET after single oral doses of haloperidol. Psychopharmacology (Berl) 1992;106(4):433–8 [Research Support, Non-US Gov't Research Support, US Gov't, P.H.S.].
29. Lima AR, Bacalcthuk J, Barnes TR, et al. Central action beta-blockers versus placebo for neuroleptic-induced acute akathisia [meta-analysis review]. Cochrane Database Syst Rev 2004;(4):CD001946.
30. Lima AR, Weiser KV, Bacaltchuk J, et al. Anticholinergics for neuroleptic-induced acute akathisia [review]. Cochrane Database Syst Rev 2004;(1): CD003727.
31. Poyurovsky M. Acute antipsychotic-induced akathisia revisited. Br J Psychiatry 2010;196(2):89–91.
32. Stryjer R, Rosenzcwaig S, Bar F, et al. Trazodone for the treatment of neuroleptic-induced acute akathisia: a placebo-controlled, double-blind, crossover study. Clin Neuropharmacol 2010;33(5):219–22.
33. Sethi KD, Patel B, Meador KJ. Metoclopramide-induced parkinsonism [case reports]. South Med J 1989;82(12):1581–2.
34. Stephen PJ, Williamson J. Drug-induced parkinsonism in the elderly. Lancet 1984;2(8411):1082–3.
35. Marti Masso JF, Poza JJ. Drug-induced or aggravated parkinsonism: clinical signs and the changing pattern of implicated drugs. Neurologia 1996;11(1): 10–5 [in Spanish].
36. Mutch WJ, Dingwall-Fordyce I, Downie AW, et al. Parkinson's disease in a Scottish city. Br Med J (Clin Res Ed) 1986;292(6519):534–6 [Research Support, Non-US Gov't].
37. Caroff SN, Hurford I, Lybrand J, et al. Movement disorders induced by antipsychotic drugs: implications of the CATIE schizophrenia trial. Neurol Clin 2011; 29(1):127–48, viii.
38. Hardie RJ, Lees AJ. Neuroleptic-induced Parkinson's syndrome: clinical features and results of treatment with levodopa. J Neurol Neurosurg Psychiatr 1988;51(6):850–4.
39. Sethi KD, Zamrini EY. Asymmetry in clinical features of drug-induced parkinsonism. J Neuropsychiatry Clin Neurosci 1990;2(1):64–6.
40. Giladi N, Kao R, Fahn S. Freezing phenomenon in patients with parkinsonian syndromes [comparative study]. Mov Disord 1997;12(3):302–5.
41. Morley JF, Duda JE. Use of hyposmia and other non-motor symptoms to distinguish between drug-induced parkinsonism and Parkinson's disease. J Parkinsons Dis 2013;4(2):169–73.
42. Brigo F, Erro R, Marangi A, et al. Differentiating drug-induced parkinsonism from Parkinson's disease: an update on non-motor symptoms and investigations [review]. Parkinsonism Relat Disord 2014;20(8):808–14.
43. Marsden CD, Tarsy D, Baldessarani RJ. Spontaneous and drug-induced movement disorders. In: Benson DF, Blumer D, editors. Psychiatric aspects of neurologic disease. New York: Grune and Stratton; 1975. p. 219–65.
44. Klawans HL Jr, Bergen D, Bruyn GW. Prolonged drug-induced parkinsonism. Confin Neurol 1973;35(6):368–77.
45. Farde L, Wiesel FA, Halldin C, et al. Central D2-dopamine receptor occupancy in schizophrenic patients treated with antipsychotic drugs. Arch Gen Psychiatry

1988;45(1):71–6 [Comparative Study Research Support, Non-US Gov't Research Support, US Gov't, P.H.S.].

46. Meltzer HY, Matsubara S, Lee JC. Classification of typical and atypical antipsychotic drugs on the basis of dopamine D-1, D-2 and serotonin2 pKi values. J Pharmacol Exp Ther 1989;251(1):238–46 [In Vitro Research Support, Non-US Gov't Research Support, US Gov't, P.H.S.].
47. Kapur S, Seeman P. Does fast dissociation from the dopamine d(2) receptor explain the action of atypical antipsychotics?: a new hypothesis. Am J Psychiatry 2001;158(3):360–9 [Research Support, Non-US Gov't Review].
48. Eichelbaum M, Kroemer HK, Mikus G. Genetically determined differences in drug metabolism as a risk factor in drug toxicity [review]. Toxicol Lett 1992; 64-65(Spec No):115–22.
49. Negrotti A, Calzetti S, Sasso E. Calcium-entry blockers-induced parkinsonism: possible role of inherited susceptibility. Neurotoxicology 1992;13(1): 261–4.
50. Forno LS. Concentric hyalin intraneuronal inclusions of Lewy type in the brains of elderly persons (50 incidental cases): relationship to parkinsonism. J Am Geriatr Soc 1969;17(6):557–75.
51. Goetz CG. Drug-induced parkinsonism and idiopathic Parkinson's disease [letter]. Arch Neurol 1983;40(5):325–6.
52. Rajput AH, Rozdilsky B, Hornykiewicz O, et al. Reversible drug-induced parkinsonism. Clinicopathologic study of two cases [case reports]. Arch Neurol 1982; 39(10):644–6.
53. Kagi G, Bhatia KP, Tolosa E. The role of DAT-SPECT in movement disorders. J Neurol Neurosurg Psychiatr 2010;81(1):5–12.
54. Tarsy D, Lungu C, Baldessarini RJ. Epidemiology of tardive dyskinesia before and during the era of modern antipsychotic drugs. Handb Clin Neurol 2011; 100:601–16.
55. Fann WE, Lake CR. Amantadine versus trihexyphenidyl in the treatment of neuroleptic-induced parkinsonism. Am J Psychiatry 1976;133(8):940–3 [Clinical Trial Controlled Clinical Trial Research Support, US Gov't, Non-P.H.S.].
56. Kelly JT, Zimmermann RL, Abuzzahab FS, et al. A double-blind study of amantadine hydrochloride versus benztropine mesylate in drug-induced parkinsonism. Pharmacology 1974;12(2):65–73 [Clinical Trial Comparative Study Controlled Clinical Trial].
57. Shoulson I. Carbidopa/levodopa therapy of coexistent drug-induced parkinsonism and tardive dyskinesia. Adv Neurol 1983;37:259–66 [Comparative Study Research Support, US Gov't, P.H.S.].
58. Tardive dyskinesia: summary of a task force report of the American Psychiatric Association. By the Task Force on Late Neurological Effects of Antipsychotic Drugs. Am J Psychiatry 1980;137(10):1163–72.
59. Jeste DV, Lacro JP, Palmer B, et al. Incidence of tardive dyskinesia in early stages of low-dose treatment with typical neuroleptics in older patients. Am J Psychiatry 1999;156(2):309–11 [Clinical Trial Comparative Study Research Support, US Gov't, Non-P.H.S. Research Support, US Gov't, P.H.S.].
60. Kane JM, Smith JM. Tardive dyskinesia: prevalence and risk factors, 1959 to 1979 [review]. Arch Gen Psychiatry 1982;39(4):473–81.
61. Correll CU, Schenk EM. Tardive dyskinesia and new antipsychotics. Curr Opin Psychiatry 2008;21(2):151–6.

62. Yassa R, Jeste DV. Gender differences in tardive dyskinesia: a critical review of the literature. Schizophr Bull 1992;18(4):701–15 [Meta-Analysis Research Support, US Gov't, Non-P.H.S. Research Support, US Gov't, P.H.S.].
63. Woerner MG, Saltz BL, Kane JM, et al. Diabetes and development of tardive dyskinesia. Am J Psychiatry 1993;150(6):966–8 [Research Support, US Gov't, P.H.S.].
64. Gardos G, Cole JO, Tarsy D. Withdrawal syndromes associated with antipsychotic drugs. Am J Psychiatry 1978;135(11):1321–4 [Research Support, US Gov't, P.H.S.].
65. Fountoulakis KN, Samara M, Siapera M, et al. Tardive Tourette-like syndrome: a systematic review. Int Clin Psychopharmacol 2011;26(5):237–42.
66. Stahl SM. Tardive Tourette syndrome in an autistic patient after long-term neuroleptic administration [case reports]. Am J Psychiatry 1980;137(10): 1267–9.
67. Little JT, Jankovic J. Tardive myoclonus [case reports]. Mov Disord 1987;2(4): 307–11.
68. Stacy M, Jankovic J. Tardive tremor. Mov Disord 1992;7(1):53–7 [Case Reports Research Support, Non-US Gov't].
69. Keegan DL, Rajput AH. Drug induced dystonia tarda: treatment with L-dopa. Dis Nerv Syst 1973;34(3):167–9.
70. Burke RE, Fahn S, Jankovic J, et al. Tardive dystonia: late-onset and persistent dystonia caused by antipsychotic drugs [case reports]. Neurology 1982;32(12): 1335–46.
71. Sethi KD, Hess DC, Harp RJ. Prevalence of dystonia in veterans on chronic antipsychotic therapy. Mov Disord 1990;5(4):319–21.
72. Yassa R, Nair V, Dimitry R. Prevalence of tardive dystonia. Acta Psychiatr Scand 1986;73(6):629–33.
73. van Harten PN, Matroos GE, Hoek HW, et al. The prevalence of tardive dystonia, tardive dyskinesia, parkinsonism and akathisia The Curacao Extrapyramidal Syndromes Study: I. Schizophr Res 1996;19(2–3):195–203 [Research Support, Non-US Gov't].
74. Chen PY, Lin PY, Tien SC, et al. Duloxetine-related tardive dystonia and tardive dyskinesia: a case report. Gen Hosp Psychiatry 2010;32(6):646.e9–11.
75. Dressler D. Tardive dystonic syndrome induced by the calcium-channel blocker amlodipine. J Neural Transm 2014;121(4):367–9.
76. Pellecchia MT, Esposito M, Cozzolino A, et al. Drug induced oromandibular dystonia: A case related to prolonged use of cetirizine. Parkinsonism Relat Disord 2014;20(5):566–7.
77. Kang UJ, Burke RE, Fahn S. Natural history and treatment of tardive dystonia. Mov Disord 1986;1(3):193–208 [Research Support, Non-US Gov't Research Support, US Gov't, P.H.S.].
78. Kiriakakis V, Bhatia KP, Quinn NP, et al. The natural history of tardive dystonia. A long-term follow-up study of 107 cases. Brain 1998;121(Pt 11):2053–66.
79. Wojcik JD, Falk WE, Fink JS, et al. A review of 32 cases of tardive dystonia [comparative study]. Am J Psychiatry 1991;148(8):1055–9.
80. Andersson U, Haggstrom JE, Levin ED, et al. Reduced glutamate decarboxylase activity in the subthalamic nucleus in patients with tardive dyskinesia. Mov Disord 1989;4(1):37–46.
81. Bressman SB, de Leon D, Raymond D, et al. Secondary dystonia and the DYTI gene. Neurology 1997;48(6):1571–7 [Research Support, Non-US Gov't Research Support, US Gov't, P.H.S.].

82. Gimenez-Roldan S, Mateo D, Bartolome P. Tardive dystonia and severe tardive dyskinesia. A comparison of risk factors and prognosis. Acta Psychiatr Scand 1985;71(5):488–94.
83. Burke RE, Kang UJ, Jankovic J, et al. Tardive akathisia: an analysis of clinical features and response to open therapeutic trials. Mov Disord 1989;4(2):157–75 [Research Support, Non-US Gov't Research Support, US Gov't, P.H.S.].
84. Schilkrut R, Duran E, Haverbeck C, et al. Course of psychopathologic and extrapyramidal motor symptoms during long-term treatment of schizophrenic patients with psycholeptic drugs (author's transl). Arzneimittelforschung 1978;28(9):1494–5 [in German, Clinical Trial].
85. Lang AE. Withdrawal akathisia: case reports and a proposed classification of chronic akathisia [case reports review]. Mov Disord 1994;9(2):188–92.
86. Sachdev P. Research diagnostic criteria for drug-induced akathisia: conceptualization, rationale and proposal. Psychopharmacology (Berl) 1994;114(1):181–6 [Research Support, Non-US Gov't Review].
87. Aquino CC, Lang AE. Tardive dyskinesia syndromes: current concepts. Parkinsonism Relat Disord 2014;20(Suppl 1):S113–7.
88. Teo JT, Edwards MJ, Bhatia K. Tardive dyskinesia is caused by maladaptive synaptic plasticity: a hypothesis. Mov Disord 2012;27(10):1205–15.
89. Gunne LM, Haggstrom JE, Sjoquist B. Association with persistent neuroleptic-induced dyskinesia of regional changes in brain GABA synthesis. Nature 1984;309(5966):347–9.
90. Ferentinos P, Dikeos D. Genetic correlates of medical comorbidity associated with schizophrenia and treatment with antipsychotics. Curr Opin Psychiatry 2012;25(5):381–90.
91. Zhang XY, Zhang WF, Zhou DF, et al. Brain-derived neurotrophic factor levels and its Val66Met gene polymorphism predict tardive dyskinesia treatment response to *Ginkgo biloba*. Biol Psychiatry 2012;72(8):700–6.
92. De Leon ML, Jankovic J. Clinical features and management of classic tardive dyskinesia, tardive myoclonus, tardive tremor and tardive tourettism. In: Sethi KD, editor. Drug-induced movement disorders. New York: Marcel Dekker; 2004. p. 77–109.
93. Jankovic J, Beach J. Long-term effects of tetrabenazine in hyperkinetic movement disorders. Neurology 1997;48(2):358–62 [Research Support, Non-US Gov't].
94. Fahn S. Long-term treatment of tardive dyskinesia with presynaptically acting dopamine-depleting agents. Adv Neurol 1983;37:267–76.
95. Klawans HL, Rubovits R. Effect of cholinergic and anticholinergic agents on tardive dyskinesia [comparative study]. J Neurol Neurosurg Psychiatr 1974;37(8):941–7.
96. Waln O, Jankovic J. An update on tardive dyskinesia: from phenomenology to treatment. Tremor Other Hyperkinet Mov (N Y) 2013;3. Available at: http://tremorjournal.org/article/view/161.
97. Bhidayasiri R, Fahn S, Weiner WJ, et al. Evidence-based guideline: treatment of tardive syndromes: report of the Guideline Development Subcommittee of the American Academy of Neurology. Neurology 2013;81(5):463–9.
98. Zhang WF, Tan YL, Zhang XY, et al. Extract of *Ginkgo biloba* treatment for tardive dyskinesia in schizophrenia: a randomized, double-blind, placebo-controlled trial. J Clin Psychiatry 2011;72(5):615–21.
99. Spindler MA, Galifianakis NB, Wilkinson JR, et al. Globus pallidus interna deep brain stimulation for tardive dyskinesia: case report and review of the literature. Parkinsonism Relat Disord 2013;19(2):141–7.

100. Tarsy D, Kaufman D, Sethi KD, et al. An open-label study of botulinum toxin A for treatment of tardive dystonia. Clin Neuropharmacol 1997;20(1):90–3 [Clinical Trial Multicenter Study Research Support, Non-US Gov't].
101. Peritogiannis V, Tsouli S. Can atypical antipsychotics improve tardive dyskinesia associated with other atypical antipsychotics? Case report and brief review of the literature. J Psychopharmacol 2010;24(7):1121–5.
102. Littrell KH, Johnson CG, Littrell S, et al. Marked reduction of tardive dyskinesia with olanzapine [case reports letter]. Arch Gen Psychiatry 1998;55(3):279–80.
103. Factor SA, Friedman JH. The emerging role of clozapine in the treatment of movement disorders. Mov Disord 1997;12(4):483–96 [Research Support, Non-US Gov't Review].
104. Lieberman JA, Saltz BL, Johns CA, et al. The effects of clozapine on tardive dyskinesia. Br J Psychiatry 1991;158:503–10 [Research Support, Non-US Gov't Research Support, US Gov't, P.H.S.].
105. Hazari N, Kate N, Grover S. Clozapine and tardive movement disorders: a review. Asian J Psychiatr 2013;6(6):439–51.
106. Albayrak Y, Hashimoto K. Beneficial effects of sigma-1 agonist fluvoxamine for tardive dyskinesia and tardive akathisia in patients with schizophrenia: report of three cases. Psychiatry Investig 2013;10(4):417–20.
107. Gardos G, Cole JO. Overview: public health issues in tardive dyskinesia. Am J Psychiatry 1980;137(7):776–81 [Research Support, US Gov't, P.H.S.].
108. Gordon MF. Toxin and drug-induced myoclonus [review]. Adv Neurol 2002;89: 49–76.
109. Klawans HL, Carvey PM, Tanner CM, et al. Drug-induced myoclonus. In: Fahn S, Marsden CD, Van Woert MH, editors. Myoclonus. New York: Raven Press; 1986. p. 251–64.
110. Lang AE. Miscellaneous drug-induced movement disorders. In: Lang AE, Weiner WJ, editors. Drug-induced movement disorders. New York: Futura Publishing; 1992. p. 339–81.
111. Treatment of ADHD in children with tics: a randomized controlled trial. Neurology 2002;58(4):527–36 [Clinical Trial Multicenter Study Randomized Controlled Trial Research Support, Non-US Gov't Research Support, US Gov't, P.H.S.].
112. Bharucha KJ, Sethi KD. Movement disorders induced by selective serotonin reuptake inhibitors and other antidepressants. In: Sethi KD, editor. Drug-induced movement disorders. New York: Marcel Dekker; 2004. p. 233–57.
113. Kellett MW, Chadwick DW. Antiepileptic drug-induced movement disorders. In: Sethi KD, editor. Drug-induced movement disorders. New York: Marcel Dekker; 2004. p. 309–56.
114. Sanchez-Ramos J. Stimulant-induced movement disorders. In: Sethi KD, editor. Drug-induced movement disorders. New York: Marcel Dekker; 2004. p. 295–308.

Wilson Disease and Other Neurodegenerations with Metal Accumulations

Petr Dusek, MD, PhD[a,b,*], Tomasz Litwin, MD, PhD[c],
Anna Czlonkowska, MD, PhD[c,d]

KEYWORDS

- Wilson disease • NBIA • Neurodegeneration with brain iron accumulation
- Manganism • Primary familial brain calcification • Chelating therapy

KEY POINTS

- Wilson disease should be suspected in young individuals presenting with movement disorder, liver abnormalities of uncertain causes, or family history of Wilson disease.
- Wilson disease can be treated effectively with D-penicillamine, trientine, or zinc, providing the treatment is started early and continued lifelong.
- Iron deposits are visualized as hypointensities in T2-weighted magnetic resonance images (MRIs), manganese deposits as hyperintensities in T1-weighted MRIs, and calcium deposits as areas of high density in computed tomography images.
- Neurodegeneration with brain iron accumulation is a heterogeneous group of disorders comprising the following core syndromes: PKAN, PLAN, MPAN, BPAN, neuroferritinopathy, and aceruloplasminemia.
- Manganese transporter deficiency manifesting as movement disorder, chronic liver disease, and polycythemia can be effectively treated by iron supplementation combined with disodium calcium edetate.

Videos of postural wing-beating, orofacial dystonia, predominant retrocollis and tongue protrusion, and spastic quadruparesis accompany this article http://www.derm.theclinics.com/

Disclosures: The authors have nothing to disclose.
Supported by Charles University in Prague PRVOUKP26/LF1/4.
[a] Department of Neurology and Centre of Clinical Neuroscience, First Faculty of Medicine and General University Hospital in Prague, Charles University in Prague, Kateřinská 30, Prague 128 21, Czech Republic; [b] Institute of Neuroradiology, University Medicine Goettingen, Robert-Koch-Street 40, Göttingen 37075, Germany; [c] 2nd Department of Neurology, Institute Psychiatry and Neurology, Sobieskiego 9, Warsaw 02-957, Poland; [d] Department of Experimental and Clinical Pharmacology, Medical University, Banacha 1b, Warsaw 02-097, Poland
* Corresponding author. Institute of Neuroradiology, University Medicine Goettingen, Robert-Koch-Street 40, Göttingen 37075, Germany.
E-mail address: pdusek@gmail.com

Neurol Clin 33 (2015) 175–204
http://dx.doi.org/10.1016/j.ncl.2014.09.006 neurologic.theclinics.com

INTRODUCTION

Trace elements, such as iron, copper, manganese, and calcium, which are essential constituents necessary for cellular homeostasis, become toxic when present in excess quantities. In this article, we describe disorders arising from endogenous dysregulation of metal homeostasis leading to their tissue accumulation. Although subgroups of these diseases lead to regional brain metal accumulation, mostly in globus pallidus (GP), which is susceptible to accumulate divalent metal ions, other subgroups cause systemic metal accumulation affecting the whole brain, as well as liver and other parenchymal organs. The latter group comprises Wilson disease, manganese transporter deficiency, and aceruloplasminemia, and responds favorably to chelation treatment.

WILSON DISEASE

Epidemiology and Pathophysiology

Wilson disease (WD) is a rare autosomal recessive (AR) disorder of copper metabolism. The prevalence of WD has not been widely studied lately. In small studies performed in Europe and the United States in the 1980s, the incidence of WD was estimated to be 1:30,000. It was also shown that in close communities, the frequency of WD was higher, probably due to lower migration rates and frequent consanguinity. These reported incidences were 1:2600 (Canary Islands), 1:7000 (Sardinia), and 1:10,000 (China and Japan).[1,2] However, a recent report from the United Kingdom demonstrated that the prevalence of WD might be 1:7000 births, which suggests that the occurrence of WD is still underestimated. In addition, from 1% (historically) to 2.5% (data from the United Kingdom) of the population are carriers of pathogenic mutations of the WD gene.[3]

WD is caused by a mutation in the *ATP7B* gene located on chromosome 13, which encodes the copper-transporting transmembrane protein ATP-ase7B that is mostly expressed in the liver. ATP-ase7B is involved in copper transport in the trans-Golgi network in hepatocytes and the incorporation of copper into the apoceruloplasmin. Functional ceruloplasmin (cp) containing 6 atoms of copper is released to the blood. Additionally, ATP-ase7B is involved in copper excretion into the bile. In WD, this protein is dysfunctional, which initially results in copper accumulation in hepatocytes leading first to mitochondrial impairment and nonspecific microsteatosis and macrosteatosis, and later on to periportal inflammation, fibrosis, and ultimately to liver cirrhosis.[1,2] Stored copper is then released into the blood, leading to its accumulation in other tissues (brain, kidney, cornea). An excess of free copper is toxic for most tissues, leading to secondary damage. The main initial mechanism of cell injuries in WD is probably mitochondrial impairment related to copper toxicosis. Copper is initially buffered by mitochondria through incorporation into cupro-enzymes. Copper progressively accumulates in mitochondrial membranes, leading to severe damage of mitochondria and defects in the respiratory cycle with failure to produce cellular energy (ATP). Mitochondrial damage and massive release of copper into the cytoplasm and other cellular compartments further increases oxidative stress and leads to cellular death (hepatocyte necrosis). In the brain, copper toxicosis leads to neuronal degeneration and astrocyte changes, probably due to hyperammonemia (in the course of Krebs cycle failure) with the occurrence of pathologic astrocytes (Opalski, Alzheimer I and II cells) and astrogliosis. Interestingly, ATP-ase7B also is expressed in the brain and its deficit may contribute to brain damage by a different mechanism.[1,2]

Currently, there are more than 500 known pathogenic mutations in the *ATP7B* gene (www.wilsondisease.med.ualberta.ca/database.asp). Several mutations are characteristic for certain geographic areas, which makes the genetic diagnosis easier. In Northern, Central, and Eastern Europe, as well as in the United States, H1069Q is the most common mutation that occurs in almost 50% to 80% of patients with WD. In other populations, different mutations occur more frequently, including R778L in China, 4193delC in Saudi Arabia, and 441/-427del in Sardinia.[3–9]

There appears to be genotype-phenotype correlation; the most common mutation described in Europe (H1069Q) seems to cause only a partial defect of ATP-ase7B and leads to milder disturbances of copper metabolism with a later onset of neurologic symptoms.[4,6] In contrast, frameshift and nonsense mutations seem to correlate with more severe impairment of copper metabolism and an earlier onset of clinical symptoms.[5] Accessible data are often conflicting, and the currently known *ATP7B* mutation does not entirely explain the different WD phenotypes, different predominant symptoms, and different ages of disease onset. Thus, other modifying factors are suggested to impact the WD phenotype, such as polymorphisms in the genes encoding methylenetetrahydrofolate reductase (*MTHFR*), apolipoprotein E (*APOE*), dopamine D2 receptors (*DRD2*), prion-related protein (*PRNP*), the copper metabolism gene *Murr1*, antioxidant-1 (*Atox-1*), and the X-linked inhibitor of apoptosis (*XIAP*), as well as iron metabolism disturbances, gender-related differences, inflammatory reactions, and oxidative stress.[1,2,10] However, all these potentially modifying factors need to be verified in larger populations before they can be used in WD management.[10]

Clinical Presentation

The clinical symptoms of WD can start at any age; however, in most patients, the age of onset is between 5 and 35 years. In almost 3% of cases, symptoms start in adulthood (even in the eighth decade of life).[11,12] There is a wide spectrum of clinical manifestations, but the most important and basic symptoms of the disease can be divided into hepatic, neurologic, and psychiatric manifestations (**Table 1**).[1,2] WD most often starts with hepatic (40%–60%), followed by neurologic (40%–50%) and psychiatric (10%–25%) symptoms.

The hepatic presentation

The hepatic presentation of WD occurs almost 10 years earlier than neurologic symptoms, with the mean age of onset 11.4 years; however, the youngest patient with WD with elevation of liver enzymes was diagnosed at 9 months old.[13] The hepatic presentation of WD can be divided into several forms:

- Asymptomatic elevation of liver enzymes (usually asymptomatic elevation of serum aminotransferases, often found accidentally).
- Acute hepatitis (in almost 25% of cases, mimicking viral hepatitis with jaundice usually with spontaneous regression of symptoms, rarely transforming into acute liver failure).
- Acute liver failure (described also as fulminant liver failure) occurs in almost 6% to 12% of patients, more often in young women (<30 years old; women-to-men ratio: 4:1). Rapidly developing liver failure is usually accompanied by severe hemolytic anemia, renal failure, encephalopathy, and hemorrhagic diathesis. It is one of the main indications for liver transplantation in WD treatment.
- Chronic hepatitis with liver cirrhosis (decompensated or compensated) is the most frequent presentation of WD (the clinical signs of liver cirrhosis include fatigue, splenomegaly, portal hypertension, coagulopathy, spider naevi); cirrhosis may develop without clinical symptoms and can be discovered accidentally when neurologic signs occur.

Table 1
The most common clinical manifestations of WD

WD Presentation	Symptoms
Hepatic	Asymptomatic elevation of liver enzymes (aminotransferases) Acute hepatitis (eg, jaundice, abdomen pain) Acute liver failure (coagulopathy, jaundice, encephalopathy) Liver cirrhosis symptoms (compensated or decompensated) (fatigue, spider naevi, portal hypertension, splenomegaly, bleeding)
Neurologic	Movement disorders (tremor, dystonia, ataxia, ballism, chorea, parkinsonian syndrome) Speech disturbances: dysarthria (extrapyramidal, dystonic, cerebellar, mixed, unclassified) Dysphagia Autonomic dysfunction (eg, salivation, electrocardiographic abnormalities, orthostatic hypotension) Gait and balance disturbances (due to involuntary movements, cerebellar ataxia, impairment of postural reflexes)
Psychiatric	Cognitive impairment (neurodegeneration due to brain copper accumulation, hepatic encephalopathy) Personality disorders (eg, abnormal, antisocial behavior, irritability, disinhibition) Mood disorders (bipolar disorders, depression, suicidal attempts) Psychosis and other psychiatric alterations (eg, rarely psychosis, anorexia, sleep disturbances)
Ophthalmologic	Kayser-Fleischer ring; sunflower cataract
Other	Renal (nephrolithiasis, aminoaciduria) Bone (osteoporosis, joint pain) Heart (cardiac arrhythmia) Skin (hyperpigmentation of lower legs) Hematopoietic system (thrombocytopenia, hemolytic anemia, leukopenia)

Besides acute liver failure with hemolytic anemia, which should immediately trigger WD diagnostic process, other hepatic manifestations of WD are not characteristic.

The neurologic presentation

The neurologic presentation occurs in almost 40% to 50% of patients,[1,2] and its mean age of onset is 19 years. However, the earliest onset of neurologic symptoms was 6 years and the latest was 72 years. The most common distinguishable neurologic presentations are (1) akinetic-rigid (parkinsonianlike), (2) tremors, (3) ataxia, and (4) dystonia.[1,2] However, in many cases it is difficult to classify the patients' neurologic symptoms because of mixed presentations. Tremor is the most frequent neurologic symptom; it occurs in almost 80% patients with the neurologic presentation.[14] We observed resting, intentional, and/or postural tremors, often with a "wing-beating" character (Video 1). Parkinsonian symptoms, such as hypomimia, drooling, micrographia, and bradykinesia, occur in almost 40% of patients with neurologic presentation. Dystonic phenotype, occurring in 10% to 30% of cases, is usually most severe and resistant to treatment. It presents as focal (risus sardonicus, orofacial dystonia [Video 2], hand dystonia [**Fig. 1**], tongue dystonia), segmental (trunk dystonia), or generalized dystonia. It is noteworthy that most neurologic patients with WD have dysarthria, which can be classified as dystonic, cerebellar, parkinsonian, or mixed.[1,2] Other movement disorders, such as chorea and ballism, as well as autonomic system impairment, are less frequent. The pyramidal signs and sensory disturbances are rare

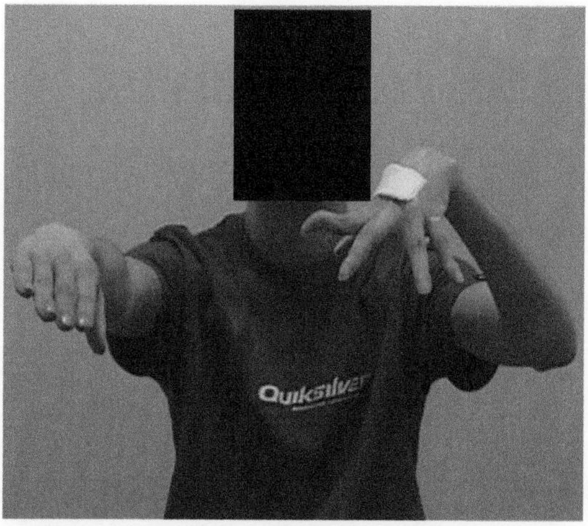

Fig. 1. Acute focal left hand dystonia in a patient with WD.

and nonspecific. They are usually caused by comorbidities or treatment complications (eg, myeloneuropathy due to copper deficiency caused by "overtreatment").[1,2] Due to the complex neurologic manifestations, the Unified Wilson's Disease Rating Score Scale was developed to objectively assess and quantify severity of symptoms.[15]

Psychiatric manifestations

Psychiatric manifestations can be the initial presentation in 25% of patients[16–19]; 65% of patients develop psychiatric symptoms during the disease progression.[16] Current classifications of WD psychiatric symptoms include (1) cognitive impairment, (2) personality disorders, (3) mood disorders, (4) psychosis, and (5) other psychiatric alterations (eg, anorexia, catatonia, substance abuse) that occur less frequently.[16] Cognitive disorders occur in up to 25% of patients, more often in those with severe neurologic symptoms. In children, decline in school performance can occur; whereas in older patients, impairment of executive functions and visuospatial processing is a common finding, rarely leading to dementia. Personality disorders occurred in 46% to 71% of patients and often included abnormal behavior, irritability, aggressiveness, and disinhibition. Mood disorders, such as depression and bipolar disorder, are reported in 30% to 60% of patients, with high prevalence of suicidal behavior (4%–16%). Psychosis used to be a commonly reported symptom, but currently it seems not to occur more frequently than in the general population. The delay between the onset of psychiatric symptoms and the disease diagnosis can reach several years; it is therefore important to increase awareness of WD among psychiatrists and possibly to perform WD screening in psychiatric patients.

Ophthalmologic manifestations

Ophthalmologic manifestations of WD include the Kayser-Fleischer ring (K-F ring) (**Fig. 2**) and sunflower cataract (SC) (**Fig. 3**), which are both pathognomonic, but reversible during treatment.[1,2] The K-F ring is caused by copper deposition in the corneal Descemet membrane; it is usually described as golden brown, green, or yellow coloration seen at the periphery of the cornea. This occurs in 90% to 100% of patients with neurologic presentation, but in only 40% to 50% of patients with hepatic presentation and in 20% to 30% of asymptomatic patients. Importantly, there are few

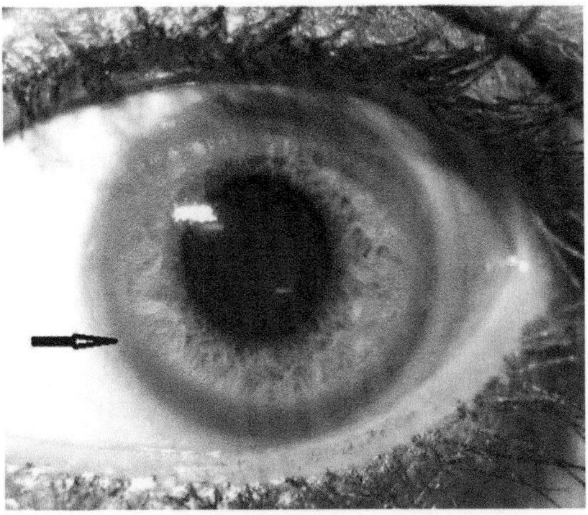

Fig. 2. The K-F ring in the right eye of a patient with WD (*arrow*).

medical conditions with eye changes similar to the K-F ring, including primary biliary cirrhosis, cryptogenic cirrhosis, cholestatic cirrhosis, as well as neoplastic disorders with high serum copper levels (multiple myeloma, leukemia) and high-dose estrogen treatment.[1,2] The occurrence of SC is estimated to be 17% to 25%, but large studies have not been done. SC is caused by copper deposits located directly under the anterior lens capsule, which resembles a sunflower (central disc with radiating petal-like spokes).

Other manifestations

Other manifestations of WD include hematologic changes (thrombocytopenia, leukopenia, hemolytic anemia), bone and joint involvement (pain, osteoporosis, spontaneous fractures), renal involvement (hypercalciuria, hyperphosphaturia, nephrocalcinosis), and skin changes, which may occur but none of them is specific for WD.[1,2]

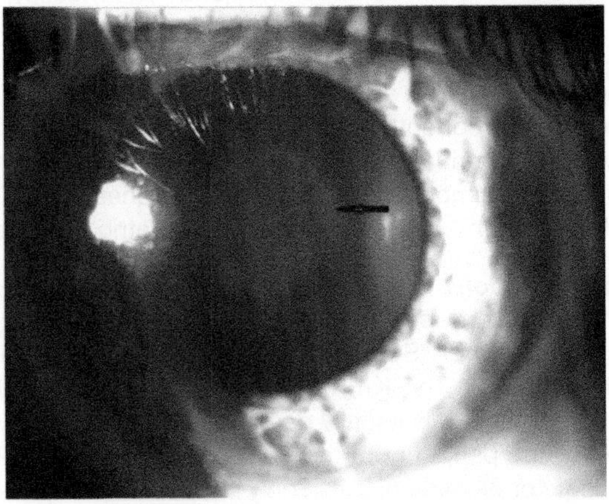

Fig. 3. The SC in the right eye of a patient with WD (*arrow*).

Diagnosis

WD should be suspected in young individuals presenting with movement disorder, liver abnormalities of uncertain causes, or family history of WD. WD diagnosis is based mainly on findings of abnormal copper metabolism. This includes (1) serum ceruloplasmin (cp) level, (2) serum copper level, and (3) 24-hour urinary copper excretion assessment. The diagnosis can be confirmed with genetic tests.

The serum ceruloplasmin level

The serum cp level is decreased to less than 0.2 g/L (normal range: 0.2–0.5 g/L) in almost 95% of patients with WD. A moderate decrease of cp is observed in approximately 20% of WD heterozygotes (carriers of a WD mutation on one chromosome). False negative, that is, normal or even increased serum cp, could be observed in almost 50% of patients with WD with decompensated liver cirrhosis or during estrogen therapy. Additionally, false-positive results (decreased level of cp) could be observed in aceruloplasminemia, sprue, protein-losing enteropathy, and nephritic syndromes. Finally, the cp level also depends on the method of examination (the immunologic assay often overestimates the protein level, whereas the nephelometric method is more accurate).[1,2,13]

The total serum copper level

The total serum copper level in patients with WD is usually decreased to less than 70 μg/dL (normal range: 70–140 μg/dL) and it mostly represents the copper bound to cp (decreases with cp). Free, non-cp–bound copper (calculated manually as difference between total and cp-bound serum copper) is increased to greater than 15 μg/dL in nontreated patients with WD. Free copper is more relevant for the WD diagnosis and treatment. The false-negative, extremely high total serum copper levels in patients with WD occur in acute liver failure with hemolytic anemia. Increased total copper level also can be observed in some neoplastic disorders (eg, leukemia, multiple myeloma) and during estrogen intake. Free-copper calculation should be performed in these cases.[1,2,13]

Daily urinary copper excretion

Daily urinary copper excretion is the best single test for WD. In patients with WD, the daily copper urinary excretion is typically increased to greater than 100 μg/24 hours (normal range: 0–50 μg/24 hours). False-negative results were observed in 16% to 23% of patients, especially in children and asymptomatic cases. False-positive results were observed in patients with acute liver failure and neoplastic disorders, such as leukemia or multiple myeloma. In pediatric patients, stimulation of urinary copper excretion by D-penicillamine (d-p) challenge test is useful (**Table 2**).[1,2,13]

Ophthalmologic examination

K-F ring and SC are pathognomonic ophthalmologic signs of WD, and their finding is helpful for the diagnosis and treatment monitoring. The ophthalmologic slit-lamp examination is more sensitive than examination by the "naked" eye and in some cases the ophthalmologist may even initiate the process of WD diagnosis.[1,2,13]

Brain imaging

Magnetic resonance imaging (MRI) is the most important neuroradiological examination for the WD diagnosis (see **Table 2**) and treatment monitoring. The typical MRI pathology is described as symmetric hyperintensity or mixed intensity in T2-weighted (T2w) images in the putamina (72%; with hyperintense peripheral putaminal rim), GP (61%), caudate nuclei (61%), thalami (58%), and pons (20%) (**Fig. 4**).[1,2,20]

Table 2
Ferenci Score: scoring system for the diagnosis of Wilson's disease developed at the 8th International Meeting on Wilson's Disease and Menkes Diseases, Leipzig 2002

K-F Rings	Present (2 Points)	Absent (0 Points)	
Neuropsychiatric symptoms suggested WD (or typical brain MRI)	Yes (2 points)	No (0 points)	
Coombs negative hemolytic anemia	Yes (1 point)	No (0 points)	
24-h urinary copper excretion (in the absence of acute hepatitis)	Normal (0 points)	1–2 × ULN (1 point)	>2 × ULN, or normal, but >5 × ULN after challenge with 2 × 0.5 g D-penicillamine (2 points)
Liver copper quantitative	Normal (−1 point)	<5 × ULN (1 point)	>5 × ULN (2 points)
Rhodanine positive hepatocytes (only in cases lacking a copper quantitative assessment)	Absent (0 points)	Present (1 point)	
Serum ceruloplasmin (nephelometric assay, normal >20 mg/dL)	Normal (0 points)	10–20 mg/dL (1 point)	<10 mg/dL (2 points)
Mutation analysis	Disease-causing mutations on both chromosomes (4 points)	Disease-causing mutations on one chromosome (1 point)	No mutation detected (0 points)

Interpretation of the WD diagnosis score: ≥4 points: diagnosis of WD highly likely; 2–3 points: diagnosis of WD probable, more investigations needed; 0–1 points: diagnosis of WD unlikely.

Abbreviations: K-F ring, Kayser-Fleischer ring; MRI, magnetic resonance imaging; ULN, upper limit of normal; WD, Wilson disease.

From Ferenci P, Caca K, Loudianos G, et al. Diagnosis and phenotypic classification of Wilson disease. Liver Int 2003;23:141; with permission.

The midbrain (49%), cerebellum (52%), corticospinal tracts, cortex, and subcortical area (atrophy in 70% of cases) are also affected.[21] The signal in T1-weighted (T1w) images is generally reduced in basal ganglia. MRI abnormalities typical for WD occurred in almost 90% to 100% of neuropsychiatric, 40% to 75% of hepatic, and 20% to 30% of asymptomatic patients.[20–24] Supposedly pathognomonic MRI findings including "the faces of the giant and miniature panda" and the bright claustrum can be seen only in fewer than 14% of cases and were also reported in other neurodegenerative disorders.[20–24] Transcranial sonography depicts lenticular nucleus hyperechogenicity even in patients with WD with normal MRI findings, but the validity of this examination in the diagnosis of WD has not been examined.[25]

Liver biopsy

Liver biopsy is used mainly in the differential diagnosis of hepatic WD cases. It includes both hepatic parenchymal copper content analysis and liver histology (with copper staining in hepatocytes). The hepatic copper content is increased in most

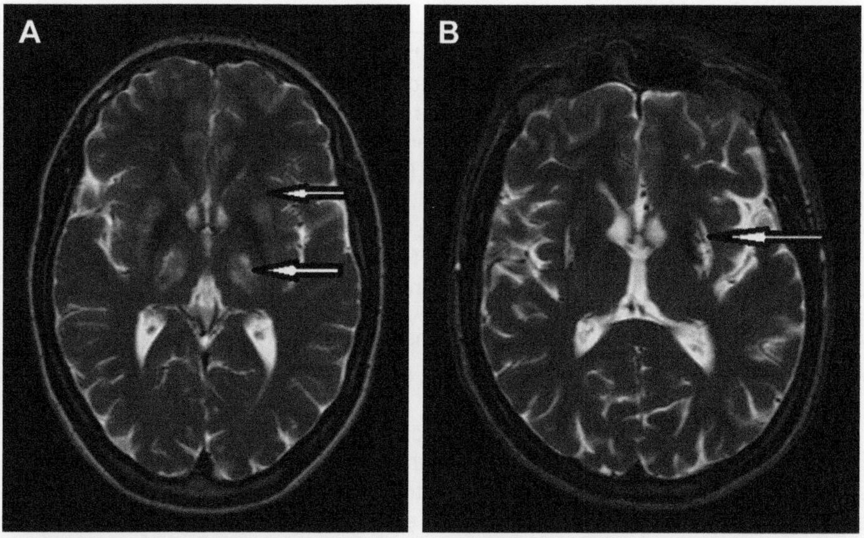

Fig. 4. The typical brain MRI in patients with WD. (*A*) Symmetrically increased signal intensity in the thalamus, GP, and caudate in both hemispheres in T2w images (*arrows*); (*B*) symmetrically increased signal intensity in the putamen in T2w images in both hemispheres (*arrows*).

patients with WD, as the pathology begins in the liver. Typically, it is elevated to greater than 250 μg/g of dry tissue.[1,2,13] The liver copper accumulation is not homogeneous, so the biopsy should include at least 1-cm length of liver core tissue. False-positive elevation of liver copper content can occur in other disorders (eg, primary liver cirrhosis). The liver histology includes noncharacteristic changes like steatosis, necrosis, fibrosis, the initial stages of liver damage, and positive copper staining.[13] If the WD diagnosis is obvious, as in neuropsychiatric patients with WD, there is no indication to perform a liver biopsy.

Genetic tests

Genetic tests confirm the WD diagnosis. The knowledge of mutations prevalent in a particular geographic region (eg, H1069Q in Europe) allows for a more effective genetic diagnosis.[3–9] In case of negative genetic screening for prevalent mutations, direct sequencing of the whole gene is possible. Genetic tests are important in the WD diagnosis algorithm, particularly in patients with inconclusive biochemical findings and in asymptomatic relatives of patients with WD (see **Table 2**).

Additional tests used in the Wilson disease diagnosis

There are 2 tests that are rarely performed today: (1) assessment of incorporation of radiocopper into cp (decreased in patients with WD) and (2) analysis of copper in cerebrospinal fluid.[1,2]

Wilson disease diagnostic score

After analyzing all of the previously mentioned WD diagnostic methods and their limitations, a scoring system for the WD diagnosis was developed at the international meeting in Leipzig in 2001 (**Table 2**).[13] It includes copper metabolism results, clinical symptoms, and genetic tests. The scoring system was named the Ferenci aka Leipzig score and is currently recommended in the guidelines for WD diagnosis and treatment.

Treatment and Prognosis

There are 2 main options for WD treatment: pharmacologic and liver transplantation. The pharmacologic treatment of WD is based on drugs leading to a negative copper balance, such as (1) chelators (d-p and trientine) inducing copper urinary excretion; (2) zinc salts, which mainly decrease the copper absorption from the digestive tract (by induction of metallothionein synthesis); and (3) "complexors" (tetrahydromolybdate, which is currently used only in clinical trials), with dual mechanism of action, that is forming complexes with copper in the digestive tract preventing its absorption and in the blood making copper unavailable for cellular uptake.[26–44] When treated correctly, liver functions and symptoms improve in 2 to 6 months in more than 90% patients. Neurologic improvement is observed less frequently (in >60% patients) and takes more time, usually 1 to 3 years.[38] The drug doses, treatment regimens, most common adverse events, and means of compliance monitoring are provided in **Table 3**.

There is a lack of prospective studies directly comparing the safety and efficacy of drugs used in WD treatment; instead, there are reports with conflicting data about the superiority of different drugs based on retrospective studies from individual WD centers, which has led to different treatment strategies in different countries.[26–44] According to the European Association for the Study of the Liver[2] and the American Association for the Study of Liver Diseases,[1] initial treatment of symptomatic patients with WD should be performed with chelators (trientine has certain advantages). Zinc salts could be used as a first line of treatment in patients without neurologic symptoms, as well as a maintenance therapy for patients with WD with neurologic symptoms.[1,2] In contrast, recently published data showed that zinc salt treatment was effective as monotherapy in hepatic patients.[43] Furthermore, recent study comparing d-p with zinc salts in the treatment of 143 symptomatic patients with WD, showed the same efficacy of d-p and zinc salts with similar frequencies of improvement of liver and neurologic parameters in both groups[29]; there was a slightly higher number of adverse events in the d-p group. It seems that choice of treatment is currently based mainly on center experience. Without prospective, multicenter, head-to-head studies comparing the drugs used in WD treatment, it is difficult to imply superiority of a particular drug; although, wide spectrum of more severe adverse events during WD treatment with d-p are reported from all WD centers (see **Table 3**).[26–44]

An extremely important adverse event affecting the patient's prognosis is paradoxic early neurologic worsening after initiating the pharmacologic treatment. It was initially reported in 50% of patients with WD treated with d-p,[1,2] suggesting that d-p should not be used in neurologic patients. Currently, neurologic worsening is reported for all kinds of WD treatments with a similar frequency (approximately 10%).[27,29,37,38] The mechanism underlying neurologic worsening is still not clear. It is partially explained by rapid mobilization of copper from tissues, which produces increased levels of free copper with associated toxicity and oxidative stress.[34,35] The mechanism of action of zinc salts theoretically protects against the rapid copper mobilization from tissues because it starts to inhibit copper absorption 2 to 3 weeks after initiating the treatment (increased metallothionein synthesis in intestinal mucosa is needed). Current treatment strategies are based on very slowly increased doses of chelators and are associated with lower occurrence of neurologic worsening; however, up to 10% of patients still neurologically deteriorate during the dose escalation.[29,32,37]

The last treatment option, used since 1971, is orthotopic liver transplantation. It is reserved only for patients with acute liver failure or decompensated liver cirrhosis.[45–49] As the genetic defect predominantly disrupts copper transport in hepatocytes, liver

Table 3
The characteristics of drugs used in WD treatment

The WD Drug	Doses	Special Treatment Regimen	Possible Adverse Events	Compliance with Treatment Examination
D-penicillamine (d-p)	• Adults: 750–1500 mg/d • Children: 20 mg/kg/d • Administration in 3 doses	• Administration 1 h before meal or 3 h after meal • Slow doses increase during initiation of treatment (to avoid neurologic worsening)	• Nephritic syndrome • Skin reaction (fever, rush, elastosis perforans serpiginosa, **Fig. 5**) • Lupuslike reaction, lymphadenopathy-aplastic anemia • Serous retinitis • Hepatotoxicity • Leukopenia, thrombocytopenia • Loss of taste • Myasthenialike syndromes	• Copper urinary excretion 200–500 μg/24 h (at the beginning of the treatment >1000 μg/24 h) • Free copper 5–15 μg/dL • Normalization of copper urinary excretion 2 d after stopping the treatment with d-p
Trientine	• 900/2700 mg/d initially (900–1500 mg/d) maintenance treatment (2–3 doses)	• Administration 1 h before meal or 3 h after meal • The treatment with iron should be avoided (iron chelation)	• Gastritis • Sideroblastic anemia • Lupuslike reactions • Loss of taste	• Copper urinary excretion 200–500 μg/24 h (at the beginning of the treatment >1000 μg/24 h) • Serum-free copper 5–15 μg/dL; normalization of copper urinary excretion 2 d after stopping the treatment with trientine
Zinc salts	• Adults: 150 mg of elemental zinc/d • Children (<50 kg): 75 mg/d • In 3 divided doses	• Administration >30 min before meals	• Gastritis • Biochemical pancreatitis • Immuno-suppression • Bone marrow depression	• Copper urinary excretion <75 μg/24 h • Serum-free copper 5–15 μg/dL (>12 mo of treatment)

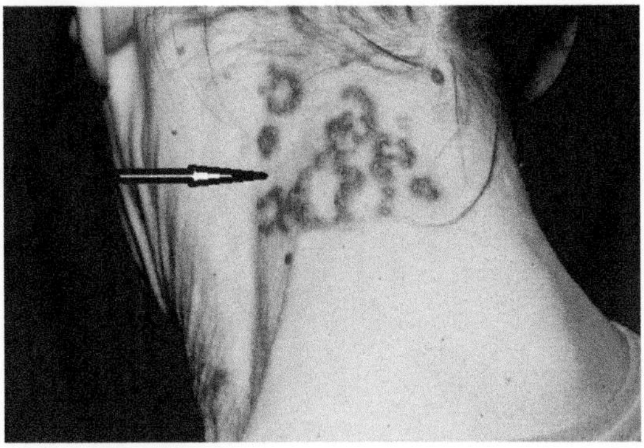

Fig. 5. Skin lesions at the neck (elastosis perforans serpiginosa) in a patient with WD after 1-year d-p treatment (*right arrow*).

transplantation corrects this defect and cures WD. Current data from transplant centers demonstrate that the survival rates vary between 78% and 90% and 65% and 75%, 1 and 5 years after the transplantations.[45,48] Liver transplantation in neurologic patients with WD is controversial and neurologic improvement unwarranted. Based on single case reports with variable results, it may not be recommended.[46,47]

Symptomatic therapy mainly addresses the symptoms of liver failure, neurologic deficits, and psychiatric symptoms.[49,50] In hepatic cases, this includes the correction of coagulopathy (vitamin K), treatment of edema (diuretics), and esophageal varices (beta-blockers, endoscopic or surgery treatment). Reports of treating neurologic symptoms are conflicting; the following treatments were reported to be beneficial in several case studies: levodopa (secondary parkinsonism), beta-blockers (tremor), anticholinergic drugs, botulinum toxin, or deep brain stimulation (dystonia).[44] When treating WD psychiatric symptoms, D2 dopamine receptor blockers should be used very carefully because of the possibility of neurologic deterioration.[28,51] In bipolar disorders, lithium treatment seems to be the safest option (not metabolized in liver; not involved in dopamine metabolism).[16]

In summary, apart from inconsistencies based on experience with different drugs in different countries, the most important conclusions regarding the WD treatment and prognosis are (1) WD can be successfully treated with pharmacologic agents if the treatment is started in the early phases of disease and is continued lifelong (long-term follow-up studies from many countries reported that the survival of patients with WD is comparable with that of general population[52–55]); (2) the siblings of patients with WD should be screened for WD and if confirmed, treatment should be started even if they have no signs of the disease; (3) the compliance and treatment monitoring seems to be more important than the choice of drug used in WD treatment; (4) during WD treatment, patients should undergo regular careful assessments of liver functions, general physical health, neurologic and psychiatric symptoms, and copper metabolism to avoid drug-related adverse events, including hypocupremia caused by "overtreatment" and to verify patients' compliance; and (5) liver transplantation in WD should be reserved only for specific indications (**Table 4**).

NEURODEGENERATION WITH BRAIN IRON ACCUMULATION

Neurodegeneration with brain iron accumulation (NBIA), formerly referred to as Hallervorden-Spatz syndrome, is a heterogeneous group of disorders with excessive

Table 4
Kings College Wilson disease prognostic index, modified by Dhawan et al

	0 Points	1 Point	2 Points	3 Points	4 Points
Serum bilirubin, μmol/L	0–100	101–150	151–200	201–300	>300
Aspartate aminotransferase, U/L	0–100	101–150	151–300	301–400	>400
International normalized ratio	0–1.29	1.3–1.6	1.7–1.9	2.0–2.4	>2.4
White blood cell count, 10^9/L	0–6.7	6.8–8.3	8.4–10.3	10.4–15.3	>15.3
Albumin, g/L	>45	34–44	25–33	21–24	<21

Score ≥11 points is associated with a high probability of death without liver transplantation and is an indication for liver transplantation.

Adapted from Dhawan A, Taylor RM, Cheeseman P, et al. Wilson's disease in children: 37-year experience and revised King's score for liver transplantation. Liver Transpl 2005;11:446; with permission.

brain iron deposition, particularly in GP and substantia nigra (SN) pars reticulata, that is recognizable as a decreased signal on routine T2w MRI images. The age of onset and clinical presentation are highly variable (**Table 5**). Combination of dystonia and/or parkinsonism with upper motor neuron signs referred to as pallido-pyramidal syndrome is fairly typical,[56] but diagnosis cannot be based solely on the clinical manifestation. The NBIA group comprises distinct genetic metabolic diseases, in some of which iron accumulation occurs only in the subgroup of affected subjects. Pantothenate-kinase–associated neurodegeneration (PKAN) and phospholipase-A2G6–associated neurodegeneration (PLAN), caused by mutations in the gene encoding pantothenate-kinase 2 (*PANK2*) and phospholipase A2 (*PLA2G6*), respectively, are long-established disorders. Neuroferritinopathy (NFP) resulting from mutations in the ferritin light-polypeptide (*FTL1*) gene and aceruloplasminemia caused by mutations in the *ceruloplasmin* gene are disorders affecting the iron metabolic pathway. Recently, several other genes causing NBIA were identified, namely *c19orf12*, causing mitochondrial membrane protein–associated neurodegeneration (MPAN); *WDR45*, causing beta-propeller protein–associated neurodegeneration (BPAN); fatty acid 2-hydroxylase (FA2H), causing fatty acid hydroxylase–associated neurodegeneration (FAHN); and CoA synthase (COASY), causing COASY protein–associated neurodegeneration (CoPAN). MRI findings suggestive of iron deposits also have been described in subgroups of patients with other rare disorders, such as Woodhouse-Sakati syndrome caused by a mutation in the *c2orf37* gene, Kufor-Rakeb syndrome caused by mutation in *ATP13A2* gene, and also in other lysosomal disorders, namely fucosidosis and GM1-gangliosidosis.[57] Although iron deposits were not confirmed histopathologically, typical MRI findings lump these diseases together with NBIA. Patients who are tested negative for mutations in the known genes receive the diagnosis of idiopathic NBIA.

Epidemiology and Pathophysiology

All NBIA variants are rare orphan diseases with an estimated prevalence up to 3:1,000,000. PKAN is the most prevalent disorder from the NBIA group, accounting for 50% of patients, whereas MPAN is probably the second most prevalent disorder, accounting for 5% to 30% of cases.[58–60] Prevalence of PKAN is approximately 1 to 3:1,000,000 and cases are reported worldwide.[61] There have been approximately 70 MPAN cases reported. Most of the patients have central European descent but patients from the Middle East, Mali, and Brazil were also reported.[62] PLAN also

Table 5
List of typical clinical and imaging findings in NBIA disorders

Disease	Mean Age at Onset (Range) in Years	Pattern of Iron Accumulation/MR Features	Characteristic CNS Features	Other Characteristic Features
PKAN	Classic 3.5 Atypical 14 (0.5–37)	GP, SN "eye-of-the-tiger" sign	Classic: Developmental delay Postural instability Dystonia Spasticity Atypical: Focal/segmental dystonia Dysarthria Parkinsonism Spasticity Psychiatric symptoms	Acanthocytosis Retinitis pigmentosa ↓ Serum beta lipoproteins ↑ Serum lactate
MPAN	10 (3–30)	GP, SN	Spasticity Cognitive dysfunction Dysarthria Movement disorders Psychiatric symptoms	Optic atrophy Axonal motor neuropathy
PLAN	Classic INAD (0.5–3.0) Atypical NAD/dystonia parkinsonism (4–30)	GP, SN Cerebellar atrophy and gliosis, white-matter lesions	Classic INAD: Developmental regression Truncal hypotonia Spasticity Strabismus Atypical NAD: Autism Gait ataxia Dysarthria Dystonia Parkinsonism Psychiatric symptoms	Axonal neuropathy with axonal spheroids in nerve biopsy Optic atrophy

Aceruloplasminemia	40–50 (16–71)	GP, caudate, putamen, SN, thalamus, dentate nuclei, cerebral cortex	Dysarthria Cerebellar ataxia Movement disorders Cognitive dysfunction	Diabetes mellitus Retinal degeneration Microcytic anemia ↓ Serum ceruloplasmin ↓ Serum iron, copper ↑ Serum ferritin
NFP	30–50 (13–63)	GP, caudate, putamen, SN, thalamus, red nuclei, dentate nuclei, motor cortex Cystic changes in putamen, GP	Dystonia Chorea Oro-linguo-mandibular dyskinesia Parkinsonism Cerebellar ataxia Dysarthria, dysphagia Cognitive decline Psychiatric symptoms	↓ Serum ferritin
BPAN	Deterioration 25 (15–37)	GP, SN Generalized atrophy Hyperintense T1w "halo" in midbrain	Developmental delay Rett-like symptoms Epilepsy Sleep disorders Dystonia-parkinsonism Cognitive dysfunction	High myopia
CoPAN	2–3	GP, SN, "eye-of-the-tiger" sign	Spastic paraparesis Dystonia Parkinsonism Psychiatric symptoms Cognitive decline	Axonal motor neuropathy
FAHN	3–10	GP, SN Cerebellar and brainstem atrophy, thinning of corpus callosum	Spastic paraparesis Dystonia Dysarthria Cognitive decline Seizures	Optic atrophy

Abbreviations: ↑, increased; ↓, decreased; BPAN, beta-propeller protein associated neurodegeneration; CNS, central nervous system; CoPan, CoA synthase protein–associated neurodegeneration; FAHN, fatty acid hydroxylase–associated neurodegeneration; GP, globus pallidus; INAD, infantile neuroaxonal dystrophy; MPAN, mitochondrial membrane protein–associated neurodegeneration; MR, magnetic resonance; NAD, atypical neuroaxonal dystrophy; NBIA, neurodegeneration with brain iron accumulation; NFP, neuroferritinopathy; PKAN, pantothenate-kinase–associated neurodegeneration; PLAN, phospholipase-A2G6–associated neurodegeneration; SN, substantia nigra; T1w, T1 weighted.

belongs to the common NBIA disorders, with an estimated prevalence of 1:1,000,000 accounting for approximately 10% to 20% of NBIA cases.[63] BPAN has only recently been described and only approximately 30 patients have been identified worldwide.[64–66] NFP was originally described in a large pedigree in northeastern England, but patients were later reported from Portugal, Australia, the United States, and Japan. More than 70 cases have been reported.[67] Aceruloplasminemia has been dominantly described in Japan, with a regional prevalence of 1:2,000,000[68]; 35 affected families worldwide have been identified.[69] FAHN has been reported in more than 30 patients with Middle Eastern, Italian, Balkan, and Asian origin.[70]

Two NBIA disorders are caused by dysfunction of proteins directly involved in iron metabolism. Disruption of normal cellular iron trafficking and storage leading to oxidative stress is presumably the cause of clinical symptoms in these diseases. In aceruloplasminemia, lack of cp ferroxidase activity prevents oxidation of ferrous ions, which is necessary for cellular iron release and binding to transferrin. This in turn leads to systemic iron accumulation affecting reticuloendothelial system, hepatocytes, pancreatic endocrine cells, myocardium, retina, and brain. Neuropathologic studies confirmed iron deposited predominantly in the perivascular spaces, terminal astrocytic processes, and neurons.[71] In NFP, dysfunctional ferritin shell is unable to protect the cellular environment from the toxic effect of labile iron and subsequent free radical production. Abnormal ferritin molecules also may contribute to neurodegeneration by inducing proteasomal activation. Neuropathologic examination in NFP reveals cavitations predominantly localized in GP, putamen, and dentate nucleus surrounded by iron-laden spherical inclusions within glial cells and neuropil.[72]

Other NBIA disorders are caused by mutation in genes involved in fatty acid/ceramide metabolism or phospholipid remodeling, both of which are important factors for cell membrane and myelin homeostasis.[57] Iron accumulation, mostly in the form of perivascular hemosiderin deposits, is largely confined to GP and SN in these disorders and its pathophysiology is poorly understood. In autopsy cases of PKAN, PLAN, and MPAN, axonal spheroids showing strong immunoreactivity for ubiquitin have been described. Neuropathological findings in MPAN and PLAN are typical for diffuse occurrence of α-synuclein–positive Lewy bodies and Lewy neurites,[58] in the latter variably accompanied by hyperphosphorylated tau deposits and neurofibrillary tangles.[73]

The third subgroup of NBIA comprises disorders caused by dysfunction of lysosomal proteins. Iron accumulation is not a universal feature of these disorders, and when present it is usually confined to GP and SN. BPAN is the well-established disorder from this group caused by mutation in *WDR45*, a protein involved in autophagy. Neuropathological findings include axonal spheroids and tau-positive tangles predominantly in SN pars compacta.

Differential Diagnosis of Neurodegeneration with Brain Iron Accumulation

Pantothenate-kinase–associated neurodegeneration

PKAN can manifest as a classic phenotype in 75% of patients and as an atypical phenotype in 25% of patients. The classic phenotype may begin with nonspecific symptoms, such as clumsiness and neurodevelopmental delay, which are later on accompanied by postural instability, lower limb spasticity, and dystonia. Visual symptoms due to pigmentary retinopathy are common (70%). Atypical phenotype often begins as focal or segmental dystonia in the cranial, cervical, or lower limb region accompanied by dysarthria, palilalia, and neuropsychiatric features, such as depression, impulsivity, and psychotic symptoms. Cognitive dysfunction is common but highly variable.[63] Retrocollis along with tongue protrusion dystonia is a fairly specific manifestation (Video 3). Parkinsonism, spasticity, and seizures are less common. Plasmatic levels of lactate may be elevated while beta lipoproteins may be decreased. Acanthocytosis is present in 8% of patients. Symptoms may progress in a stepwise manner leading to loss of ambulation, typically within 15 years of diagnosis. The "eye-of-the-tiger" sign (**Fig. 6**) is a specific MRI marker for PKAN. It may, however, not be apparent early and very late in the disease course as well as in some genetic subtypes. Findings similar to eye-of-the-tiger sign have been described in other NBIAs, as well as in WD, multiple system atrophy, or progressive supranuclear palsy.[74] The mode of inheritance is AR; the most common mutation, c.1561G>A, consistently leads to the classic phenotype.[63]

Mitochondrial membrane protein–associated neurodegeneration

MPAN typically manifests as a combination of central and peripheral nervous system dysfunction. It is an AR disorder and currently approximately 30 mutations have been identified. In a group of 67 patients, the most frequent symptoms were upper motor neuron signs (88%), cognitive dysfunction (86%), dysarthria (82%), optic atrophy (75%), dystonia (67%), psychiatric symptoms (64%), motor neuropathy (56%), dysphagia (56%), and parkinsonism (45%) (Video 4).[62] Brain MRI universally shows iron deposits in GP and SN (**Fig. 7**). In some patients, hyperintense streaking of the internal medullary lamina of GP can be observed in T2w images.[58] Clinical presentation resembles PKAN, but the average age at onset of 10 years is higher and the rate of progression slower. The most distinctive clinical feature of MPAN is the presence of lower motor neuron signs, which, in combination with upper motor neuron signs, may mimic juvenile amyotrophic lateral sclerosis.[75] Predominance of upper motor neuron signs may lead to a spastic paraparesis phenotype.[76]

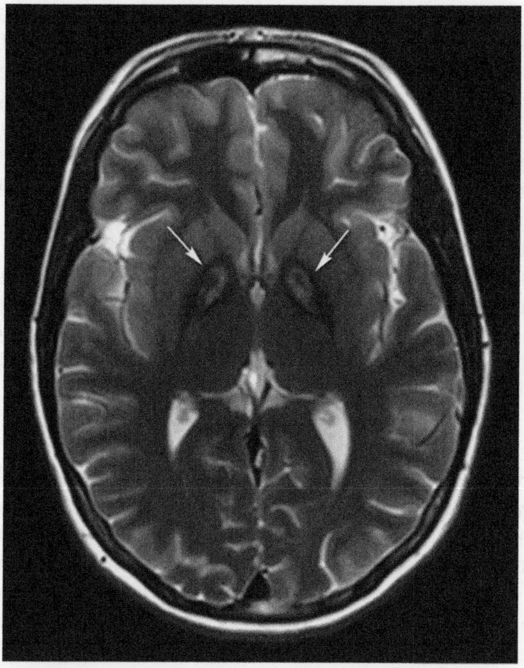

Fig. 6. Typical brain MRI in a patient with PKAN showing eye-of-the-tiger sign (central hyperintensity surrounded by hypointensity in GP) in T2w image (*arrows*). (*Courtesy of* Dr M. Dezortova, ZRIR, IKEM, Prague.)

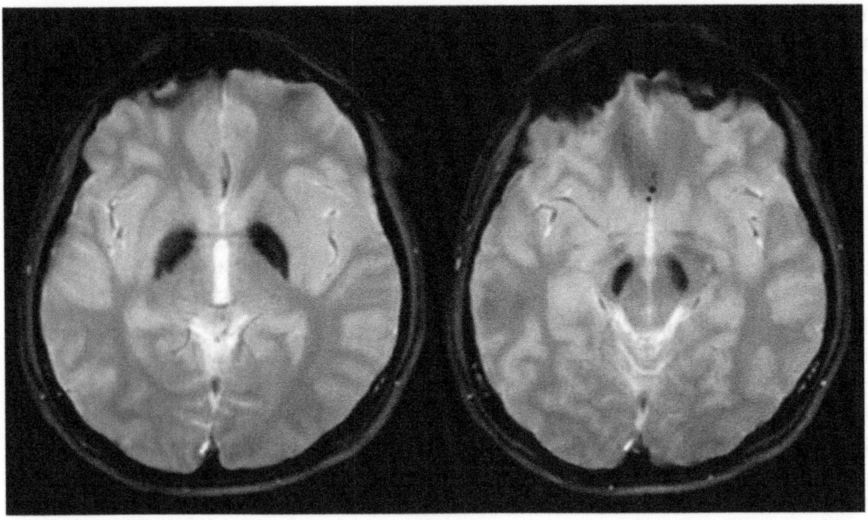

Fig. 7. Typical brain MRI in a patient with MPAN showing hypointensity in GP (*left image*) and SN (*right image*) in T2*w images. (*Courtesy of* Dr A. Burgetova, Department of Radiology, 1.LFUK a VFN, Prague.)

Phospholipase-A2G6–associated neurodegeneration

PLAN comprises a continuum of 3 overlapping phenotypes: classic infantile neuroaxonal dystrophy (INAD), atypical neuroaxonal dystrophy (NAD), and adult-onset dystonia-parkinsonism. INAD typically manifests within the first years of life as psychomotor regression, loss of ambulation, axial hypotonia, upper motor neuron signs, and strabism. Atypical NAD and dystonia-parkinsonism phenotypes have a wide range of presentation, including gait ataxia, dystonia, parkinsonism, spastic paresis, and dysarthria, often accompanied by psychiatric symptoms, such as autistic traits, impulsivity, psychosis, emotional instability, and cognitive dysfunction.[63] INAD and atypical NAD may be accompanied by axonal neuropathy with axonal spheroids that can be documented in peripheral nerve biopsy. Optic atrophy is a common finding in later stages, and can be diagnosed by ophthalmologic examination or visual evoked potentials. Brain MRI shows cerebellar atrophy in most and iron deposits in GP and SN in 40% to 50% of patients. White-matter changes are common. PLAN is an AR disorder with more than 70 reported mutations. Genotype-phenotype correlations exist and patients with the dystonia-parkinsonism phenotype harbor mutations that do not impair catalytic activity of the enzyme.[77]

Beta-propeller protein–associated neurodegeneration

BPAN is the only X-linked dominant NBIA and mutations in the *WDR45* gene in most cases arise de novo. Most affected individuals are female. Affected male individuals with phenotype indistinguishable from female individuals are suspected to harbor postzygotic mutations, as hemizygotic *WDR45* mutations are likely lethal. Clinical symptoms begin as a static global developmental delay with a disproportionate expressive language disorder in early childhood. Other symptoms include stereotypies, epileptic seizures, sleep dysfunction, high myopia, and other ocular defects. Patients with BPAN are frequently diagnosed as atypical Rett syndrome. Marked worsening usually begins in early adulthood, manifesting as levodopa-responsive dystonia-parkinsonism and progressive cognitive decline.[65] The benefit of levodopa is within several years overshadowed by development of severe dyskinesias. Brain MRI is usually unremarkable before the onset of parkinsonism. Once clinical worsening occurs, iron deposits become apparent in GP and SN, along with generalized brain atrophy. A hypointense band surrounded by a hyperintense "halo" in the SN region in T1w images is a characteristic finding.[78]

Aceruloplasminemia

Aceruloplasminemia is a systemic disorder affecting erythropoiesis, pancreatic endocrine cells, and the central nervous system. Adult-onset neurologic symptoms are frequently preceded by diabetes mellitus (70%) and microcytic anemia (80%) unresponsive to iron supplements. The spectrum of neurologic symptoms in a group of 71 patients consisted of dysarthria; cerebellar ataxia (71%); movement disorders (64%) manifesting as a combination of blepharospasm, oromandibular dystonia, chorea, tremor, and parkinsonism accompanied by cognitive dysfunction (60%); and retinal degeneration (76%).[69] General fatigue and chronic asthenia also are commonly reported complaints. Iron deposits in liver may be demonstrated by abdominal MRI showing diffuse hypointensity in T2w sequences and by liver biopsy showing increased liver iron concentration (>1200 μg/g dry weight) without signs of cirrhosis or fibrosis. Brain MRI is distinctive, invariably showing profound iron deposits in basal ganglia, thalamus, cerebellum, and variably also in the cerebral cortex.[79] The typical pattern of laboratory findings consists of undetectable serum cp, low serum copper, high serum ferritin, and low serum iron concentrations. Most of the more than 50 described mutations are unique to individual families.[80] Although regarded as an AR disorder, a small proportion of heterozygotes may become symptomatic manifesting with cerebellar ataxia.[81]

Neuroferritinopathy

NFP, also referred to as hereditary ferritinopathy, is an adult-onset disorder manifesting with movement disorders, cerebellar ataxia, cognitive dysfunction, and psychiatric symptoms.[67] In a series of 41 patients, prevalence of symptoms was as follows: dystonia (82%), chorea (70%), orofacial dyskinesia (65%), parkinsonism (45%), cognitive or psychiatric disturbances (42%), and tremor (5%).[82] Iron accumulation has been variably reported in kidney, liver, muscle, and skin, but its clinical significance is uncertain. Laboratory tests reveal low serum ferritin in 65% of male individuals and 85% of female individuals.[67] Brain MRI typically shows iron deposits surrounding T2-hyperintense lesions in basal ganglia representing cystic changes, gliosis, and edema.[79] Overt iron deposition has been documented in the presymptomatic stage.[83] NFP is the only NBIA with an autosomal dominant (AD) mode of inheritance and there are 7 known pathogenic mutations. The most widely reported mutation is 460InsA, manifesting typically with choreodystonia and dysarthria.[82] The 458dupA genotype typically manifests with rapidly progressive cerebellar ataxia,[84] whereas the 498InsTC genotype by postural tremor and slowly progressive ataxia in combination with extrapyramidal symptoms.[85] Hereditary hyperferritinemia-cataract syndrome, allelic to NFP, is caused by mutations in the untranslated regulatory iron-responsive element of the *FTL1* gene. It manifests as early-onset cataract with positive family history and elevated serum ferritin without neurologic symptoms or signs of iron overload.[86]

Coenzyme A synthase protein–associated neurodegeneration

CoPAN is a recently described disorder affecting the same metabolic pathway as PKAN, leading to decreased synthesis of Coenzyme A. Only 2 patients, with Italian origin, have been described. The clinical manifestation resembles typical PKAN phenotype with early-onset development of spastic-dystonic gait and subsequent progression of gait impairment, dysarthria, cognitive decline, and psychiatric symptoms (obsessive-compulsive and mood disorders). Motor axonal neuropathy was described in both affected subjects.[87]

Fatty acid hydroxylase–associated neurodegeneration

FAHN presents as childhood onset of spastic paraparesis (also designated SPG35), familial leukodystrophy, or NBIA. Although complicated spastic paraparesis (100%) usually dominates, the clinical picture is a spectrum of these distinct phenotypes. Dystonia (80%), dysarthria (90%), optic atrophy (70%), cognitive decline (90%), and seizures (30%) are common.[88,89] Brain MRI shows white-matter changes, cerebellar atrophy, and thin corpus callosum. Iron deposits in GP are not a universal finding but occur in most patients. Approximately 10 disease-causing mutations have been reported without clear genotype-phenotype correlation.[89]

Several clinical, imaging, and laboratory findings may help in the differential diagnosis (see **Table 5**). The "eye-of-the-tiger" sign is suggestive of PKAN, but was described also in NFP. Profound iron accumulation in basal ganglia, thalamus, dentate nuclei, and cortex is suggestive of aceruloplasminemia or NFP, accompanied by striatal cystic changes in the latter. Confluent white-matter changes, cerebellar atrophy, and hypoplastic corpus callosum may be especially apparent in FAHN and PLAN. Classic PLAN and BPAN begins within the first or second year of life. Symptom onset in early childhood is a typical for PKAN, but at the same age, FAHN or atypical variant of PLAN may also begin. Adult-onset disorders are typically NFP and aceruloplasminemia. The latter may be diagnosed sooner based on the presence of diabetes and microcytic anemia. Laboratory findings may show low ferritin in NFP, high ferritin along with low iron and copper concentration in aceruloplasminemia, and acanthocytes in PKAN. Motor neuropathy is common in MPAN, PLAN, and CoPAN.

Treatment Possibilities

Chelating treatment in NBIA is best advocated in aceruloplasminemia, particularly when initiated in the presymptomatic phase. Several weeks to months of treatment with deferasirox 500 to 1000 mg per day led to neurologic improvement in several cases,[90,91] whereas no improvement during treatment lasting up to 5 months was reported by others.[92] Treatment with intravenous deferoxamine 500 mg once weekly led to mild improvement in a single case study, but other reports did not find any clinical improvement on the dose of 500 to 2000 mg 2 to 5 times weekly.[80] Deferiprone 75 mg/kg per day administered for 6 months was ineffective in 1 case study.[93] Most importantly, patients who started treatment with deferasirox 500 to 1000 mg per day in the presymptomatic phase remained without neurologic symptoms during follow-up.[94–96] Other treatment strategies reported to be effective in individual patients with aceruloplasminemia are administration of fresh frozen plasma[97] to replenish cp levels, and oral zinc therapy to decrease iron absorption and improve antioxidative defense.[98]

The clinical experience with chelation treatment in other NBIA has yielded mixed results so far. In symptomatic patients with NFP, 4000 mg desferrioxamine weekly for 14 months, 2000 mg deferiprone 3 times a day for 2 months, and regular monthly venesections for 6 months did not lead to clinical improvement.[67] In PKAN, clinical benefit was not observed in a phase-II pilot study in 9 patients despite 30% reduction of iron content in the GP after 6 months of 25 mg/kg per day deferiprone treatment.[99] In another study, 15 mg/kg per day deferiprone treatment was mildly effective in 2 of 4 PKAN and 1 of 2 idiopathic NBIA patients. Clinical improvement and stabilization of symptoms in these patients was apparent after 1 year and persisted at 4 years of follow-up.[100,101] Other case studies with idiopathic NBIA and PKAN patients reported beneficial effect of 15 to 30 mg/kg per day deferiprone.[102] Because of potential side effects, long-term treatment with chelator must be closely monitored (blood count, renal parameters, and clinical symptoms). In the case of deferasirox treatment, gastrointestinal disturbances and skin rashes must be monitored.

High-dose pantothenate (vitamin B5) treatment is used in some centers in patients with atypical PKAN phenotype in whom residual PANK2 activity can be expected.[61] Pantothene derivates, such as pantethine or phosphopantothenate, capable of circumventing the metabolic defect are being developed.

Symptomatic treatment of NBIA disorders involves application of botulinum toxin into dystonic or spastic muscles, and medication capable of inhibiting dyskinesia (eg, anticholinergic drugs, benzodiazepines, baclofen, or tetrabenazine). In case of severe dystonia and spasticity, a baclofen pump may be useful.[102] Physiotherapy, occupational therapy, and hand surgery may be beneficial in case of limb dystonia, spasticity, or contractures. Speech therapy is indicated in dysarthria and in management of swallowing difficulties. Severe dysphagia may be managed by feeding via gastric tube.

Deep brain stimulation (DBS) of GPi is an effective symptomatic treatment option for dystonia in PKAN and possibly in other NBIA. It may be a life-saving procedure in medication-refractory status dystonicus and should be considered in severe pharmacoresistent, preferentially axial, and mobile, generalized dystonia.[74] A retrospective study in 23 patients with PKAN confirmed improvement of more than 20% in two-thirds of patients treated by DBS-GPi. At 9 to 15 months' follow-up, the mean improvement of dystonia and global quality-of-life rating was 26% and 83%, respectively.[103]

DISORDERS WITH BRAIN MANGANESE AND CALCIUM ACCUMULATION

Neurodegeneration Associated with Manganese Accumulation

Manganese transporter deficiency

Manganese transporter deficiency due to recessive mutation in the *SLC30A10* gene causes childhood-onset chronic liver disease and movement disorder.[104] Neurologic symptoms typically begin during the first decade as dystonia, with a characteristic high-stepping (cock-walk) gait variably accompanied by dysarthria, spastic paraparesis, parkinsonism, psychiatric symptoms, and motor neuropathy.[105] Two cases with adult-onset parkinsonism were also reported.[106] Severity of liver involvement is highly variable, ranging from mildly elevated liver transaminases to liver failure due to cirrhosis.[107]

MRI is specific for manganese deposits showing only mild abnormalities in T2w images, whereas T1w images show hyperintensities predominantly in GP, extending also to striatum, cerebellum, pituitary, and white matter. Liver biopsy confirms increased hepatic manganese concentration, whereas common laboratory findings are polycythemia (hemoglobin may exceed 20 g/dL) and low serum ferritin and iron levels.[108] More than 10 mutations have been identified worldwide in more than 20 patients.[108,109]

Iron supplementation combined with chelation therapy is the treatment of choice, leading to clinical improvement in most patients. Chelation therapy, usually using monthly 5-day courses of intravenous disodium calcium edetate (Na_2Ca-EDTA) 20 mg/kg twice a day, enhances manganese excretion, and iron supplementation reduces intestinal manganese absorption.[108] Serum level of zinc and copper should be monitored during Na_2Ca-EDTA treatment.

The differential diagnosis involves manganism caused by manganese overexposure, which has similar clinical and imaging features (**Fig. 8**) except for liver cirrhosis and

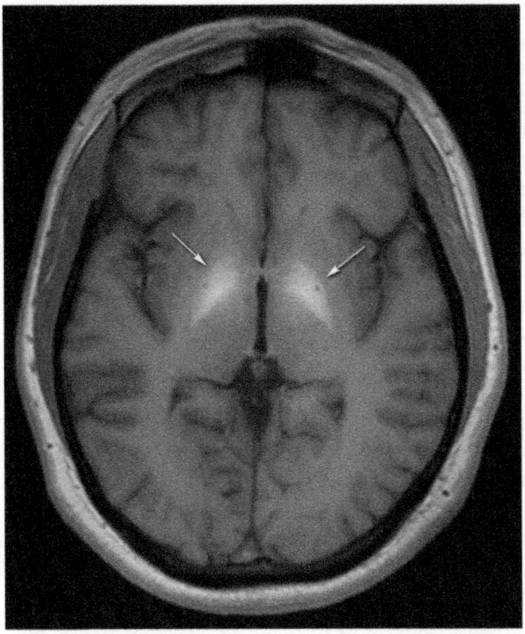

Fig. 8. Typical brain MRI in manganism (due to ephedrone abuse) showing bilateral hyperintensities in GP in T1w image (*arrows*). (*Courtesy of* Dr M. Okujava, Institute of Medical Research, Tbilisi.)

polycythemia. It has been described largely in workers in mining, welding, and smelting industries, but it also may arise from intravenous manganese intake, as in long-term parenteral nutrition or in methcathinone (ephedrone) abusers who use potassium permanganate for the synthesis of the drug. The mainstay of treatment is removal from exposure, which may be sufficient. In severe cases, Na_2Ca-EDTA treatment has proven beneficial.[105] Similar clinical symptoms and imaging features have been described in acquired hepatocerebral degeneration in end-stage liver disease.[105]

Primary Familial Brain Calcification

Primary familial brain calcification (PFBC), formerly referred to as Fahr disease or idiopathic basal ganglia calcifications, is a genetically heterogeneous syndrome with extensive calcifications in GP and other locations, including basal ganglia, thalamus, cerebellum, brainstem, capsula interna, cerebral cortex, and subcortical white matter. The phenotypic spectrum in a large PFBC cohort of different genetic backgrounds comprised movement disorders (33%–71%), including parkinsonism, postural tremor, chorea, focal or generalized dystonia, and ataxia (0%–36%) accompanied by dysarthria (14%–46%), pyramidal signs (14%–26%), cognitive decline (33%–71%), seizures (0%–10%), and psychiatric symptoms.[110] Psychiatric symptoms, including mood disorders and psychosis, are common, affecting 50% to 83% of patients and they may be also the presenting symptom.[110] Age at onset is highly variable, ranging from the first to seventh decades and some subjects with profound calcium deposits may be asymptomatic. Computerized tomography (CT) is the most helpful neuroimaging method for depicting calcifications as hyperdense areas (**Fig. 9**). MRI is less reliable because calcifications may be depicted as hypointense, isointense, or hyperintense areas. The most common picture is hypointensities in T2w images, similar to iron deposits. CT is thus necessary to distinguish iron from calcium deposits in these cases. White-matter hyperintensities of presumed vascular origin are common.[111] The most frequent cause of PFBC, accounting for approximately 40% to 50% of cases, is mutation in the *SLC20A2* gene encoding the inorganic phosphate transporter PiT2. To date, more than 30 mutations in families of various ethnicities have been reported.[112,113] Mutation in the *PDGFRB* gene encoding the platelet-derived growth factor receptor family type β (PDGFRβ) has been reported in 2 families and 1 sporadic case with PFBC from France and the United States.[111,114] Approximately 10 PFBC cases were found to harbor mutations in the *PDGFB* gene encoding platelet-derived growth factor B, which is a ligand for PDGFRβ.[115,116] All known PFBC mutations are AD disorders. It is likely that other causative genes will be identified in the near future.[117]

In the differential diagnosis, it is important to exclude secondary causes, namely endocrine disorders, such as hypoparathyroidism, pseudohypoparathyroidism, or autoimmune polyglandular syndrome. Other secondary causes are inflammatory (systemic lupus erythematosus), infectious (brucellosis, toxoplasmosis), and neoplastic (leukemia), as well as chemotherapy and radiotherapy. Calcifications may be present in several neurodegenerative and hereditary disorders, such as Cockayne syndrome, Aicardi-Goutieres syndrome, and polycystic lipomembranous osteodysplasia with sclerosing encephalopathy.[117] The laboratory routine should include serum phosphorus, calcium, electrolytes, renal and liver function tests, and parathormone and thyroid hormone levels. Calcifications limited to GP found incidentally in elderly subjects are prevalent (5.5%–20.0%) but likely have no clinical significance.[115,118]

There is currently no established therapy. Improvement of symptoms after bisphosphonate treatment (etidronate disodium 15 mg/kg divided twice daily for 6 months) was documented in a few case studies.[119]

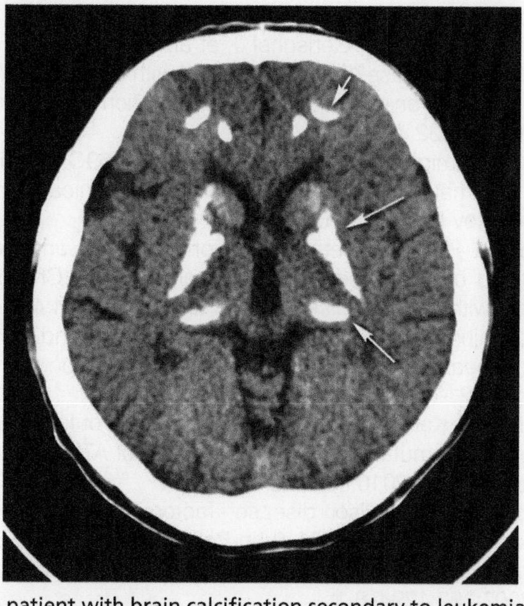

Fig. 9. CT scan of a patient with brain calcification secondary to leukemia and cranial radiotherapy. Arrows indicate calcifications in basal ganglia, thalamus, and white matter. (*Courtesy of* Dr A. Burgetova, Department of Radiology, 1.LFUK a VFN, Prague.)

SUMMARY

Disorders with brain metal accumulation are rare but important from the therapeutic perspective. Metal accumulation advances insidiously, and may be asymptomatic for a long time. When diagnosis is made and chelation therapy initiated, already profound metal accumulation and irreversible brain damage has been done. This is true especially for systemic metal overload disorders, such as WD, manganese transporter deficiency, and aceruloplasminemia. One cannot stress enough the importance of timely diagnosis and initiation of chelation therapy. Imaging biomarkers and availability of genetic examination can improve prognosis of these disorders by facilitating chelation therapy in the presymptomatic stage.

SUPPLEMENTARY DATA

Supplementary data related to this article can be found online at http://dx.doi.org/10.1016/j.ncl.2014.09.006

REFERENCES

1. Roberts EA, Schilsky ML, American Association for Study of Liver Diseases. Diagnosis and treatment of Wilson disease: an update. Hepatology 2008;47:2089–111.
2. European Association for Study of Liver. EASL Clinical Practice Guidelines: Wilson's disease. J Hepatol 2012;56:671–85.
3. Coffey AJ, Durkie M, Hague S, et al. A genetic study of Wilson's disease in the United Kingdom. Brain 2013;136:1476–87.
4. Stapelbroek JM, Bollen CW, van Amstel JK, et al. The H1069Q mutation in ATP7B is associated with late and neurologic presentation in Wilson disease: results of a meta-analysis. J Hepatol 2004;41:758–63.
5. Gromadzka G, Schmidt HH, Genschel J, et al. Frameshift and nonsense mutations in the gene for ATPase7B are associated with severe impairment of copper metabolism and with an early clinical manifestation of Wilson's disease. Clin Genet 2005;68:524–32.
6. Gromadzka G, Schmidt HH, Genschel J, et al. p.H1069Q mutation in ATP7B and biochemical parameters of copper metabolism and clinical manifestation of Wilson's disease. Mov Disord 2006;21:245–8.
7. Gu YH, Kodama H, Du SL, et al. Mutation spectrum and polymorphisms in ATP7B identified on direct sequencing of all exons in Chinese Han and Hui ethnic patients with Wilson's disease. Clin Genet 2003;64:479–84.
8. Al Jumah M, Majumdar R, Al Rajeh S, et al. A clinical and genetic study of 56 Saudi Wilson disease patients: identification of Saudi-specific mutations. Eur J Neurol 2004;11:121–4.
9. Okada T, Shiono Y, Kaneko Y, et al. High prevalence of fulminant hepatic failure among patients with mutant alleles for truncation of ATP7B in Wilson's disease. Scand J Gastroenterol 2010;45:1232–7.
10. Litwin T, Czlonkowska A. Wilson disease - factors affecting clinical presentation. Neurol Neurochir Pol 2013;47:161–9 [in Polish].
11. Ferenci P, Czlonkowska A, Merle U, et al. Late-onset Wilson's disease. Gastroenterology 2007;132:1294–8.
12. Ala A, Borjigin J, Rochwarger A, et al. Wilson disease in septuagenarian siblings: raising the bar for diagnosis. Hepatology 2005;41:668–70.

13. Ferenci P, Caca K, Loudianos G, et al. Diagnosis and phenotypic classification of Wilson disease. Liver Int 2003;23:139–42.
14. Litwin T, Gromadzka G, Czlonkowska A. Gender differences in Wilson's disease. J Neurol Sci 2012;312:31–5.
15. Czlonkowska A, Tarnacka B, Moller JC, et al. Unified Wilson's disease rating scale - a proposal for the neurological scoring of Wilson's disease patients. Neurol Neurochir Pol 2007;41:1–12.
16. Carta M, Mura G, Sorbello O, et al. Quality of life and psychiatric symptoms in Wilson's disease: the relevance of bipolar disorders. Clin Pract Epidemiol Ment Health 2012;8:102–9.
17. Dening TR, Berrios GE. Wilson's disease. Psychiatric symptoms in 195 cases. Arch Gen Psychiatry 1989;46:1126–34.
18. Srinivas K, Sinha S, Taly AB, et al. Dominant psychiatric manifestations in Wilson's disease: a diagnostic and therapeutic challenge! J Neurol Sci 2008;266:104–8.
19. Svetel M, Potrebic A, Pekmezovic T, et al. Neuropsychiatric aspects of treated Wilson's disease. Parkinsonism Relat Disord 2009;15:772–5.
20. Litwin T, Gromadzka G, Czlonkowska A, et al. The effect of gender on brain MRI pathology in Wilson's disease. Metab Brain Dis 2013;28:69–75.
21. Magalhaes AC, Caramelli P, Menezes JR, et al. Wilson's disease: MRI with clinical correlation. Neuroradiology 1994;36:97–100.
22. King AD, Walshe JM, Kendall BE, et al. Cranial MR imaging in Wilson's disease. AJR Am J Roentgenol 1996;167:1579–84.
23. da Costa Mdo D, Spitz M, Bacheschi LA, et al. Wilson's disease: two treatment modalities. Correlations to pretreatment and posttreatment brain MRI. Neuroradiology 2009;51:627–33.
24. Prayer L, Wimberger D, Kramer J, et al. Cranial MRI in Wilson's disease. Neuroradiology 1990;32:211–4.
25. Walter U, Krolikowski K, Tarnacka B, et al. Sonographic detection of basal ganglia lesions in asymptomatic and symptomatic Wilson disease. Neurology 2005;64:1726–32.
26. Medici V, Di Leo V, Lamboglia F, et al. Effect of penicillamine and zinc on iron metabolism in Wilson's disease. Scand J Gastroenterol 2007;42:1495–500.
27. Czlonkowska A, Gajda J, Rodo M. Effects of long-term treatment in Wilson's disease with D-penicillamine and zinc sulphate. J Neurol 1996;243:269–73.
28. Czlonkowska A, Tarnacka B, Litwin T, et al. Wilson's disease-cause of mortality in 164 patients during 1992-2003 observation period. J Neurol 2005;252:698–703.
29. Czlonkowska A, Litwin T, Karlinski M, et al. D-penicillamine versus zinc sulfate as first-line therapy for Wilson's disease. Eur J Neurol 2014;21:599–606.
30. Dziezyc K, Karlinski M, Litwin T, et al. Compliant treatment with anti-copper agents prevents clinically overt Wilson's disease in pre-symptomatic patients. Eur J Neurol 2014;21:332–7.
31. Walshe JM. Penicillamine, a new oral therapy for Wilson's disease. Am J Med 1956;21:487–95.
32. Hoogenraad TU, Van Hattum J, Van den Hamer CJ. Management of Wilson's disease with zinc sulphate. Experience in a series of 27 patients. J Neurol Sci 1987;77:137–46.
33. Brewer GJ, Terry CA, Aisen AM, et al. Worsening of neurologic syndrome in patients with Wilson's disease with initial penicillamine therapy. Arch Neurol 1987; 44:490–3.
34. Brewer GJ. Penicillamine should not be used as initial therapy in Wilson's disease. Mov Disord 1999;14:551–4.

35. Brewer GJ. Neurologically presenting Wilson's disease: epidemiology, pathophysiology and treatment. CNS Drugs 2005;19:185–92.
36. Brewer GJ. Zinc and tetrathiomolybdate for the treatment of Wilson's disease and the potential efficacy of anticopper therapy in a wide variety of diseases. Metallomics 2009;1:199–206.
37. Weiss KH, Gotthardt DN, Klemm D, et al. Zinc monotherapy is not as effective as chelating agents in treatment of Wilson disease. Gastroenterology 2011;140:1189–98.e1.
38. Weiss KH, Thurik F, Gotthardt DN, et al. Efficacy and safety of oral chelators in treatment of patients with Wilson disease. Clin Gastroenterol Hepatol 2013;11:1028–35.e1–2.
39. Wiggelinkhuizen M, Tilanus ME, Bollen CW, et al. Systematic review: clinical efficacy of chelator agents and zinc in the initial treatment of Wilson disease. Aliment Pharmacol Ther 2009;29:947–58.
40. Kim B, Chung SJ, Shin HW. Trientine-induced neurological deterioration in a patient with Wilson's disease. J Clin Neurosci 2013;20:606–8.
41. Medici V, Trevisan CP, D'Inca R, et al. Diagnosis and management of Wilson's disease: results of a single center experience. J Clin Gastroenterol 2006;40:936–41.
42. Kalita J, Kumar V, Chandra S, et al. Worsening of Wilson disease following penicillamine therapy. Eur Neurol 2014;71:126–31.
43. Ranucci G, Di Dato F, Spagnuolo MI, et al. Zinc monotherapy is effective in Wilson's disease patients with mild liver disease diagnosed in childhood: a retrospective study. Orphanet J Rare Dis 2014;9:41.
44. Aggarwal A, Bhatt M. The Pragmatic Treatment of Wilson's Disease. Mov Disord Clin Pract 2014;1:14–23.
45. Dhawan A, Taylor RM, Cheeseman P, et al. Wilson's disease in children: 37-year experience and revised King's score for liver transplantation. Liver Transpl 2005;11:441–8.
46. Litwin T, Gromadzka G, Czlonkowska A. Neurological presentation of Wilson's disease in a patient after liver transplantation. Mov Disord 2008;23:743–6.
47. Stracciari A, Tempestini A, Borghi A, et al. Effect of liver transplantation on neurological manifestations in Wilson disease. Arch Neurol 2000;57:384–6.
48. Weiss KH, Schafer M, Gotthardt DN, et al. Outcome and development of symptoms after orthotopic liver transplantation for Wilson disease. Clin Transplant 2013;27:914–22.
49. Weiss KH, Stremmel W. Clinical considerations for an effective medical therapy in Wilson's disease. Ann N Y Acad Sci 2014;1315:81–5.
50. Hedera P. Treatment of Wilson's disease motor complications with deep brain stimulation. Ann N Y Acad Sci 2014;1315:16–23.
51. Litwin T, Chabik G, Czlonkowska A. Acute focal dystonia induced by a tricyclic antidepressant in a patient with Wilson disease: a case report. Neurol Neurochir Pol 2013;47:502–6.
52. Merle U, Schaefer M, Ferenci P, et al. Clinical presentation, diagnosis and long-term outcome of Wilson's disease: a cohort study. Gut 2007;56:115–20.
53. Bruha R, Marecek Z, Pospisilova L, et al. Long-term follow-up of Wilson disease: natural history, treatment, mutations analysis and phenotypic correlation. Liver Int 2011;31:83–91.
54. Svetel M, Pekmezovic T, Petrovic I, et al. Long-term outcome in Serbian patients with Wilson disease. Eur J Neurol 2009;16:852–7.

55. Beinhardt S, Leiss W, Stattermayer AF, et al. Long-term outcomes of patients with Wilson disease in a large Austrian cohort. Clin Gastroenterol Hepatol 2014;12:683–9.
56. Kruer MC, Salih MA, Mooney C, et al. C19orf12 mutation leads to a pallido-pyramidal syndrome. Gene 2014;537:352–6.
57. Dusek P, Jankovic J, Le W. Iron dysregulation in movement disorders. Neurobiol Dis 2012;46:1–18.
58. Hogarth P, Gregory A, Kruer MC, et al. New NBIA subtype: genetic, clinical, pathologic, and radiographic features of MPAN. Neurology 2013;80:268–75.
59. Hartig MB, Iuso A, Haack T, et al. Absence of an orphan mitochondrial protein, c19orf12, causes a distinct clinical subtype of neurodegeneration with brain iron accumulation. Am J Hum Genet 2011;89:543–50.
60. Panteghini C, Zorzi G, Venco P, et al. C19orf12 and FA2H mutations are rare in Italian patients with neurodegeneration with brain iron accumulation. Semin Pediatr Neurol 2012;19:75–81.
61. Gregory A, Polster BJ, Hayflick SJ. Clinical and genetic delineation of neurodegeneration with brain iron accumulation. J Med Genet 2009;46:73–80.
62. Hartig M, Prokisch H, Meitinger T, et al. Mitochondrial membrane protein-associated neurodegeneration (MPAN). Int Rev Neurobiol 2013;110:73–84.
63. Kurian MA, Hayflick SJ. Pantothenate kinase-associated neurodegeneration (PKAN) and PLA2G6-associated neurodegeneration (PLAN): review of two major neurodegeneration with brain iron accumulation (NBIA) phenotypes. Int Rev Neurobiol 2013;110:49–71.
64. Saitsu H, Nishimura T, Muramatsu K, et al. De novo mutations in the autophagy gene WDR45 cause static encephalopathy of childhood with neurodegeneration in adulthood. Nat Genet 2013;45:445–9, 449e1.
65. Hayflick SJ, Kruer MC, Gregory A, et al. beta-Propeller protein-associated neurodegeneration: a new X-linked dominant disorder with brain iron accumulation. Brain 2013;136:1708–17.
66. Haack TB, Hogarth P, Kruer MC, et al. Exome sequencing reveals de novo WDR45 mutations causing a phenotypically distinct, X-linked dominant form of NBIA. Am J Hum Genet 2012;91:1144–9.
67. Keogh MJ, Morris CM, Chinnery PF. Neuroferritinopathy. Int Rev Neurobiol 2013;110:91–123.
68. Miyajima H, Kohno S, Takahashi Y, et al. Estimation of the gene frequency of aceruloplasminemia in Japan. Neurology 1999;53:617–9.
69. Kono S. Aceruloplasminemia: an update. Int Rev Neurobiol 2013;110:125–51.
70. Rupps R, Hukin J, Balicki M, et al. Novel mutations in FA2H-associated neurodegeneration: an underrecognized condition? J Child Neurol 2013;28:1500–4.
71. Gonzalez-Cuyar LF, Perry G, Miyajima H, et al. Redox active iron accumulation in aceruloplasminemia. Neuropathology 2008;28:466–71.
72. Curtis AR, Fey C, Morris CM, et al. Mutation in the gene encoding ferritin light polypeptide causes dominant adult-onset basal ganglia disease. Nat Genet 2001;28:350–4.
73. Paisan-Ruiz C, Li A, Schneider SA, et al. Widespread Lewy body and tau accumulation in childhood and adult onset dystonia-parkinsonism cases with PLA2G6 mutations. Neurobiol Aging 2012;33:814–23.
74. Schneider SA, Dusek P, Hardy J, et al. Genetics and pathophysiology of neurodegeneration with brain iron accumulation (NBIA). Curr Neuropharmacol 2013;11:59–79.

75. Deschauer M, Gaul C, Behrmann C, et al. C19orf12 mutations in neurodegeneration with brain iron accumulation mimicking juvenile amyotrophic lateral sclerosis. J Neurol 2012;259:2434–9.
76. Landoure G, Zhu PP, Lourenco CM, et al. Hereditary spastic paraplegia type 43 (SPG43) is caused by mutation in C19orf12. Hum Mutat 2013;34:1357–60.
77. Engel LA, Jing Z, O'Brien DE, et al. Catalytic function of PLA2G6 is impaired by mutations associated with infantile neuroaxonal dystrophy but not dystonia-parkinsonism. PLoS One 2010;5:e12897.
78. Haack TB, Hogarth P, Gregory A, et al. BPAN: the only X-linked dominant NBIA disorder. Int Rev Neurobiol 2013;110:85–90.
79. McNeill A, Birchall D, Hayflick SJ, et al. T2* and FSE MRI distinguishes four subtypes of neurodegeneration with brain iron accumulation. Neurology 2008;70:1614–9.
80. McNeill A, Pandolfo M, Kuhn J, et al. The neurological presentation of ceruloplasmin gene mutations. Eur Neurol 2008;60:200–5.
81. Miyajima H, Kono S, Takahashi Y, et al. Cerebellar ataxia associated with heteroallelic ceruloplasmin gene mutation. Neurology 2001;57:2205–10.
82. Chinnery PF, Crompton DE, Birchall D, et al. Clinical features and natural history of neuroferritinopathy caused by the FTL1 460InsA mutation. Brain 2007;130:110–9.
83. Keogh MJ, Jonas P, Coulthard A, et al. Neuroferritinopathy: a new inborn error of iron metabolism. Neurogenetics 2012;13:93–6.
84. Devos D, Tchofo PJ, Vuillaume I, et al. Clinical features and natural history of neuroferritinopathy caused by the 458dupA FTL mutation. Brain 2009;132:e109.
85. Ory-Magne F, Brefel-Courbon C, Payoux P, et al. Clinical phenotype and neuroimaging findings in a French family with hereditary ferritinopathy (FTL498-499InsTC). Mov Disord 2009;24:1676–83.
86. Girelli D, Corrocher R, Bisceglia L, et al. Molecular basis for the recently described hereditary hyperferritinemia-cataract syndrome: a mutation in the iron-responsive element of ferritin L-subunit gene (the "Verona mutation"). Blood 1995;86:4050–3.
87. Dusi S, Valletta L, Haack TB, et al. Exome sequence reveals mutations in CoA synthase as a cause of neurodegeneration with brain iron accumulation. Am J Hum Genet 2014;94:11–22.
88. Alderson NL, Rembiesa BM, Walla MD, et al. The human FA2H gene encodes a fatty acid 2-hydroxylase. J Biol Chem 2004;279:48562–8.
89. Cao L, Huang XJ, Chen CJ, et al. A rare family with Hereditary Spastic Paraplegia Type 35 due to novel FA2H mutations: a case report with literature review. J Neurol Sci 2013;329:1–5.
90. Suzuki Y, Yoshida K, Aburakawa Y, et al. Effectiveness of oral iron chelator treatment with deferasirox in an aceruloplasminemia patient with a novel ceruloplasmin gene mutation. Intern Med 2013;52:1527–30.
91. Skidmore FM, Drago V, Foster P, et al. Aceruloplasminaemia with progressive atrophy without brain iron overload: treatment with oral chelation. J Neurol Neurosurg Psychiatry 2008;79:467–70.
92. Finkenstedt A, Wolf E, Hofner E, et al. Hepatic but not brain iron is rapidly chelated by deferasirox in aceruloplasminemia due to a novel gene mutation. J Hepatol 2010;53:1101–7.
93. Mariani R, Arosio C, Pelucchi S, et al. Iron chelation therapy in aceruloplasminaemia: study of a patient with a novel missense mutation. Gut 2004;53:756–8.

94. Rusticeanu M, Zimmer V, Schleithoff L, et al. Novel ceruloplasmin mutation causing aceruloplasminemia with hepatic iron overload and diabetes without neurological symptoms. Clin Genet 2014;85:300–1.
95. Tai M, Matsuhashi N, Ichii O, et al. Case of presymptomatic aceruloplasminemia treated with deferasirox. Hepatol Res 2013. http://dx.doi.org/10.1111/hepr.12292.
96. Roberti Mdo R, Borges Filho HM, Goncalves CH, et al. Aceruloplasminemia: a rare disease - diagnosis and treatment of two cases. Rev Bras Hematol Hemoter 2011;33:389–92.
97. Yonekawa M, Okabe T, Asamoto Y, et al. A case of hereditary ceruloplasmin deficiency with iron deposition in the brain associated with chorea, dementia, diabetes mellitus and retinal pigmentation: administration of fresh-frozen human plasma. Eur Neurol 1999;42:157–62.
98. Kuhn J, Bewermeyer H, Miyajima H, et al. Treatment of symptomatic heterozygous aceruloplasminemia with oral zinc sulphate. Brain Dev 2007;29:450–3.
99. Zorzi G, Zibordi F, Chiapparini L, et al. Iron-related MRI images in patients with pantothenate kinase-associated neurodegeneration (PKAN) treated with deferiprone: results of a phase II pilot trial. Mov Disord 2011;26:1756–9.
100. Abbruzzese G, Cossu G, Balocco M, et al. A pilot trial of deferiprone for neurodegeneration with brain iron accumulation. Haematologica 2011;96:1708–11.
101. Cossu G, Abbruzzese G, Matta G, et al. Efficacy and safety of deferiprone for the treatment of pantothenate kinase-associated neurodegeneration (PKAN) and neurodegeneration with brain iron accumulation (NBIA): Results from a four years follow-up. Parkinsonism Relat Disord 2014;20:651–4.
102. Zorzi G, Nardocci N. Therapeutic advances in neurodegeneration with brain iron accumulation. Int Rev Neurobiol 2013;110:153–64.
103. Timmermann L, Pauls KA, Wieland K, et al. Dystonia in neurodegeneration with brain iron accumulation: outcome of bilateral pallidal stimulation. Brain 2010;133:701–12.
104. Tuschl K, Clayton PT, Gospe SM Jr, et al. Syndrome of hepatic cirrhosis, dystonia, polycythemia, and hypermanganesemia caused by mutations in SLC30A10, a manganese transporter in man. Am J Hum Genet 2012;90:457–66.
105. Tuschl K, Mills PB, Clayton PT. Manganese and the brain. Int Rev Neurobiol 2013;110:277–312.
106. Quadri M, Federico A, Zhao T, et al. Mutations in SLC30A10 cause parkinsonism and dystonia with hypermanganesemia, polycythemia, and chronic liver disease. Am J Hum Genet 2012;90:467–77.
107. Delnooz CC, Wevers RA, Quadri M, et al. Phenotypic variability in a dystonia family with mutations in the manganese transporter gene. Mov Disord 2013;28:685–6.
108. Stamelou M, Tuschl K, Chong WK, et al. Dystonia with brain manganese accumulation resulting from SLC30A10 mutations: a new treatable disorder. Mov Disord 2012;27:1317–22.
109. Ribeiro RT, dos Santos-Neto D, Braga-Neto P, et al. Inherited manganism. Clin Neurol Neurosurg 2013;115:1536–8.
110. Nicolas G, Pottier C, Charbonnier C, et al. Phenotypic spectrum of probable and genetically-confirmed idiopathic basal ganglia calcification. Brain 2013;136:3395–407.
111. Nicolas G, Pottier C, Maltete D, et al. Mutation of the PDGFRB gene as a cause of idiopathic basal ganglia calcification. Neurology 2013;80:181–7.

112. Yamada M, Tanaka M, Takagi M, et al. Evaluation of SLC20A2 mutations that cause idiopathic basal ganglia calcification in Japan. Neurology 2014;82: 705–12.
113. Wang C, Li Y, Shi L, et al. Mutations in SLC20A2 link familial idiopathic basal ganglia calcification with phosphate homeostasis. Nat Genet 2012;44:254–6.
114. Sanchez-Contreras M, Baker MC, Finch NA, et al. Genetic Screening and Functional Characterization of PDGFRB Mutations Associated with Basal Ganglia Calcification of Unknown Etiology. Hum Mutat 2014;35:964–71.
115. Nicolas G, Richard AC, Pottier C, et al. Overall mutational spectrum of SLC20A2, PDGFB and PDGFRB in idiopathic basal ganglia calcification. Neurogenetics 2014;15:215–6.
116. Nicolas G, Jacquin A, Thauvin-Robinet C, et al. A de novo nonsense PDGFB mutation causing idiopathic basal ganglia calcification with laryngeal dystonia. Eur J Hum Genet 2014. http://dx.doi.org/10.1038/ejhg.2014.9.
117. Lemos RR, Ferreira JB, Keasey MP, et al. An update on primary familial brain calcification. Int Rev Neurobiol 2013;110:349–71.
118. Yamada M, Asano T, Okamoto K, et al. High frequency of calcification in basal ganglia on brain computed tomography images in Japanese older adults. Geriatr Gerontol Int 2013;13:706–10.
119. Loeb JA, Sohrab SA, Huq M, et al. Brain calcifications induce neurological dysfunction that can be reversed by a bone drug. J Neurol Sci 2006;243:77–81.

Psychogenic Movement Disorders

Mary Ann Thenganatt, MD*, Joseph Jankovic, MD

KEYWORDS

• Psychogenic • Movement disorders • Tremor • Dystonia • Myoclonus
• Parkinsonism • Tics • Paroxysmal dyskinesia

KEY POINTS

- Psychogenic movement disorders (PMDs) can present with a broad spectrum of phenomenology that may resemble but can be differentiated from organic movement disorders by careful history and examination, sometimes supplemented by ancillary tests.
- PMDs often have an abrupt onset with a rapid progression to maximum severity and spontaneous remissions and exacerbations.
- PMDs share several characteristic findings on examination, such as variability, distractibility, entrainment, and suggestibility.
- Ancillary tests, including functional imaging, electroencephalography, electromyography, and other neurophysiologic techniques, are primarily used in a research setting but may be helpful in some cases where the diagnosis is in doubt.
- There are no evidence-based guidelines for the diagnosis and treatment of PMDs but they may include a multidisciplinary approach involving a neurologist, psychiatrist, psychologist, and physical, occupational, and speech therapist.
- The pathogenesis of PMDs is not well understood but psychological stress and physical trauma often trigger or are associated with the onset of the movement disorder.

Videos of convergence spasm, psychogenic tremor, psychogenic dystonia, psychogenic myoclonus, psychogenic parkinsonism, psychogenic tics, psychogenic paroxysmal dyskinesia, psychogenic gait, psychogenic chorea, and psychogenic facial spasm accompany this article at http://www.neurologic.theclinics.com/

INTRODUCTION

PMDs represent one of the largest categories of psychogenic neurologic disorders. Traditionally, PMDs have been considered a manifestation of an underlying psychological stressor and have been evaluated and managed by both neurologists and

Department of Neurology, Parkinson's Disease Center and Movement Disorders Clinic, Baylor College of Medicine, The Smith Tower, Suite 1801, 6550 Fannin, Houston, Texas 77030, USA
* Corresponding author.
E-mail address: mary.thenganatt@bcm.edu

Neurol Clin 33 (2015) 205–224
http://dx.doi.org/10.1016/j.ncl.2014.09.013 neurologic.theclinics.com
0733-8619/15/$ – see front matter

psychiatrists. Despite the increasing recognition of PMDs and the considerable distress and disability they can cause patients, family members, and caregivers, physicians are largely unfamiliar with this group of disorders. Often patients are evaluated by numerous specialists and undergo multiple investigations prior to diagnosis, usually at a tertiary care movement disorders center. It is important to keep in mind that patients with a PMD can have a coexisting organic disorder, and distinguishing the 2 within a given patient may be challenging. Early diagnosis and treatment are essential for improving outcomes and reducing socioeconomic burden on patients and society. This review discusses advancing knowledge of various PMDs, including epidemiology, clinical characteristics, ancillary testing, pathophysiology, therapeutic options, and prognosis.

NOMENCLATURE AND DIAGNOSTIC CRITERIA

This review uses the term, *psychogenic movement disorder (PMD)*, acknowledging that there is considerable debate about the appropriate nomenclature. Several other terms have been used in the literature, including *hysteria*, *functional*, *nonorganic*, *medically unexplained*, and *conversion disorder* (**Box 1**).[1,2] The authors prefer the term *psychogenic* to *functional* because the latter term seems vague and patients perceive themselves as dysfunctional rather than functional. When the term psychogenic is introduced to patients in a sensitive and tactful way and patients are reassured that there is no evidence of neurologic damage, they are more willing to

Box 1
Psychogenic movement disorders terminology

Psychogenic

Although it suggests a purely psychological etiology, it is widely used among neurologists, implying biopsychosocial pathogenesis.

Functional

It does not address disability because patients perceive themselves unable to function (dysfunctional rather than functional).

Nonorganic

"Organic" is not well defined. It implies a nondiagnosis.

Conversion disorder

According to the *Diagnostic and Statistical Manual of Mental Disorders*, it requires an identifiable trigger.

Psychosomatic

In its true intended sense, it implies an interaction between mind and body manifested by multiple physical symptoms.

Medically unexplained

It may become obsolete as better understanding is gained of the underlying pathogenesis. Also it is impractical when conveying the diagnosis to patients.

Dissociative motor disorder

There is a lack of evidence that dissociation is the underlying mechanism.

Hysterical

It suggests a link between symptoms and uterus and carries substantial stigma.

accept the role of psychodynamic factors, such as stress, in their condition and are more amenable to psychological and psychiatric intervention. Most patients understand that stress can cause elevation in blood pressure, palpitations, and tremors, so they can also accept that dystonia or other movement disorders can be a manifestation of stress or other psychological factors.[2]

PMDs are distinguished from factitious disorder and malingering in that the latter 2 involve intentional deception.[3] Factitious disorder involves the fabrication of physical or psychological symptoms; the patients presenting themselves as ill without an obvious external reward. Malingering, on the other hand, involves the falsification of symptoms for secondary gain, such as avoiding employment or obtaining financial compensation. Fabricated or induced illness imposed on another, typically a child, was previously known as Munchausen syndrome by proxy.[4] It involves deception on the part of the caregiver regarding physical or mental illness of the child to obtain excessive medical testing and care. Up to 10% of patients with factitious disorders have Munchausen syndrome or Munchausen by proxy, characterized by simulated illness, pathologic living (pseudologia fantastica), and wandering from place to place (peregrination). These individuals may also have underlying organic illness. Early recognition of the features suggesting a fabricated illness is important to prevent a child from undergoing unnecessary invasive testing and procedures.

Although there are no evidence-based guidelines or gold standard for the diagnosis of PMDs, there are 2 main diagnostic criteria described in the literature. The Fahn-Williams diagnostic criteria are the most widely used and categorize patients into 4 categories: documented, clinically established, probably, and possible (**Box 2**).[5] Shill and Gerber[6] modified these diagnostic criteria, which place greater emphasis on historical information. The inter-rater reliability of diagnosis using the Fahn-Williams and Shill-Gerber criteria was evaluated among movement disorder neurologists and general neurologists.[7] Based on video evaluation of phenomenology alone, there was a low level of diagnostic agreement among raters, and diagnosis relied heavily on clinical history and diagnostic work-up. A survey about the diagnostic and treatment practices for PMDs of 509 neurologists who were members of the Movement Disorders Society found that even when patients showed definite signs of a PMD, only

Box 2
Fahn-Williams criteria for the diagnosis of psychogenic movement disorders

Documented

Persistent relief by psychotherapy, suggestion, or placebo has been demonstrated, which may be helped by physiotherapy, or the patient was seen without the movement disorder when believing himself or herself unobserved.

Clinically established

The movement disorder is incongruent with a classical movement disorder or there are inconsistencies in the examination, plus at least 1 of the following 3: other psychogenic signs, multiple somatizations, or an obvious psychiatric disturbance.

Probable

The movement disorder is incongruent or inconsistent with typical movement disorders or there are psychogenic signs or multiple somatizations.

Possible

Evidence of an emotional disturbance.

From Fahn S, Williams DT. Psychogenic dystonia. Adv Neurol 1988;50:431–55; with permission.

20% of neurologists informed patients of the diagnosis without additional diagnostic testing[8]; 50% reported conducting additional diagnostic testing to rule out organic causes. This practice often reflects limited experience of the neurologists because it was associated with fewer years of fellowship training and a smaller PMD population in their practice.

PREVALENCE AND RISK FACTORS

The reported prevalence of PMDs at movement disorders clinic varies from 2% to 20%.[9] These disorders are associated with marked disability and distress, reported to be similar to or greater than those reported by patients with neurodegenerative disease, such as Parkinson disease.[10] A study evaluating the social impact of disease in patients with psychogenic neurologic disorders found these patients to have worse physical and mental health status compared with controls.[11] They were also more likely to be unemployed due to medical reasons and to be obtaining disability benefits.

Although the underlying cause of PMDs is not well understood, there are several risk factors associated with this group of disorders. Nearly all studies have shown that PMDs are more common in women, accounting for 70% to 80% of all cases.[12] Although PMDs are most common in young adults, before age 50, they have also been reported in children and the elderly.[13–16] Among reports of PMDs in children, girls were more frequently affected, but there was no female predominance with onset prior to age 13.[13] Two-thirds of children demonstrated multiple phenotypes with the most common being tremor, dystonia, and myclonus. Children experienced marked disability with prolonged absences from school and underwent unnecessary surgical procedures. PMDs in children should be differentiated from several childhood disorders that are often misdiagnosed as psychogenic (**Box 3**). On the other end of the spectrum, in a retrospective review of PMDs in patients with an age at onset greater than 60 years, tremor was the most common PMD and gait abnormalities and psychogenic seizures were more common compared with younger patients.[16] Besides female gender, other risk factors associated with PMDs include history of childhood trauma, such as emotional, physical, and sexual abuse.[17] Not all patients with PMDs, however, report a psychological stressor. Recent physical events may also be associated with the development of PMDs, including physical injury, infection, neurologic illness, drug reaction, surgery, and vasovagal syncope.[18] Although a positive family history may suggest organic disease, a report of 10 cases of PMDs from 5

Box 3
Childhood organic disorders commonly misdiagnosed as psychogenic movement disorders

- Paroxysmal dyskinesia
- Episodic ataxia
- Dopa-responsive dystonia
- Rapid-onset dystonia-parkinsonism
- Task-specific dystonia
- Acute drug-induced dystonia
- Tourette syndrome
- Sandifer syndrome
- Stereotypic masturbatory behavior

families showed similar phenomenology in affected family members.[19] Thus, a detailed examination of affected family members can help with diagnosis and a family history of a PMD may be a risk factor. PMDs occurring in large groups of individuals have also been reported in the media (http://www.nytimes.com/2012/01/29/opinion/sunday/adolescent-girl-hysteria.html; http://www.nytimes.com/2009/07/30) and in the scientific literature as manifestations of "mass hysteria."[20]

CLINICAL FEATURES

The clinical history and neurologic examination provide the essential information needed to arrive at a clinical diagnosis. It is important to inquire about the circumstances regarding the onset of symptoms, the progression of symptoms, and variation over time. Additional history about other unexplained medical conditions, investigations, and procedures as well as social and family history can provide important contextual information regarding a patient's clinical and social environment.

HISTORICAL FEATURES

PMDs typically have an abrupt onset with a rapid progression to maximum severity. Patients often recall the exact moment symptoms started and what they were doing at the time. The movements may be paroxysmal or episodic with spontaneous remissions and recurrences.[21] Patients may describe a change in phenomenology over time. In addition to their motor symptoms, many have marked somatization and present a long list of other unexplained medical symptoms, such as atypical chest pain, fibromyalgia, chronic fatigue, and irritable bowel syndrome. Some of them use a variety of devices, such as canes, crutches, and sunglasses, and may even show regressive behavior, such as forming attachments with stuffed animals.[22] Most PMD patients have seen multiple medical professionals and some have undergone numerous investigations and surgical procedures before the correct diagnosis is made. There may be impending litigation, which may be a source of secondary gain and may be associated with more severe and persistent disability.[23] Patients may assume the "sick role" and become dependent on friends and family for assistance with activities of daily living.

GENERAL CLINICAL FINDINGS

Many features of PMDs can be noted through careful observation throughout the encounter in addition to focused examination (**Box 4**). The neurologic examination of PMDs often demonstrates variability of phenomenology in terms of direction, amplitude, and frequency. There can be distractibility of movements when focusing on other motor or mental tasks. Distractibility can be demonstrated by asking the patient to focus on motor tasks, such as finger tapping with the opposite hand, or more complex patterns of tapping, such as "1st finger, 3rd finger, 5th finger." There can also be distractibility with mental tasks, such as "serial sevens" or reciting the months of the year backwards. Suggestibility is another typical feature of PMDs. Thus, the movements may be either triggered or suppressed when a vibrating tuning fork is applied to the affected body part or even at a distant site along with a powerful suggestion that "vibration" has been known to cause or help abnormal movements. Entrainability refers to the adoption of a similar frequency as that of movements performed with the opposite limb, such as finger tapping or flexion-extension of the wrist. The movements may not necessarily entrain to the exact frequency but may adopt a harmonic of the frequency.

Box 4
Physical examination findings supportive of a diagnosis of psychogenic movement disorders

- Variability of direction, frequency, and amplitude
- Distractibility when focusing on other motor or mental tasks
- Entrainment
- Nonpatterned abnormal postures and spasms
- Suggestibility to sensory stimuli, such as a vibrating tuning fork or pressure applied to "trigger points"
- Giveway weakness
- Nonanatomic sensory findings
- Excessive startle to sensory stimuli
- Exaggerated response to minimal pull backwards
- Astasia-abasia, knee buckling, bouncing gait, monoplegic dragging gait
- Convergence spasm
- Deliberate slowness demonstrating excessive effort when performing rapid successive movements
- Abnormal speech pattern (hesitant and slow, bursts of verbal gibberish, changing dialects and accents)
- Facial grimacing, alternating facial contractions
- La belle indifference
- Demonstration of exhaustion and extreme effort to perform tasks

In addition to neurologic findings specific to the PMD, other physical findings can support a diagnosis of PMDs. Patients may demonstrate la belle indifference, not appearing concerned about their illness, and often smiling and giggling during the examination. They may embellish their symptoms, out of proportion to their mild neurologic deficits on examination; some use a cane or become confined to a wheelchair. Giveway weakness is manifested by a patient's initial resistance against an examiner's attempt to move a limb, followed by sudden loss of the active resistance (giveway). Other psychogenic features, including nonanatomic sensory loss, such as splitting the midline with vibratory sense, may be present. There may be an exaggerated (but often delayed) startle response to a sudden sound or exaggerated loss of balance on a pull test. Patients with PMDs may have convergence spasm (ocular convergence, miosis, and accommodation causing dysconjugate gaze), which has been shown to be more common in PMD patients than controls (Video 1).[24] Identifying the presence of these additional features on examination can support a diagnosis of a PMD. No one feature, however, is diagnostic and should be taken into consideration in the context of the entire clinical picture.

PSYCHOGENIC TREMOR

Psychogenic tremor comprises the largest subcategory of PMDs, reported to represent approximately 50% of cases.[25] Psychogenic tremor is often present in all states (rest, posture, and kinetic), which is not typical of organic tremor. Tremor may spread to different body parts, especially when 1 limb is restrained or occupied with another activity. There are several classic clinical features of psychogenic tremor that can be demonstrated in the clinic or at the bedside (Video 2).[26] Tremor variability may present as a change in direction, frequency, or amplitude. Tremor can be entrainable to the frequency of voluntary movements of the opposite limb, such as finger tapping or flexion-extension of the wrist. Tremor can be distractible, often with almost complete cessation of tremor, when focusing on another physical or mental task. Psychogenic tremor may be suggestible, either increasing or decreasing in severity to certain stimuli, such as an application of a tuning fork accompanied by a suggestion that the vibration may trigger, enhance, or suppress the tremor. There can be tremor coherence—the simultaneous presence of tremor in multiple body parts with similar frequency. Sometimes, physical restraint by an examiner of a limb tremor may trigger tremor in an anatomically distant body part. Episodic, especially total body, tremor is also suggestive of psychogenic tremor. These various clinical features have been evaluated for their sensitivity and specificity in discriminating psychogenic tremor from essential tremor involving 45 patients at Baylor College of Medicine.[27] Psychogenic tremor patients were more likely to report a sudden onset, spontaneous remission, and shorter duration of tremor whereas family history was more common in essential tremor. Psychogenic tremor was significantly associated with moderate–marked distractibility with alternate finger tapping and mental tasks compared with essential tremor. Suggestibility with a vibrating tuning fork and exacerbation with hyperventilation were associated with psychogenic tremor. Entrainability did not differ between psychogenic and essential tremor.

Although laboratory testing is often not necessary for the diagnosis of psychogenic tremor, neurophysiologic testing, including accelerometers and surface electromyography (EMG), can provide objective information, supporting a diagnosis of psychogenic tremor. Quantitative analysis demonstrated that in contrast to organic tremor, which decreases in amplitude with weight loading, psychogenic tremor paradoxically increases in tremor amplitude with weighting of the limb.[28] An early study demonstrated that the coactivation sign and absence of finger tremor were distinguishing features of psychogenic tremor from organic tremor.[28] The coactivation sign in psychogenic tremor refers to the coactivation of antagonistic muscles that underlies psychogenic tremor. Thus, when assessing muscle tone through passive range of motion about a joint, there is variability in tone and when completely relaxed the tremor also resolves. Thus the tremor requires coactivation of muscles to occur. With EMG, the coactivation sign can be demonstrated as a tonic contraction of antagonistic muscles prior to a burst of tremor. The coherence entrainment test, which evaluates the ability of a patient to tap at a frequency different from the tremor in the opposite limb, was evaluated in 25 patients with psychogenic or dystonic tremor and 10 controls.[29] Coherence of tremor frequency in multiple limbs, as well as tremor entrainment to the frequency of voluntary movements with the opposite limb, distinguished psychogenic tremor from organic tremor. Tremor may not entrain to the exact frequency of the contralateral limb movements but to a harmonic of that frequency.[30] One study demonstrated that tapping at a lower frequency of 3 Hz was more effective at eliciting entrainment than a faster frequency of 5 Hz.[30] Distractibility can be evaluated by asking patients to perform a ballistic movement with the contralateral limb. One study demonstrated a significant reduction of tremor amplitude or cessation of contralateral tremor in psychogenic tremor patients but not in patients with Parkinson disease or essential tremor.[31] Psychogenic patients are more likely to demonstrate dual-task interference when asked to perform a task while tremor is present. Delayed reaction times have been demonstrated in psychogenic patients compared with essential tremor and Parkinson disease patients when asked to perform a simple reaction time task.[32] Various neurophysiologic tests in patents with psychogenic tremor have shown that although psychogenic tremor is characterized by marked variability in tremor frequency, entrainability is rare.[33] Although no 1 neurophysiologic test has sufficient sensitivity and specificity to reliably differentiate between psychogenic and organic tremor, the overall performance on the group of tests could distinguish the 2 forms of tremor.

PSYCHOGENIC DYSTONIA

Psychogenic dystonia may present as fixed or mobile dystonia. Patient with psychogenic dystonia generally do not describe alleviating maneuvers or sensory tricks that are typically used by patients with organic dystonia to correct the abnormal posture.[34] Although the posture is fixed at rest, an examiner may be able to easily passively move the joint, or active resistance to passive range of motion may be detected. There may be variability of the abnormal posture in different states, without demonstrating a pattern to the abnormal movement. Psychogenic dystonia can also be suggestible with resolution of symptoms to a vibrating tuning fork or pressure applied to trigger points (Video 3). In contrast to mobile dystonia seen in patients with organic dystonia, psychogenic dystonia commonly presents as fixed dystonia affecting a limb. In contrast, organic dystonia is often action induced at onset and does not present with a fixed posture. Fixed dystonia is often preceded by a peripheral injury and is the most common presentation of peripherally induced movement disorders described in the literature.[35] In the largest reported series of patients with fixed dystonia, 84% of 103 patients were female, with a mean age at onset of 29.7 years.[36] The limbs were most commonly affected with rare involvement of the shoulders, neck, and jaw. In this series, 37% of patients met criteria for psychogenic dystonia, 29% somatization disorder, and 20% complex regional pain syndrome; 63% of patients had a preceding peripheral injury and 41% reported pain as a major complaint. After a structured neuropsychiatric interview, patients with fixed dystonia more commonly demonstrated features of dissociative and affective disorders compared with patients with classic dystonia. A follow-up study on 41 patients from this cohort at a mean of 7.6 years found that only 23% had improved, 31% worsened, and 6% achieved major remission. A baseline diagnosis of complex regional pain syndrome was associated with a poor outcome. Patients with fixed dystonia and complex regional pain syndrome, manifested by sensory, autonomic, and trophic features, have been shown to have a greater association with early traumatic experiences, general psychopathology, and somatoform dissociative experiences compared with normative data in the general population.[37] Although organic peripherally induced movement disorders have been well documented, some have argued that they are mostly psychogenic in origin and should not be considered a separate diagnostic entity.[38] The relationship between PMDs, peripherally induced movement disorders, and complex regional pain syndrome is not well understood and controversial.[39]

Although fixed dystonia is a characteristic manifestation of psychogenic dystonia, there are other presentations of psychogenic dystonia, including intermittent or paroxysmal dystonia.[21]

Neurophysiologic studies have not been able to reliably distinguish organic from psychogenic dystonia.[40] Short intercortical inhibition and contralateral silent period were found to be abnormal in patients with fixed dystonia, similar to organic dystonia, suggesting the underlying impairment of cortical excitability may predispose some patients to dystonia.[41] But similar abnormalities were also found in patients with psychogenic dystonia (discussed later).[42]

PSYCHOGENIC MYOCLONUS

Psychogenic myoclonus can be challenging to distinguish from organic myoclonus, which is characterized by intermittent random jerks. Patients with psychogenic myoclonus, however, can show distractibility when concentrating on other tasks or may have episodes of myoclonic jerks (Video 4). These patients may also demonstrate an excessive startle response to sensory stimuli, such as loud sounds. The largest reported series of 76 patients with psychogenic axial myoclonus described flexor spasms, similar to what has been reported in patients with propriospinal myoclonus, as the most common presentation.[43] In 42.1% of patients, the jerks were multifocal without a stereotyped pattern. More than half of patients had a prolonged muscle contraction after the jerks or additional features, such as psychogenic tremor or a psychogenic gait pattern. A preceding event, such as a minor surgical procedure, was identified in more than one-third of all patients. A delay in diagnosis was associated with a worse prognosis.

Neurophysiologic testing can demonstrate several features that help distinguish psychogenic myoclonus from organic myoclonus. Psychogenic myoclonus typically has an EMG burst duration longer than 75 ms, whereas organic myoclonus usually has a duration of less than 75 ms.[44] Furthermore, EMG bursts in psychogenic myoclonus often consist of a well organized triphasic pattern of activation of agonist and antagonist muscles.[44] Reflex latency to external stimuli demonstrates a longer latency (>100 ms) in psychogenic myoclonus compared with organic myoclonus.[44] Giant somatosensory evoked potentials, EEG spikes occurring approximately 20 ms prior to jerks, are present in cortical myoclonus but are not seen in psychogenic myoclonus. EEG-EMG back-averaging measures cortical activity (referred to as the Bereitschaftspotential) prior to movements with a slow rising potential more than 1.5 seconds prior to voluntary movements.[45] This reflects a premotor cortical potential seen in voluntary movement and in psychogenic myoclonus but not organic myoclonus. Studies have shown that a Bereitschaftspotential is often present in cases of spinal myoclonus and thus can help distinguish psychogenic from organic cases.[46]

A clinical diagnosis of axial myoclonus is often unreliable, as reported in several recent large case series. The largest cohort of propriospinal myoclonus described 65 patients who had electrophysiologic evidence of psychogenic myoclonus, including an incongruent EMG pattern in 84% of patients and a Bereitschaftspotential in 86% of patients.[47]

Palatal myoclonus, which is characterized by rhythmic contractions of the soft palate, also has been described as a PMD. In a retrospective evaluation of 10 patients with isolated palatal myoclonus, 7 had a clinical diagnosis of psychogenic palatal myoclonus.[48] In contrast to patients with organic palatal myoclonus, psychogenic palatal myoclonus was variable, entrainable, and distractible, and all psychogenic patients reported ear clicking. Psychogenic palatal myoclonus had an abrupt onset with a preceding physical event (most commonly a minor viral respiratory infection) and had a static course. Additionally, most patients had multiple somatizations and underlying psychiatric conditions.

PSYCHOGENIC PARKINSONISM

Psychogenic parkinsonism presents with a variety of clinical signs, including tremor, slowness, and abnormalities of speech and gait.[49] The tremor often involves the dominant hand and is variable and distractible. There may be spread of tremor to other body parts when the affected limb is restricted. The slowness of movement is characterized by effortful rapid successive movements often associated with grimacing and sighing without a clear decrement of amplitude when performing rapid successive movements. There may be normal speed of other movements when distracted. Active resistance to passive range of motion is detected and can be distractible. Speech abnormalities may be characterized by excessive slowness, stuttering, and whispering. There may be an exaggerated response even to a mild pull test (Video 5). The largest reported series of 32 patients with psychogenic parkinsonism had a mean age at onset of 48 years and 54% were female, which is in contrast to Parkinson disease, where there is usually 3:2 male predominance.[49] A precipitating event was identified in 56% of patients, including occupational and personal stressors as well as physical trauma; 56% of patients had a history of psychiatric illness, most commonly depression. Response to placebo was assessed in 50% of patients, including carbidopa, tuning fork, and saline injection. Six patients had mild improvement and 4 had marked improvement in symptoms. Between 1995 and 2011 there have been 7 reports published on psychogenic parkinsonism, describing a total of 84 patients, with mean age of 48.8 years, mean duration of symptoms of 5.2 years, and a vast majority having abrupt onset. In contrast to Parkinson disease, in which approximately two-thirds of affected individuals are men, there was 43:38 female preponderance (in 1 report of 4 cases no gender was noted).[25,49–54] Although several of these features can help distinguish psychogenic parkinsonism from organic parkinsonism, the 2 conditions may also coexist in the same patient.[55]

PSYCHOGENIC TICS

Psychogenic tics can be challenging to discriminate from organic tics, which can demonstrate features classically associated with PMDS, such as distractibility, suggestibility, and a fluctuating course with spontaneous remissions. One study identified 9 patients with psychogenic motor tics.[56] No patients had a family or childhood history of organic tics. Compared with Tourette syndrome, patients presenting to the same center during the study period, those with psychogenic tics had an older age at presentation and a female predominance. Patients with psychogenic tics represented 4.9% of all patients with PMDs during the study period and there was no significant difference in age or gender compared with other PMDs. Only 1 psychogenic patient was able to suppress tics; a premonitory sensation, a characteristic feature of organic tics seen in patients with Tourette syndrome,[34,57] was described in only 2 patients. These patients had other associated PMDs and pseudoseizures. Four of 7 patients had moderate improvement with psychotherapy and stress management (Video 6).

Although the Bereitschaftspotential has been reported in a small proportion of patients with simple organic tics, those with psychogenic jerks have a significantly higher proportion of jerks preceded by the Bereitschaftspotential and with a significantly earlier onset prior to jerks compared with those with organic tics.[58]

PSYCHOGENIC PAROXYSMAL DYSKINESIA

PMDs often include movements that occur intermittently and episodically and can be categorized as psychogenic paroxysmal dyskinesias. The largest series of psychogenic paroxysmal dyskinesias, involving 26 cases, predominantly women, had a mean age at onset of 38.6 years, later than the typical childhood onset in organic paroxysmal dyskinesias.[21] The clinical presentation for psychogenic paroxysmal dyskinesia was commonly dystonia in isolation but 69.2% had a combination of movements. Although most subjects had long attacks, there was marked variability of episodes in terms of duration, frequency and phenomenology. Identifiable triggers, atypical of organic paroxysmal dyskinesia, were noted in 50% of patients, and

42.3% had unusual alleviating strategies. Furthermore, 34.6% of patients had additional psychogenic signs in-between episodes. Precipitating physical or emotional stressors were identified in most cases and 26.9% had psychiatric comorbidities. An additional organic movement disorder was present in 19.2%, highlighting the importance of recognizing the coexistence of organic and psychogenic disease (Video 7).

PSYCHOGENIC GAIT DISORDERS

Psychogenic gait disorders can have various clinical presentations and are frequently associated with other PMDs. Psychogenic gait disorders need to be distinguished from complex gait patterns than can be seen in dystonia and Huntington disease. Psychogenic patients may have astasia-abasia, characterized by the ability to maintain good balance and even perform tandem gait, despite bizarre contortions and side-to-side swaying of their bodies, without falling (Video 8). They may also have buckling at the knees, a bouncing stance, or a seemingly effortful gait, with 1 leg dragging behind with the medial aspect of the foot sweeping the ground and the leg externally rotated. Abnormal gait patterns were studied in a series of 279 patients with PMDs.[59] In those patients with a pure psychogenic gait disorder, buckling at the knees was most common whereas in those patients with a coexisting PMD, slowness of gait was more common. A fear of falling gait, which is not classified as a psychogenic gait, is most commonly seen in elderly women after a fall.[60] It is characterized by a sliding or shuffling gait, with a need to hold on for support as if walking on ice. Often misdiagnosed as Parkinson disease, this gait disorder is often treatable with education, physical therapy, reassurance, and psychological and pharmacologic treatment of underlying anxiety.

Gait analysis in the laboratory can also help identify a psychogenic gait. A trained automated neural network system analyzed gait patterns in psychogenic gait patients and normal controls on repeated occasions 3 months apart.[61] None of the psychogenic gait patients maintained their gait pattern on follow-up objective testing, a variation not detected or fully appreciated based only on clinical assessments. Such gait analysis may provide helpful information in challenging cases.

OTHER PSYCHOGENIC MOVEMENT DISORDERS

Psychogenic chorea has been rarely reported in the literature, in 1 series representing 0.6% of patients with PMDs (Video 9).[62] A single case report of psychogenic chorea in a patient with a strong family history of Huntington disease highlighted the importance of “anticipation” in patients with this hereditary disease.[63] She had choreic movements of the head, arms, and legs that were distractible, markedly diminishing when performing voluntary repetitive movements. She did not have other characteristic signs of Huntington disease, such as abnormal saccades. Genetic testing for Huntington disease showed normal 16 and 17 CAG repeats in the Huntington disease gene.

PMDs can also manifest as psychogenic facial movements (Video 10).[64,65]

A retrospective review, including 7 movement disorders centers, identified 87 patients with psychogenic facial movements, representing 16.3% of all patients with PMDs[66]; 61 patients were included in the study with a female predominance and a mean age at onset of 37.0 years. The most common movement was unilateral, tonic, lateral, or downward contraction of the lower lip with ipsilateral jaw deviation (84.3%). Blepharospasm or spasms of the platysma was present in 60.7%, either in isolation or in combination with lip contraction. There was abrupt onset in 80.3% with an identified psychological stress/trauma in 57.4%. These patients had a fluctuating course with spontaneous remission and exacerbations in 60%. In contrast to elevation of the ipsilateral eyebrow, known as the other Babinski sign,[67] patients with psychogenic hemifacial spasm had a depression in the ipsilateral eyebrow.

A movement disorder called jumpy stump occurs after limb amputation and is characterized by tremor and spasms of the stump often associated with pain. Although considered a typical example of peripherally induced movement disorder,[35] a report of psychogenic jumpy stump described a man with rapid, rhythmic jerks of a stump that was episodic, worsening with excitement and resolving with distraction.[68] Neurophysiologic testing demonstrated reciprocal contraction of the hamstrings and quadriceps during the jerks and variation of the amplitude and frequency of recordings when tapping with a finger. Furthermore, EMG activity increased when the limb was immobilized. These features suggested psychogenic etiology for the movement disorder in this patient.

PATHOPHYSIOLOGY

The pathophysiology of PMDs is not well understood but the traditional view has suggested the contribution of an underlying psychological or physical stress to the development of abnormal movements. Not all patients with PMDs, however, report an underlying stressor. Some investigators have suggested the chief mechanism of psychogenic disorders involves repression of memories and conversion to somatic symptoms.[69]

Structural imaging, such as CT and MRI, are generally unremarkable in patients with a classic presentation of a PMD. Functional neuroimaging, however, is sometimes used, especially in research settings, to evaluate PMDs.[70] Single-photon emission CT can distinguish patients with organic and psychogenic parkinsonism by evaluating striatal dopamine transporters.[53] A normal scan does not distinguish, however, between psychogenic parkinsonism and other forms for parkinsonism, such as drug-induced parkinsonism. Psychogenic parkinsonism and organic parkinsonism may also coexist within the same patient.[54] A small study involving 5 patients, each with psychogenic tremor, essential tremor, and controls, demonstrated a distinct pattern of cerebral perfusion in psychogenic tremor with reduced cerebral blood flow in the ventral medial prefrontal cortex and anterior cingulate region, which corresponds to the anterior portion of the default mode network.[71] Deactivation of the default mode network during motor tasks that provoked tremor in psychogenic patients, suggests that more attention and effort was required to provoke the tremor compared with ET patients.

Positron emission tomography (PET) imaging comparing psychogenic and organic dystonia has shown both overlapping and distinguishing features. One study comparing 6 patients with psychogenic and 5 patients with organic dystonia of the right leg and 6 healthy controls demonstrated increased blood flow in the primary motor cortex in organic dystonia as opposed to increased blood flow in the cerebellum and basal ganglia in patients with psychogenic dystonia.[72] These patterns suggest involvement of cortical structures in organic dystonia and greater involvement of subcortical structures in psychogenic dystonia. Common to both organic and psychogenic dystonia, as opposed to controls, was activation of the right dorsolateral prefrontal cortex. Functional MRI (fMRI) studies can provide insight into underlying neural circuits involved in PMDs. Studies have suggested the involvement of areas outside of the primary motor cortex, including the prefrontal, supplementary motor, and anterior cingulate cortex in psychogenic compared with organic movement disorders.[70,73,74] An fMRI study evaluating brain activation during the recall of stressful life events demonstrated enhanced connectivity between the amygdala and motor areas and impaired regulation by the right inferior frontal cortex in patients with conversion disorder.[69] The findings suggest that the processing of emotional stressors contributes to the physical manifestation of conversion disorder.

Studies involving transcranial magnetic stimulation (TMS) have demonstrated similar cortical excitability in patients with fixed dystonia and organic dystonia compared with normal controls.[41,42] Another study demonstrated that although impaired cortical excitability was present in organic and psychogenic dystonia patients, increased plasticity was a hallmark feature of organic dystonia.[75]

Based on recent research studies, 3 key processes have been in implicated in the neurobiology of PMDs: abnormal beliefs, abnormal self-focus, and an abnormal sense of agency.[76] The proposed models suggest that excessive self-focus triggers movements that are not associated with the normal sense of agency associated with involuntary movements. In a study involving 9 patients with psychogenic tremor and normal controls, psychogenic patients reported a delayed sense of intention prior to voluntary movements.[77] These findings support the hypothesis of an impaired sense of volition in patients with PMDs and suggest that movements that are physiologically voluntary are experienced as involuntary by these patients.

TREATMENT

Although there is no standard protocol for the treatment of PMDs, several approaches have been suggested, including open and candid communication with patients about the diagnosis at the initiation of treatment.[78,79] Because patients who are accepting of their diagnosis at the onset are more likely to have long-term successful outcomes,[80] appropriate education is critical. In addition to providing insight to the psychodynamics of the PMD, the authors provide patients with educational materials about psychogenic disorders and refer them to the following Web site for additional information: www.neurosymptoms.org. Some suggest that sharing the supporting physical signs of PMDs with patients may have therapeutic benefit and help them understand their diagnosis.[81]

Treatment programs may require a multidisciplinary approach, involving neurologists, psychologist, psychiatrists, and occupational, speech, and physical therapists. A small, single-blind study involving 10 patients with PMDs evaluated the efficacy of 12 weeks of 1 hour/week psychotherapy.[82] Anxiolytics and antidepressants were also prescribed by the treating psychiatrist. At the end of 12 weeks, there was significant improvement in the Psychogenic Movement Disorder Rating Scale (PMDRS) from a baseline score of 71.2 to 29.0 ($P = .0195$) after treatment. There were also significant improvements in the Hamilton Depression Rating Scale score ($P = .009$), Beck anxiety inventory score ($P = .002$), and the Global Assessment of Functioning ($P = .0083$) score after treatment. One study evaluated the outcome in patients receiving psychotherapy versus neurologic observation and support in a randomized, crossover study.[83] Fifteen patients were randomized to early psychotherapy versus neurologic observation for 3 months and then switched groups for 3 months. At the end of the study there was significant improvement in PMDs as measured by Clinical Global Impression severity ($P = .04$) as well as improvement in the Hamilton Depression Rating Scale ($P = .001$) and Beck Anxiety Inventory ($P<.0005$) compared with baseline but no significant difference in improvement between groups at 3 ($P = .46$) or 6 months ($P = .15$). The similar improvement suggests that continued neurologic support can be just as effective for treatment of PMDs as psychiatric care. Consistent neurologic follow-up, reinforcing the diagnosis and addressing patient concerns and questions, is important for good outcome. This relationship between the neurologist and patient should be maintained, rather than simply referring to a psychiatrist, and following up as needed. A randomized trial of cognitive behavioral therapy (CBT) compared the efficacy of usual care and CBT-based guided self-help with usual care alone in 127 patients with psychogenic symptoms.[84] The guided self-help included a manual and face-to-face sessions. The primary outcome at 3 months demonstrated a 13% absolute difference in the proportion of patients that were "better" or "much better" on the Clinical Global Improvement Rating Scale in favor of those randomized to the CBT; however, this difference was not significant at 6 months.

The largest study evaluating physical therapy for PMDs consisted of a 1-week intensive outpatient physical therapy program that focused on reversing abnormal learned patterns of movement in 60 patients with PMDs.[85] At 1 week, a rating of markedly improved or almost completely normal/in remission was seen in 68.8% as reported by patients and in 73.3% based on physician assessment. At long-term follow-up at a median of 33 months, PMD patients reported marked improvement or almost completely normal/in remission in 60.4% of PMD patients compared with 21.9% in 60 controls who did not undergo the rehabilitation program. Another study evaluated a low-intensity (walking) exercise program in 16 PMD patients for 12 weeks.[86] At the end of 12 weeks there was a mean improvement from baseline of approximately 70% on the PMDRS. A randomized controlled trial compared the effects of 3 weeks of inpatient therapy with no treatment in 60 patients with psychogenic gait disorder.[87] Treatment consisted of physical activity as well as education and CBT. At 4 weeks, compared with the controls, the treated group had a mean difference of 8.4 Functional Independence Measure units ($P<.001$) and 6.9 Functional Mobility Scale units ($P<.001$). A majority of patients returned to independent living and many returned to work. Tremor "retrainment" was evaluated in a small proof-of-concept study in 5 patients with psychogenic tremor.[88] Via visual computer feedback, patients were instructed to "retrain" their tremor to a different frequency during 1 to 3 consecutive sessions. There was a significant improvement in the tremor subscale of the Rating Scale for Psychogenic Movement Disorders from a baseline score of 22.2 ± 13.39 to 4.3 ± 5.51 ($P = .0019$) at the end of treatment. At 6 months, 6 patients had marked improvement and 4 had relapsed. Successful treatment with physical therapy can be challenging with many barriers to care. A survey of physical therapists revealed that although therapists are interested in treating patients with PMDs, inadequate service structure and knowledge and support from colleagues in other disciplines were thought to limit successful treatment with physical therapy.[89]

The use of transcutaneous electrical nerve stimulation (TENS) devices, which deliver low-voltage electrical current to the skin, has been studied as a treatment of PMDs.[90] In a study of 19 patients with PMDs treated with TENS, only 5 patients had greater than 50% improvement on the PMDRS score immediately afterward. Two patients had 20% to 30% improvement, 2 had transient worsening and 10 had less than 5% improvement from baseline. At mean follow-up of 6.9 months, there was a significant improvement in the PMDRS and self-rated outcome compared with baseline. The 5 patients with greater than 50% improvement during their initial session had no movements at follow-up. There were no side effects except a transient worsening of the PMD in 2 patients. Repetitive low-intensity TMS, which transiently modifies cortical excitability, has shown mixed results for the treatment of PMDs. A study involving 24 PMDs conducted a blinded evaluation of movements before and immediately after low-frequency TMS[91]; 75% of patients had greater than 50% improvement in the clinical rating scale and among those patients one-third had complete resolution of symptoms. At median follow-up of 19.8 months, 71% reported some degree of persistent improvement. There were no side effects reported.

The treatment of patients with severe PMDs, especially those with fixed dystonia who are unable to participate in physical therapy, is challenging. A retrospective study evaluated the efficacy of therapeutic sedation with propofol administered via standardized protocol for psychogenic neurologic symptoms, including paralysis, dystonia, mutism, and coma.[92] This treatment was focused on highly motivated patients who were accepting of their diagnosis. Subjects were sedated to a level where they were still able to verbally interact with others and follow commands. While sedated, patients underwent passive and active movements with encouragement or through painful stimulation. The session lasted 30 to 60 minutes. Within 24 hours of sedation, 3 patients became asymptomatic, 3 had major improvement, and 2 had minor improvement. At a median follow-up of 30 months, 2 patients were asymptomatic, 3 had major improvement, and 1 had minor improvement. There were no adverse events.

PROGNOSIS

Early diagnosis and treatment of PMDs is associated with improved outcome; however, the long-term outcome in PMDs is often poor. In 1 study on the long-term outcome of psychogenic tremor, after a median follow-up of 5.1 years, 64% of patients reported moderate to severe tremor.[93] Those with mild or no tremor at follow-up had a shorter duration of symptoms prior to diagnosis. A systematic review of the literature of the prognosis of patients with psychogenic motor symptoms found highly variable reported outcomes.[94] In 4 studies, 66% to 100% of patients had similar or worse symptoms at follow-up; in 14 studies, 33% to 66% had similar or worse symptoms, and in 5 studies, 33% or less of patients had similar or worse symptoms at follow-up. Delayed diagnosis and personality disorder were associated with a poor outcome whereas short duration of symptoms, early diagnosis, and high satisfaction with patient care was associated with good outcome. At Baylor College of Medicine, long-term prognosis of PMD patients at a mean follow-up of 3.4 years was reported as improved in 57% of patients, worse in 22% of patients, and static symptoms in 21%. Factors associated with improved outcomes included shorter duration of symptoms, stronger physical health, positive social life perceptions, elimination of stressors, and patients' perception of receiving effective treatment, including medication.

SUMMARY

PMDs represent a group of disorders that are challenging to diagnose and treat. There are many characteristic features of the history as well as classic findings on physical examination that can help clinicians arrive at an accurate diagnosis and avoid unnecessary testing. The diagnosis is not one of exclusion but should be based on supporting features of PMDs. It is important to recognize that PMDs can coexist with organic disease and a skilled clinician must discern between the 2. Ancillary testing can be helpful, although it is largely used for research purposes and is not needed for diagnosis. Early diagnosis and treatment is important, because a delay is associated with poor prognosis. Treatment of PMDs may and, in some cases should, include a multidisciplinary approach with continued follow-up and support for patients. Although a neurologist should be responsible for making the diagnosis, a psychiatrist experienced in psychogenic disorders can be helpful in providing insight to patients about the psychodynamic factors that may be playing a role as well as long-term psychotherapy. The psychiatrist should, however, refrain from challenging a neurologist's diagnosis or expressing doubt in front of a patient because this may likely undermine the neurologist–patient relationship. Further research into the underlying pathophysiology of PMDs is important to develop more effective, enduring therapies.

SUPPLEMENTARY DATA

Supplementary data related to this article can be found online at http://dx.doi.org/10.1016/j.ncl.2014.09.013.

REFERENCES

1. Edwards MJ, Stone J, Lang AE. From psychogenic movement disorder to functional movement disorder: it's time to change the name. Mov Disord 2014;29:849–52.
2. Fahn S, Olanow CW. "Psychogenic movement disorders": they are what they are. Mov Disord 2014;29:853–6.
3. Bass C, Halligan P. Factitious disorders and malingering: challenges for clinical assessment and management. Lancet 2014;383:1422–32.
4. Bass C, Glaser D. Early recognition and management of fabricated or induced illness in children. Lancet 2014;383:1412–21.
5. Fahn S, Williams DT. Psychogenic dystonia. Adv Neurol 1988;50:431–55.
6. Shill H, Gerber P. Evaluation of clinical diagnostic criteria for psychogenic movement disorders. Mov Disord 2006;21:1163–8.
7. Morgante F, Edwards MJ, Espay AJ, et al. Diagnostic agreement in patients with psychogenic movement disorders. Mov Disord 2012;27:548–52.
8. Espay AJ, Goldenhar LM, Voon V, et al. Opinions and clinical practices related to diagnosing and managing patients with psychogenic movement disorders: an international survey of movement disorder society members. Mov Disord 2009;24:1366–74.
9. Edwards MJ, Bhatia KP. Functional (psychogenic) movement disorders: merging mind and brain. Lancet Neurol 2012;11:250–60.
10. Anderson KE, Gruber-Baldini AL, Vaughan CG, et al. Impact of psychogenic movement disorders versus Parkinson's on disability, quality of life, and psychopathology. Mov Disord 2007;22:2204–9.
11. Carson A, Stone J, Hibberd C, et al. Disability, distress and unemployment in neurology outpatients with symptoms 'unexplained by organic disease'. J Neurol Neurosurg Psychiatry 2011;82:810–3.
12. Edwards MJ, Schrag A. Hyperkinetic psychogenic movement disorders. Handb Clin Neurol 2011;100:719–29.
13. Ferrara J, Jankovic J. Psychogenic movement disorders in children. Mov Disord 2008;23:1875–81.
14. Schwingenschuh P, Pont-Sunyer C, Surtees R, et al. Psychogenic movement disorders in children: a report of 15 cases and a review of the literature. Mov Disord 2008;23:1882–8.
15. Canavese C, Ciano C, Zibordi F, et al. Phenomenology of psychogenic movement disorders in children. Mov Disord 2012;27:1153–7.
16. Batla A, Stamelou M, Edwards MJ, et al. Functional movement disorders are not uncommon in the elderly. Mov Disord 2013;28:540–3.
17. Kranick S, Ekanayake V, Martinez V, et al. Psychopathology and psychogenic movement disorders. Mov Disord 2011;26:1844–50.

18. Parees I, Kojovic M, Pires C, et al. Physical precipitating factors in functional movement disorders. J Neurol Sci 2014;338:174–7.
19. Stamelou M, Cossu G, Edwards MJ, et al. Familial psychogenic movement disorders. Mov Disord 2013;28:1295–8.
20. Mink JW. Conversion disorder and mass psychogenic illness in child neurology. Ann N Y Acad Sci 2013;1304:40–4.
21. Ganos C, Aguirregomozcorta M, Batla A, et al. Psychogenic paroxysmal movement disorders–clinical features and diagnostic clues. Parkinsonism Relat Disord 2014;20:41–6.
22. Hoerth MT, Wellik KE, Demaerschalk BM, et al. Clinical predictors of psychogenic nonepileptic seizures: a critically appraised topic. Neurologist 2008;14:266–70.
23. Scarano VR, Jankovic J. Post-traumatic movement disorders: effect of the legal system on outcome. J Forensic Sci 1998;43:334–9.
24. Fekete R, Baizabal-Carvallo JF, Ha AD, et al. Convergence spasm in conversion disorders: prevalence in psychogenic and other movement disorders compared with controls. J Neurol Neurosurg Psychiatry 2012;83:202–4.
25. Factor SA, Podskalny GD, Molho ES. Psychogenic movement disorders: frequency, clinical profile, and characteristics. J Neurol Neurosurg Psychiatry 1995;59:406–12.
26. Thenganatt MA, Jankovic J. Psychogenic tremor: a video guide to its distinguishing features. Tremor Other Hyperkinet Mov (N Y) 2014;4:253.
27. Kenney C, Diamond A, Mejia N, et al. Distinguishing psychogenic and essential tremor. J Neurol Sci 2007;263:94–9.
28. Deuschl G, Koster B, Lucking CH, et al. Diagnostic and pathophysiological aspects of psychogenic tremors. Mov Disord 1998;13:294–302.
29. McAuley J, Rothwell J. Identification of psychogenic, dystonic, and other organic tremors by a coherence entrainment test. Mov Disord 2004;19:253–67.
30. Zeuner KE, Shoge RO, Goldstein SR, et al. Accelerometry to distinguish psychogenic from essential or parkinsonian tremor. Neurology 2003;61:548–50.
31. Kumru H, Valls-Sole J, Valldeoriola F, et al. Transient arrest of psychogenic tremor induced by contralateral ballistic movements. Neurosci Lett 2004;370:135–9.
32. Kumru H, Begeman M, Tolosa E, et al. Dual task interference in psychogenic tremor. Mov Disord 2007;22:2077–82.
33. Schwingenschuh P, Katschnig P, Seiler S, et al. Moving toward "laboratory-supported" criteria for psychogenic tremor. Mov Disord 2011;26:2509–15.
34. Patel N, Jankovic J, Hallett M. Sensory aspects of movement disorders. Lancet Neurol 2014;13:100–12.
35. Jankovic J. Peripherally induced movement disorders. Neurol Clin 2009;27: 821–32, vii.
36. Schrag A, Trimble M, Quinn N, et al. The syndrome of fixed dystonia: an evaluation of 103 patients. Brain 2004;127:2360–72.
37. Reedijk WB, van Rijn MA, Roelofs K, et al. Psychological features of patients with complex regional pain syndrome type I related dystonia. Mov Disord 2008;23: 1551–9.
38. Hawley JS, Weiner WJ. Psychogenic dystonia and peripheral trauma. Neurology 2011;77:496–502.
39. van Rooijen DE, Geraedts EJ, Marinus J, et al. Peripheral trauma and movement disorders: a systematic review of reported cases. J Neurol Neurosurg Psychiatry 2011;82:892–8.
40. Hallett M. Physiology of psychogenic movement disorders. J Clin Neurosci 2010; 17:959–65.

41. Avanzino L, Martino D, van de Warrenburg BP, et al. Cortical excitability is abnormal in patients with the "fixed dystonia" syndrome. Mov Disord 2008;23: 646–52.
42. Espay AJ, Morgante F, Purzner J, et al. Cortical and spinal abnormalities in psychogenic dystonia. Ann Neurol 2006;59:825–34.
43. Erro R, Edwards MJ, Bhatia KP, et al. Psychogenic axial myoclonus: Clinical features and long-term outcome. Parkinsonism Relat Disord 2014;20(6):596–9.
44. Brown P, Thompson PD. Electrophysiological aids to the diagnosis of psychogenic jerks, spasms, and tremor. Mov Disord 2001;16:595–9.
45. Terada K, Ikeda A, Van Ness PC, et al. Presence of Bereitschaftspotential preceding psychogenic myoclonus: clinical application of jerk-locked back averaging. J Neurol Neurosurg Psychiatry 1995;58:745–7.
46. Esposito M, Edwards MJ, Bhatia KP, et al. Idiopathic spinal myoclonus: a clinical and neurophysiological assessment of a movement disorder of uncertain origin. Mov Disord 2009;24:2344–9.
47. Erro R, Bhatia KP, Edwards MJ, et al. Clinical diagnosis of propriospinal myoclonus is unreliable: an electrophysiologic study. Mov Disord 2013;28: 1868–73.
48. Stamelou M, Saifee TA, Edwards MJ, et al. Psychogenic palatal tremor may be underrecognized: reappraisal of a large series of cases. Mov Disord 2012;27: 1164–8.
49. Jankovic J. Diagnosis and treatment of psychogenic parkinsonism. J Neurol Neurosurg Psychiatry 2011;82:1300–3.
50. Lang AE, Koller WC, Fahn S. Psychogenic parkinsonism. Arch Neurol 1995;52: 802–10.
51. Booij J, Speelman JD, Horstink MW, et al. The clinical benefit of imaging striatal dopamine transporters with [123I]FP-CIT SPET in differentiating patients with presynaptic parkinsonism from those with other forms of parkinsonism. Eur J Nucl Med 2001;28:266–72.
52. Gaig C, Marti MJ, Tolosa E, et al. 123I-Ioflupane SPECT in the diagnosis of suspected psychogenic Parkinsonism. Mov Disord 2006;21:1994–8.
53. Benaderette S, Zanotti Fregonara P, Apartis E, et al. Psychogenic parkinsonism: a combination of clinical, electrophysiological, and [(123)I]-FP-CIT SPECT scan explorations improves diagnostic accuracy. Mov Disord 2006;21:310–7.
54. Felicio AC, Godeiro-Junior C, Moriyama TS, et al. Degenerative parkinsonism in patients with psychogenic parkinsonism: a dopamine transporter imaging study. Clin Neurol Neurosurg 2010;112:282–5.
55. Hallett M. Psychogenic parkinsonism. J Neurol Sci 2011;310:163–5.
56. Baizabal-Carvallo JF, Jankovic J. The clinical features of psychogenic movement disorders resembling tics. J Neurol Neurosurg Psychiatry 2014;85:573–5.
57. Jankovic J, Kurlan R. Tourette syndrome: evolving concepts. Mov Disord 2011; 26:1149–56.
58. van der Salm SM, Tijssen MA, Koelman JH, et al. The bereitschaftspotential in jerky movement disorders. J Neurol Neurosurg Psychiatry 2012;83:1162–7.
59. Baik JS, Lang AE. Gait abnormalities in psychogenic movement disorders. Mov Disord 2007;22:395–9.
60. Kurlan R. "Fear of falling" gait: a potentially reversible psychogenic gait disorder. Cogn Behav Neurol 2005;18:171–2.
61. Merello M, Ballesteros D, Rossi M, et al. Lack of maintenance of gait pattern as measured by instrumental methods suggests psychogenic gait. Funct Neurol 2012;27:217–24.

62. Thomas M, Jankovic J. Psychogenic movement disorders: diagnosis and management. CNS Drugs 2004;18:437–52.
63. Fekete R, Jankovic J. Psychogenic chorea associated with family history of Huntington disease. Mov Disord 2010;25:503–4.
64. Tan EK, Jankovic J. Psychogenic hemifacial spasm. J Neuropsychiatry Clin Neurosci 2001;13:380–4.
65. Yaltho TC, Jankovic J. The many faces of hemifacial spasm: differential diagnosis of unilateral facial spasms. Mov Disord 2011;26:1582–92.
66. Fasano A, Valadas A, Bhatia KP, et al. Psychogenic facial movement disorders: clinical features and associated conditions. Mov Disord 2012;27:1544–51.
67. Stamey W, Jankovic J. The other Babinski sign in hemifacial spasm. Neurology 2007;69:402–4.
68. Zadikoff C, Mailis-Gagnon A, Lang AE. A case of a psychogenic "jumpy stump". J Neurol Neurosurg Psychiatry 2006;77:1101.
69. Aybek S, Nicholson TR, Zelaya F, et al. Neural correlates of recall of life events in conversion disorder. JAMA Psychiatry 2014;71:52–60.
70. Mehta AR, Rowe JB, Schrag AE. Imaging psychogenic movement disorders. Curr Neurol Neurosci Rep 2013;13:402.
71. Czarnecki K, Jones DT, Burnett MS, et al. SPECT perfusion patterns distinguish psychogenic from essential tremor. Parkinsonism Relat Disord 2011;17:328–32.
72. Schrag AE, Mehta AR, Bhatia KP, et al. The functional neuroimaging correlates of psychogenic versus organic dystonia. Brain 2013;136:770–81.
73. Voon V, Brezing C, Gallea C, et al. Emotional stimuli and motor conversion disorder. Brain 2010;133:1526–36.
74. Voon V, Gallea C, Hattori N, et al. The involuntary nature of conversion disorder. Neurology 2010;74:223–8.
75. Quartarone A, Rizzo V, Terranova C, et al. Abnormal sensorimotor plasticity in organic but not in psychogenic dystonia. Brain 2009;132:2871–7.
76. Edwards MJ, Fotopoulou A, Parees I. Neurobiology of functional (psychogenic) movement disorders. Curr Opin Neurol 2013;26:442–7.
77. Edwards MJ, Moretto G, Schwingenschuh P, et al. Abnormal sense of intention preceding voluntary movement in patients with psychogenic tremor. Neuropsychologia 2011;49:2791–3.
78. Jankovic J, Cloninger CR, Fahn S, et al. Therapeutic approaches to psychogenic movement disorders. In: Hallett M, Fahn S, Jankovic J, et al, editors. Psychogenic movement disorders: neurology and neuropsychiatry. Philadelphia: AAN Enterprises and Lippincott Williams and Wilkins; 2006. p. 323–8.
79. Ricciardi L, Edwards MJ. Treatment of functional (psychogenic) movement disorders. Neurotherapeutics 2014;11:201–7.
80. Jankovic J, Vuong KD, Thomas M. Psychogenic tremor: long-term outcome. CNS Spectr 2006;11:501–8.
81. Stone J, Edwards M. Trick or treat? Showing patients with functional (psychogenic) motor symptoms their physical signs. Neurology 2012;79:282–4.
82. Hinson VK, Weinstein S, Bernard B, et al. Single-blind clinical trial of psychotherapy for treatment of psychogenic movement disorders. Parkinsonism Relat Disord 2006;12:177–80.
83. Kompoliti K, Wilson B, Stebbins G, et al. Immediate vs. delayed treatment of psychogenic movement disorders with short term psychodynamic psychotherapy: randomized clinical trial. Parkinsonism Relat Disord 2014;20:60–3.
84. Sharpe M, Walker J, Williams C, et al. Guided self-help for functional (psychogenic) symptoms: a randomized controlled efficacy trial. Neurology 2011;77:564–72.

85. Czarnecki K, Thompson JM, Seime R, et al. Functional movement disorders: successful treatment with a physical therapy rehabilitation protocol. Parkinsonism Relat Disord 2012;18:247–51.
86. Dallocchio C, Arbasino C, Klersy C, et al. The effects of physical activity on psychogenic movement disorders. Mov Disord 2010;25:421–5.
87. Jordbru AA, Smedstad LM, Klungsoyr O, et al. Psychogenic gait disorder: a randomized controlled trial of physical rehabilitation with one-year follow-up. J Rehabil Med 2014;46:181–7.
88. Espay AJ, Edwards MJ, Oggioni GD, et al. Tremor retrainment as therapeutic strategy in psychogenic (functional) tremor. Parkinsonism Relat Disord 2014; 20(6):647–50.
89. Edwards MJ, Stone J, Nielsen G. Physiotherapists and patients with functional (psychogenic) motor symptoms: a survey of attitudes and interest. J Neurol Neurosurg Psychiatry 2012;83:655–8.
90. Ferrara J, Stamey W, Strutt AM, et al. Transcutaneous electrical stimulation (TENS) for psychogenic movement disorders. J Neuropsychiatry Clin Neurosci 2011;23:141–8.
91. Garcin B, Roze E, Mesrati F, et al. Transcranial magnetic stimulation as an efficient treatment for psychogenic movement disorders. J Neurol Neurosurg Psychiatry 2013;84:1043–6.
92. Stone J, Hoeritzauer I, Brown K, et al. Therapeutic sedation for functional (psychogenic) neurological symptoms. J Psychosom Res 2014;76:165–8.
93. McKeon A, Ahlskog JE, Bower JH, et al. Psychogenic tremor: long-term prognosis in patients with electrophysiologically confirmed disease. Mov Disord 2009;24: 72–6.
94. Gelauff J, Stone J, Edwards M, et al. The prognosis of functional (psychogenic) motor symptoms: a systematic review. J Neurol Neurosurg Psychiatry 2014;85: 220–6.

Ataxia

Umar Akbar, MD, Tetsuo Ashizawa, MD*

KEYWORDS

- Ataxia • Inherited • Sporadic • Autosomal dominant • Autosomal recessive
- Mitochondrial • Diagnosis • Treatment

KEY POINTS

- Balance and coordination are products of complex circuitry involving the basal ganglia, cerebellum, and cerebral cortex, as well as peripheral motor and sensory pathways.
- Malfunction of any part of this intricate circuitry can lead to imbalance and incoordination, or ataxia, of gait, the limbs, or eyes, or a combination thereof.
- Ataxia can be a symptom of a multisystemic disorder, or it can manifest as the major component of a disease process.
- Ongoing discoveries of genetic abnormalities suggest the role of mitochondrial dysfunction, oxidative stress, abnormal mechanisms of DNA repair, possible protein misfolding, and abnormalities in cytoskeletal proteins.
- Few ataxias are fully treatable, and most are symptomatically managed.

INTRODUCTION

Complex circuitry connecting the basal ganglia, cerebellum, and cerebral cortex is involved in producing coordinated movements of the eyes and limbs. Malfunction of any part of this intricate circuitry can lead to incoordination, or ataxia, of gait, the limbs, or eyes, or a combination thereof. Afferent inputs into the motor circuitry are also critical in production of coordinated movements, and disruptions in sensory pathways can produce incoordination known as sensory ataxia. Ataxia can be acquired, inherited, or sporadic (lacking a definite genetic defect or acquired etiology). This review focuses on the inherited ataxias, their clinical presentation, pathophysiology, and available treatments, with a quick overview of acquired ataxias.

ACQUIRED ATAXIAS

Vascular insults, including strokes and global anoxic events, tumors, trauma, and demyelinating disease (ie, multiple sclerosis) are common causes of acquired ataxia.

Department of Neurology, Center for Movement Disorders and Neurorestoration College of Medicine, McKnight Brain Institute, University of Florida, 1149 South Newell Drive, L3-100, Gainesville, FL 32611, USA
* Corresponding author.
E-mail address: tetsuo.ashizawa@neurology.ufl.edu

Neurol Clin 33 (2015) 225–248
http://dx.doi.org/10.1016/j.ncl.2014.09.004 **neurologic.theclinics.com**

Other causes include congenital anomalies, infection, autoimmunity, and vitamin deficiencies. Detailed history and examination, imaging studies, and other corroborating tests often confirm the etiology in these cases. Hypothyroidism can occasionally cause mild disequilibrium and gait ataxia with pathology in the midline cerebellar structures.[1] Symptoms can be dramatically improved with timely recognition and thyroid replacement.[2] Alcohol is a major toxic cause of ataxia and excessive use leads to degeneration of the midline cerebellum. Progressive trunk and gait ataxia is characteristic, with little involvement of upper limbs, eyes, or speech (a corollary of relative cerebellar hemispheric sparing). More than 1 year of abstinence can improve ataxia drastically.[3] Chemotherapy agents, especially 5-fluorouracil and cytosine arabinoside, can cause a cerebellar syndrome, particularly when given in higher than conventional doses.[4] Supratherapeutic serum levels of antiepilepsy drugs, particularly phenytoin, are associated with acute reversible dose-dependent cerebellar signs, and permanent ataxia may emerge with chronic use. All but 2 antiepilepsy drugs (gabapentin and levetiracetam) were shown in a meta-analysis to have a higher and dose-dependent risk of imbalance.[5] Heavy metals can also cause ataxia. Paresthesias, ataxia, and visual field defect can be seen in organic mercury exposure. Lead poisoning, particularly in children, is typically associated with encephalopathy and abdominal colic, but ataxia can be a prominent presenting feature. Chelation therapy has been reported to successfully restore neurologic function.[6] Excessive use of bismuth subsalicylate (eg, Pepto-Bismol) can cause bismuth toxicity, which is associated with ataxic gait, myoclonus, and confusion.[7] Abuse of paint products that contain toluene may lead to persistent ataxia, cognitive impairment, and pyramidal tract signs.[8]

Ataxia can be caused by infectious or postinfectious syndromes involving the cerebellum, brainstem, or both. Neuroimaging, serology, and cerebrospinal fluid analysis can help to identify the etiology. Combination of ophthalmoplegia, ataxia, and other cranial nerve deficits is suggestive of Bickerstaff encephalitis.[9] Ataxia can be one of many neurologic symptoms in human immunodeficiency virus infection. Rapidly progressive ataxia and dementia can be seen in Creutzfeldt–Jakob disease. Ataxia is a more common neurologic symptom of Whipple's disease than the pathognomonic feature of oculomasticatory myorhythmia.[10] The condition, which is otherwise fatal, should be promptly diagnosed using brain imaging, cerebrospinal fluid assays, and duodenal biopsies, and treated with antibiotics.[10]

Paraneoplastic cerebellar degeneration is one of several autoimmune causes of ataxia, and can be associated with other neurologic signs, including dysarthria, oscillopsia, dementia, and extrapyramidal signs.[11] Thorough neoplasia workup should be performed, because cancer treatment can improve the ataxia. Anti-Purkinje cell antibodies, such as anti-Yo, Hu, and Ri antibodies, may be detectable. The combination of ataxia, hyperreflexia, and peripheral neuropathy is seen in celiac disease owing to gluten sensitivity. Dietary restriction of gluten can improve symptoms once the diagnosis is confirmed with antibody testing and small bowel biopsy.[12]

Anti-Glutamic Acid Decarboxylase Ataxia

Antibodies against glutamic acid decarboxylase have been reported in patients with progressive ataxia.[13] The affected are typically adult women who present with ataxia, nystagmus, and dysarthria, and develop antibodies against thyroid, parietal cells, and pancreatic islet cells, the latter leading to insulin-dependent diabetes. Glutamic acid decarboxylase is instrumental in synthesizing gamma-aminobutyric acid from glutamate, and the antibodies are thought to pathologically bind to gamma-aminobutyric acid terminals. Antibody testing is commercially available and symptoms may be improved with intravenous immunoglobulins (Igs) and immunosuppressive agents.[14–17]

Superficial Siderosis

Concealed bleeding in the brain can lead to iron and hemosiderin accumulation in the pial and subpial areas, causing superficial siderosis, which manifests with ataxia, deafness, and cognitive dysfunction.[18] T2-weighted MRI shows characteristic hypointensity over the brain structures. Treatment of the source of bleeding can control the disease.[19]

INHERITED ATAXIAS

Autosomal-Recessive Ataxias

Most autosomal-recessive ataxias begin during childhood or early adulthood, but onset later in life is also possible. Two defective copies of the gene (one from each parent) are required to manifest symptoms; thus, parents as carriers are usually asymptomatic. Parental consanguinity increases the risk of heritability, but is not a requisite. Most patients present singly, without other affected family members. Advances in whole-exome and whole-genome sequencing provide an opportunity for the identification of causative recessive genes, especially in cases of consanguinity.

Friedrich Ataxia

Nicholas Friedrich described siblings with an ataxia syndrome in the late 19th century and recognized the possibility of a genetic cause.[20] That syndrome, now called Friedrich ataxia (FA), is the most common inherited ataxia, typically beginning in childhood, and presenting with gait ataxia, clumsiness, sensory neuropathy, areflexia, and eye movement abnormalities.[21] As the disease progresses, dysarthria, dysphagia, and lower extremity weakness become more apparent, and complete loss of ambulation occurs 9 to 15 years after symptom onset. Skeletal deformities and hypertrophic cardiomyopathy are common extraneurologic symptoms, and glucose intolerance, deafness, and optic atrophy occur less frequently.[21] This clinical picture results from the degeneration of dorsal root ganglion cells, dorsal column and spinocerebellar tracts, dentate nucleus, and corticospinal tract. Cerebellar Purkinje cells are spared. No abnormalities of the cerebellum are seen on MRI, but atrophy of the upper cervical cord and density changes of the posterior columns may be seen.[22]

In FA, the nuclear *FXN* gene on chromosome 9q13–21.1, which codes for the mitochondrial protein frataxin, is mutated by a homozygous expansion of the GAA repeat in intron 1.[23] The mutation decreases the transcription of *FXN*, which results in reduced levels of the frataxin protein.[24] Normal alleles have 5 to 33 GAA repeats, whereas 66 to over 1000 repeats are seen in expanded alleles. Before the discovery of the FA gene mutation, onset before age 25 years and presence of reflexes were considered exclusionary diagnostic criteria, but late-onset FA and FA with retained reflexes have been recognized.[25] Other phenotypic variations have been documented, including chorea, myoclonus, pure sensory ataxia, and isolated cardiomyopathy, but their mechanisms remain unknown.[26,27]

Although its exact role is unclear, frataxin is thought to be involved in transfer of iron from the mitochondria to various proteins, which contain iron–sulfur clusters. Iron–sulfur cluster biogenesis depends strongly on frataxin, whose deficiency leads to iron accumulation in the mitochondria, respiratory chain dysfunction and increased oxidative stress.[21]

Symptomatic and supportive treatments are the mainstay for patients with FA. The risk of aspiration owing to dysphagia, glucose intolerance and diabetes, and cardiomyopathy require routine screening and close monitoring. Several antioxidants and iron chelators have been studied in FA. Idebenone has been shown to improve cardiomyopathy in 1 study,[28] but had no effect on cardiac function in another study.[29] A 6-month, phase III study of idebenone showed no improvement in neurologic function, although the longer follow up open-label data demonstrated significant improvement.[30,31] Alpha-tocopherolquinone is an antioxidant that has shown dose-dependent neurologic improvement in FA.[30] Erythropoeietin in a pilot study demonstrated safety and tolerability, but failed to show any neurologic improvement.[31] Idebenone combined with deferipone in an open-label study did not show neurologic improvement.[32] An open-label pilot study of resveratrol did not show improvement in frataxin levels, but the high-dose group showed improvement in neurologic and speech functions.[33] In an 8-week follow-up study, riluzole showed a modest improvement in ataxia scores in a mixed population of patients with various ataxias, including a small number of FA patients.[34] Two single doses of epoetin alpha administered in FA patients demonstrated no acute effects of frataxin levels, but did show delayed elevation of frataxin, along with safety and tolerability.[35] Most recently, a trial of nicotinamide (vitamin B_3) showed no clinical improvement in FA symptoms, but did show increase in the levels of frataxin proportional to dose escalation.[36]

Trials of the following agents are underway or have been recently completed and are as yet unpublished (ClinicalTrials.gov): Carbamylated erythropeitin, deferiprone, acetyl-L-carnitine, EPI-743 (redox modulating agent), pioglitazone, epoetin alpha, interferon-gamma 1b, EGb761, VP20629 (a naturally occurring antioxidant), and RG2833.[37]

Ataxia with Isolated Vitamin E Deficiency

Ataxia with isolated vitamin E deficiency is related to mutation in the gene encoding the alpha-tocopherol transfer protein (*TTP1*) on chromosome 8.[38] The deficiency of vitamin E is not owing to poor intestinal absorption, but rather related to dysfunction of hepatic processing. Vitamin E has antioxidant properties and its deficiency can cause neurodegeneration with ataxia. Similar to FA, patients present with ataxia, areflexia, and polyneuropathy, but glucose intolerance and cardiomyopathy occur less frequently than in FA.[24,39] Owing to the role of vitamin E in vision, retinitis pigmentosa and visual loss can also be seen. Childhood-onset sporadic ataxia should trigger testing of vitamin E level, and the level is typically less than 1.8 mg/L. Replacement of vitamin E with large doses can stabilize neurologic function and even prevent the onset of neurologic symptoms, particularly with early initiation of therapy.[40,41]

Abetalipoproteinemia (Bassen Kornzweig Disease)

The *MTTP* gene on chromosome 4 encodes a large subunit of microsomal triglyceride transfer protein. Mutations in this gene, as seen in abetalipoproteinemia, cause malabsorption of lipid and lipid-soluble vitamins (ie, vitamins A, D, E, K); thus, the clinical presentation is similar to ataxia with isolated vitamin E deficiency, but with evidence of malabsorption.[42] Blood levels reveal low vitamin E and cholesterol, absent apolipoprotein B, presence of acanthocytes in peripheral smear, and elevated transaminases and International Normalized Ratio. Modifying the diet and replacing vitamins may prevent neurologic deterioration.

Cayman Ataxia

Cayman ataxia was first identified in the Grand Cayman Island and is related to a mutation in the *ATCAY* gene on chromosome 19, encoding for the caytaxin protein, which plays a role in synaptogenesis of cerebellar granular and Purkinje cells and glutamate synthesis. Affected patients carry 2 homozygous mutations,[43] and present with developmental delay, early-onset hypotonia, and nonprogressive axial cerebellar ataxia. Treatment is supportive.

Ataxia–Telangiectasia

With an estimated prevalence of 1 in 20,000 to 100,000 live births,[44] ataxia-telangiectasia (AT) is the most common cause of recessive ataxia in patients under age 5 years. Children typically present during the first decade of life with progressive ataxia and oculocutaneous telangiectasias. Polyneuropathy, hypotonia, areflexia, and oculomotor apraxia develop as disease progresses. Telangiectasias are found most frequently on the conjunctivae and can also occur in other locations, including the earlobes and popliteal fossa. AT patients can have immunodeficiency, which often manifests as recurrent bronchopulmonary infections. AT is also associated with radiation sensitivity and increased risk of malignancies, especially of hematologic origin.

Numerous recognized mutations of the *ATM* gene on chromosome 11 have been associated with AT. Although defective DNA repair of double-strand breaks is thought to be the main cause of AT,[45] the exact role of *ATM* in pathogenesis of ataxia in unknown. The *ATM* protein, a serine–threonine kinase, responds to DNA damage by initiating phosphorylation of downstream proteins in the signal cascade.[46,47]

Atrophy of the cerebellum can be seen on brain imaging and blood tests reveal low levels of IgA, IgM, and IgE, lymphocytopenia, and elevated alpha fetoprotein (AFP). The confirmatory test of choice is immunoblot analysis for the *ATM* protein, which shows no or trace amounts of protein in AT patients.

Clinical management is supportive and includes thorough screening and close monitoring for infections and malignancies, and avoiding radiation exposure. Chronic intermittent infusions of Igs can be tried in patients with recurrent infections, along with other experimental therapeutic agents, including antioxidants,[48–50] betamethasone,[51] and dexamethasone.[52]

Ataxia–Telangiectasia-like Disorder

Mutation of another protein involved in repair of DNA double-strand breaks, *MRE11*, located on chromosome 11 in proximity to the *ATM* gene,[53] can cause a rare disorder called AT-like disorder. Clinical presentation is of early onset with slowly progressive ataxia and oculomotor apraxia. The disease course is milder than in AT. Elevation of serum AFP and telangiectasias are typically absent in AT-like disorder.[54,55]

Ataxias with Oculomotor Apraxia

Ataxias with oculomotor apraxia (AOAs) are the most common recessive ataxias with childhood onset and typically present with characteristic eye movement abnormality. Oculomotor apraxia is the impairment of saccade initiation and cancellation of vestibular–ocular reflex, resulting in hypometric saccades and defective control of voluntary eye movements. To date, no disease-specific treatments are available.

Ataxia with Oculomotor Apraxia, Type 1

Onset of type 1 AOA (AOA1) is usually less than 10 years of age with motor symptoms similar to AT. Slowly progressive ataxia of gait, oculomotor apraxia, polyneuropathy, and areflexia followed by dysarthria and upper extremity ataxia are seen in AOA1. Impaired cognition, choreoathetosis, and dystonia may also be seen. Gradual progression of axonal neuropathy eventually leads to severe motor disability with weakness and wasting. Skeletal deformities may ensue. Most children become wheelchair bound by adolescence with loss of independent ambulation 7 to 10 years after onset. It is the most common recessive ataxia in Japan and second most frequent (after FA) in Portugal.[56,57]

AOA1 is related to mutations in the aprataxin (*APTX*) gene, which encodes a protein involved in DNA single-strand break repair.[58] Despite the role of *APTX* in DNA repair, AOA1 patients are not at greater risk for malignancies or hypersensitive to radiation.[59] Laboratory studies demonstrate hypoalbuminemia and hypercholesterolemia, increased creatine kinase, and no elevation in AFP.

Ataxia with Oculomotor Apraxia, Type 2

Oculomotor apraxia is seen in about half of the cases of type 2 AOA (AOA2),[56,58] which is also called spinocerebellar ataxia (SCA), recessive 1. Other features associated with AOA2 include axonal neuropathy, cerebellar atrophy, and elevated AFP.[56] Dystonia, chorea, upper motor neuron signs, head tremor, and strabismus can also be seen. Elevated serum creatine kinase and hypogonadotropic hypogonadism is rare. Other extraneurologic involvement is not present. Disease onset is usually in the teens and progresses to loss of independent ambulation within 15 years.

AOA2 is associated with mutations in *SETX* gene on chromosome 9, which encodes the senataxin protein.[58] Senataxin is a DNA/RNA helicase involved in coordinating DNA replication, transcription, homologous recombination, meiotic sex chromosome inactivation, and DNA damage response.[60] In general, defective *SETX* gene leads to the disruption of genomic integrity. A less severe form of AOA2 can be seen with missense mutations in the helicase domain than in other mutations, whereas truncating and missense mutations outside of the helicase domain may be related to severe motor neuropathy.[56] Particular dominant mutations in the *SETX* gene can lead to a familial form of juvenile amyotrophic lateral sclerosis, and 2 missense mutations can cause a dominant ataxia syndrome.[61] AOA was also seen in a family with a homozygous missense mutation in the *PIK3R5* gene.[62]

Autosomal-Recessive Spastic Ataxia of Charlevoix-Saguenay

In 1978, Bouchard was the first to identify a recessive spastic ataxia in children in the Charlevoix-Sanguenay region of Quebec, Canada.[63] Since that description, autosomal-recessive spastic ataxia of Charlevoix-Saguenay has been reported in Japan, Europe, the United States, Brazil, North Africa, and Turkey.[64,65] Disease onset is usually in the first decade and presents with spasticity followed by ataxia, polyneuropathy, and amyotrophy of distal muscles.[66] Because progression is slow, patients often live into their 50s. autosomal-recessive spastic ataxia of Charlevoix-Saguenay is caused by over 70 mutations of the *SACS* gene on chromosome 13, which encodes a large chaperone protein, sacsin. The involvement of sacsin in the ubiquitin–proteasome pathway is suggested by its extensive homology with heat shock protein 90 and the *N*-terminus containing a ubiquitinlike domain.[67] Sacsin is also noted to localize to the mitochondria and plays a role in mitochondrial fission by interacting with dynamin-related protein 1.[68] In addition to the central nervous system, sacsin is highly expressed in skin, skeletal muscle, and pancreas. Variations in phenotype have occurred with association of unusual features including epilepsy,[69] supranuclear ophthalmoplegia, skin lipofuscin deposits,[70] autonomic dysfunction,[71] straightening of the dorsal spine,[72] and cognitive–behavioral dysfunction.[73]

Cervical spinal cord, cerebral cortex, and vermian atrophy is seen on MRI, with hyperintensities in the lateral pons with middle cerebellar peduncle thickening.[74] Tractography reveals axonal degeneration of the pyramidal tracts and widespread demyelination of the white matter.[75] Treatment is limited to supportive therapies. Muscle relaxants orally or by intrathecal delivery can be used for spasticity.

Infantile-Onset Spinocerebellar Ataxia

Infantile-onset SCA is a severe ataxia syndrome presenting soon after the first year of life with ataxia, hypotonia, athetosis, and areflexia. Similar to Alpers–Huttenlocher syndrome caused by *POLG* mutations, infantile-onset SCA can present with early-onset encephalopathy with liver dysfunction.[76] With progression, ophthalmoplegia, sensorineural hearing loss, axonal neuropathy, epilepsy, and optic atrophy may emerge. White matter changes, cerebellar cortical atrophy, thinning of the cervical spinal cord, and hyperintensities in the dentate nuclei and surrounding the fourth ventricle are seen on MRI.[77]

The culprit in infantile-onset SCA is a mutation in the gene *C10orf2*, which codes the twinkle protein, a mitochondrial helicase that participates in DNA replication, and a splice variant known as *twinky* on chromosome 10.[78] Twinkle catalyzes adenosine triphosphate–dependent $5' \rightarrow 3'$ unwinding of the duplex DNA,[79] and pairs with the mitochondrial DNA (mtDNA) polymerase gamma to create a processive replication machinery for single-stranded DNA synthesis.[80] The carboxy terminal part of Twinkle is crucial for mtDNA helicase function,[81] and the *N*-terminal portion is essential for efficient binding to ssDNA.[82] Defects in these regions disrupt both helicase activity and functional efficacy of the mtDNA replisome.[82] Dominant mutations of the C10orf2 gene have been reported with autosomal-dominant progressive external ophthalmoplegia[83] and sensory ataxic neuropathy, dysarthria and ophthalmoparesis.[84]

Refsum Disease

Buildup of phytanic acid, a branched chain fatty acid, in blood and other tissues leads to a peroxisomal disorder called Refsum's disease. Refsum's disease is distinct from infantile Refsum's disease (peroxisome biogenesis disorder), which manifests with sensorineural deafness, mental and growth retardation, hypotonia, atypical retinitis pigmentosa, facial dysmorphism, and hepatomegaly.[85] Refsum's disease, on the other hand, is caused by mutation in the gene encoding phytanoyl coenzyme A hydroxylase (*PHYH*) on chromosome 10 and is characterized by cerebellar ataxia, retinitis pigmentosa, sensorineural deafness, polyneuropathy, anosmia, skeletal abnormalities, ichthyosis, renal failure, elevated cerebrospinal fluid protein, and cardiac myopathy and arrhythmias.[86,87] Symptoms typically begin in childhood or adolescence, but adulthood onset can also be seen. Dietary modifications can decrease attacks and acute attacks can be treated with plasma exchange to lower plasma phytanic acid levels.[87,88]

Cerebrotendinous Xanthomatosis

Cerebrotendinous xanthomatosis is a rare lipid storage disease caused by mutations in the *CYP27A1* gene on chromosome 2, which codes for sterol 27-hydroxylase.[89,90] The deficiency of this enzyme leads to elevated plasma levels of cholestanol, a cholesterol derivative, and its accumulation in tissues, including the brain, tendons, and lungs. During the first decade of life, children present with diarrhea, hepatitis, jaundice, pale optic disk, cataracts, premature retinal senescence, and hypermyelinated retinal nerve fibers. By their teens and 20s, patients develop xanthomas, typically on the Achilles tendon or patella, hand, elbow and neck tendons, and neurologic symptoms including pyramidal signs, ataxia, epilepsy, polyneuropathy, cognitive impairment, and psychiatric problems. Rare features include myoclonus, dystonia, and parkinsonism.[91–93] Cerebellar ataxia is seen in most patients.[94] The xanthomas and early atherosclerosis can be distinguished from other conditions by the presence of cataracts and progressive neurologic symptoms.[95] Elevated levels of cholestanol in the serum and tendons can help with confirming the diagnosis. Serum cholesterol levels are in the low-to-normal range in cerebrotendinous xanthomatosis. Clinical deterioration can be prevented by prompt treatment with cholic acid, or chenodeoxycholic acid. A 3-hydroxy-3-methylglutaryl coenzyme A reductase inhibitor can be used alone or in combination with cholic acid.[96,97]

Marinesco–Sjogren Syndrome

Marinesco–Sjogren syndrome (MSS) is a recessive disorder characterized primarily by cerebellar ataxia, congenital cataracts, delayed psychomotor maturation, and myopathy associated with progressive muscle weakness.[98] Other associated features are skeletal deformities, short stature, and hypogonadotropic hypogonadism.[99] The responsible gene is *SIL1* on chromosome 5, which encodes a nucleotide exchange factor for the heat shock protein 70 chaperone HSPA5.[100] A defect in *SIL1* function leads to the accumulation of potentially cytotoxic unfolded proteins.[101] Although *SIL1* is the only gene associated with MSS, some patients with the typical MSS phenotype have been reported without *SIL1* mutations.[102] A genetically distinct entity, congenital cataracts, facial dysmorphism, and neuropathy is caused by mutation in *CTDP1* gene on chromosome 18. The 2 disorders share common features, including cataracts, ataxia, and psychomotor delay.[103] Brain MRI in MSS reveals vermian atrophy and hyperintensities of the cerebellar cortex.[104,105] Cerebellar cortical atrophy is seen on brain pathology, along with vacuolated Purkinje cells. Muscle pathology demonstrates myopathic changes and electronmicroscopic findings of autophagic vacuoles, membranous whorls, and electron-dense double-membrane structures associated with nuclei.[106–108] Clinical management is symptomatic, and includes surgical removal of the cataracts and hormonal replacement for the hypogonadism.

Seizures, Sensorineural Deafness, Ataxia, Mental Retardation, and Electrolyte Imbalance Syndrome

Seizures, sensorineural deafness, ataxia, mental retardation, and electrolyte imbalance (SeSAME) syndrome is characterized by infancy-onset generalized seizures, sensorineural hearing loss, ataxia, and psychomotor developmental delay associated with electrolyte abnormalities.[109] Intention tremor, lower extremity weakness, and axonal neuropathy can also be seen. Deafness typically manifests by 18 months. K^+ channel mutation of the *KCNJ10* gene on chromosome 1 is responsible for this rapidly progressive disorder, which causes complete loss of ambulation in children by age 6 years.[109,110] Cerebellar atrophy is visible on brain imaging and laboratory studies demonstrate abnormalities of potassium, pH, magnesium, calcium, plasma renin and aldosterone levels, and urinary loss of potassium, sodium, and magnesium.

SYNE1 ataxia (also known as spinocerebellar ataxia, autosomal recessive 8, recessive ataxia of Beauce, autosomal-recessive cerebellar ataxia 1)

In multiple French–Canadian families from the Beauce region of Quebec, affected members were found to have mutations in the *SYNE1* gene on chromosome 6 encoding a structural protein, which is a member of the spectrin family.[111] Symptoms begin in young adulthood with progressive ataxia, mild eye movement abnormalities, hyperreflexia, and dysarthria. Four unique homozygous mutations in *SYNE1* were seen in a Japanese family of consanguineous parents. Their phenotype was similar to that of the Canadian families with pure cerebellar atrophy on neuroimaging, and electromyeography and nerve conduction studies were unremarkable. One of the Japanese patients developed a slowly progressive upper and lower motor neuron disease at 6 years and developed ataxia at age 19 years.[112] Electromyeography of this patient showed chronic denervation throughout and MRI revealed atrophy of the cerebellum and brain stem.

Coenzyme Q10 Deficiency (Also Known as Autosomal-Recessive Cerebellar Ataxia 2)

Coenzyme Q10 (CoQ10) deficiency is a rare, clinically heterogenous disorder caused by a mutation in any gene associated with synthesis of coenzyme Q. Five major phenotypes have been described, including encephalomyopathy with seizures and ataxia; a multisystemic infantile type with encephalopathy, cardiomyopathy, and renal syndrome; an ataxic type with cerebellar atrophy; Leigh syndrome with growth retardation; and a myopathic form.[113] In the ataxic form, ataxia and cerebellar atrophy beginning in childhood is seen with markedly low levels of CoQ10 in muscle biopsy, along with lactic academia, elevated serum creatine kinase, and episodic myoglobulinemia. Other features include myoclonus, seizures, mental retardation, muscle weakness, fatigability, hyporeflexia, and pyramidal signs. Oral CoQ10 replacement causes dramatic improvement.[114,115] The role of CoQ10 in the pathogenesis of AOA1 is suspected in a family with a homozygous aprataxin gene mutation, accompanied by presumed secondary CoQ10 deficiency and ataxia.[116] Several gene mutations have been reported in CoQ10 deficiency, including *PDSS2* on chromosome 6 (COQ10D3), *PDSS1* on chromosome 10 (COQ10D2), *COQ2* on chromosome 4, *COQ4* on chromosome 9, *COQ6* on chromosome 14 (COQ10D6), *COQ8* on chromosome 1 (COQ10D4), and *COQ9* on chromosome 16 (COQ10D5).[113,117]

Posterior Column Ataxia and Retinitis Pigmentosa

Posterior column ataxia and retinitis pigmentosa presents in childhood with visual field narrowing and proprioceptive loss. By their 20s, patients are blind and have severe ataxia owing to sensory loss, develop scoliosis, achalasia, and weakness.[118] Hyperintensities of the spinal cord are seen on MRI.[119] The responsible gene is *FLVCR1* on chromosome 1,[120] whose mutation causes mislocalization of the *FLVCR1* protein in cells and decreases its half-life.[121] Treatment is supportive.

Late-Onset Tay–Sachs Disease

Mutation of the *HEXA* gene on chromosome 15 leads to a deficiency of β-hexosaminidase causing GM2 gangliosidosis,[122] which affects the thalamus, brainstem, substantia nigra, and cerebellum.[123] The late-onset syndrome is characterized by areflexia, proximal muscle weakness, fasciculations, cerebellar ataxia, and psychiatric and behavioral problems. Late-onset Tay–Sachs disease is reported to have presented with FA phenotype.[24]

Spinocerebellar Ataxia, Autosomal Recessive 1–13

These are rare autosomal-recessive ataxias, often reported in a single family. As gene loci become known, the disorders are named successively with the SCAR prefix. SCA, recessive 1 (AOA2), SCAR8 (SYNE1), and SCAR9 (COQ10D4) have already been discussed. **Table 1** summarizes the major features of the SCARs.

Table 1
Spinocerebellar ataxia, autosomal recessive (SCAR)

	Other Designations	Locus	Gene	Major Features
SCAR1	AOA2, SCAN2	9q34.13	*SETX*	Ataxia, hyperkinesia, peripheral neuropathy and areflexia beginning in the second decade. Oculomotor apraxia in ~20%. Skeletal and foot deformities. Elevated α-fetoprotein, gamma-globulin, and CK levels in the serum.
SCAR2	Cerebelloparenchymal disorder III (Norman type, CPD3), cerebellar ataxia 1 (autosomal recessive; CLA1)	9q34-qter	*SCAR2*	Nonprogressive cerebellar ataxia and cognitive impairment with severe granule cell loss beginning in childhood.
SCAR3	Spinocerebellar ataxia with blindness and deafness (SCABD)	6p23-p21	*SCAR3*	Ataxia with blindness and deafness.
SCAR4	Spinocerebellar ataxia with saccadic intrusions (SCASI; formerly SCA24)	1p36	*SCASI*	Progressive ataxia with difficulty in reading, pyramidal signs, myoclonus, axonal neuropathy and *pes cavus*. Onset in third decade.
SCAR5	Cerebellar ataxia with mental retardation, optic atrophy, and skin abnormalities (CAMOS)	15q25.3	*ZNF592*	Congenital spastic ataxia, developmental delay, microcephaly, optic atrophy, skin vessel changes and cerebellar atrophy.
SCAR6	Norwegian infantile-onset ataxia	20q11-q13	*CLA3*	Infancy-onset ataxia, hypotonia, mild spasticity, slow motor and speech development in early childhood, short stature, and *pes cavus.*
SCAR7	Classic late-infantile neuronal ceroid lipofuscinosis 2 (CLN2) disease	11p15	*TPP1*	Slowly progressive ataxia in childhood with cerebellar atrophy and occasional pyramidal and posterior column signs.
SCAR8	Beauce ataxia, SYNE1 ataxia	6q25.1-q25.2	*SYNE1*	Pure cerebellar ataxia with occasional lower limb hyperreflexia beginning in middle age.

SCAR9	COQ10D4, coenzyme Q10 deficiency	1q42.13	*COQ8*	Ataxic form beginning in childhood with ataxia associated with pyramidal signs, mild cognitive decline, and seizures. Muscle biopsy with ragged red fibers, and high lactic acid and CK levels. Other forms include myopathic, infantile, and Leigh syndrome.
SCAR10		3p22.1	*ANO10*	Cerebellar ataxia, LMN signs, and severe cerebellar atrophy beginning in the 3rd decade
SCAR11		1q32.2	*SYT14*	Cerebellar ataxia with psychomotor retardation; onset in childhood.
SCAR12	Spinocerebellar ataxia with mental retardation and epilepsy	16q21-q23	*SCAR12*	Childhood-onset cerebellar ataxia with generalized seizures, delayed psychomotor development, and mild cerebellar atrophy.
SCAR13		6q24.3	*GRM1*	Infancy-onset gait ataxia with delayed psychomotor development, profound mental retardation, poor speech, hyperreflexia, seizures, eye movement abnormalities, and cerebellar atrophy, ventriculomegaly on MRI.
SCAR14	Infantile-onset spinocerebellar ataxia and psychomotor delay	11q13	*SPTBN2*	Nonprogressive ataxia, psychomotor delay, tremor, and UMN signs beginning in first year of life
SCAR15		3q29	*KIAA0226*	Slowly progressive cerebellar syndrome, generalized epilepsy starting in first year of life.
SCAR16		16p13	*STUB1*	Variable age at onset with cerebellar syndrome; cognitive dysfunction, hypogonadism, spasticity, eye movement abnormalities in some patients.

Abbreviations: CK, creatine kinase; LMN, lower motor neuron; SCAR, spinocerebellar ataxia, autosomal recessive; UMN, upper motor neuron.

AUTOSOMAL-DOMINANT ATAXIAS

Autosomal-dominant ataxias occur in every generation of a pedigree, with a 50% risk of inheritance of the mutation from the affected parent, and without a gender predilection. Depending on the disease course, autosomal-dominant ataxias can be divided into the progressive, SCAs, and the episodic ataxias (EAs). Each entity in these categories is consecutively numbered to distinguish between various gene loci. SCA1 through SCA37 have been recognized and the list continues to grow. Dentatorubral-pallidoluysian atrophy (DRPLA)[124] belongs to the SCA group despite the unique nomenclature. There have been excellent recent reviews of SCAs in the literature.[125–128] Remarkably, SCA1-3, 6-8, 10, 12, 17, 31, and 36, and DRPLA are caused by expanded microsatellite repeats. Of these, SCA1-3, 6, 7, and 17, and DRPLA are caused by an expansion of polyglutamine-coding CAG repeats, whereas an expansion of noncoding repeats consisting of different repeat units causes SCA8 (CTG/CAG), 10 (ATTCT), 12 (CAG), 31 (TGGAA), and 36 (GGCCTG). Remaining SCAs are caused by point mutations. **Table 2** highlights the major features of the SCAs along with their gene mutations and loci gleaned from a recent consensus statement about the pathologic mechanisms of inherited ataxias.[128] It should be noted that there is no SCA9, because it was initially designated but not substantiated; mutations in the same gene are seen in SCA15 and SCA16; SCA19 and SCA22 are considered allelic disease; SCA24 is now assigned to a family of recessive ataxias (SCAR).

The EAs are characterized by transient reversible spells of ataxia, often associated with other features of variable duration. Brief attacks (seconds to minutes) of ataxia associated with tremor and dysarthria with childhood onset is seen in EA1. Interictal myokymia can be seen clinically or detected electrophysiologically. Some children have been reported with partial epilepsy, postural abnormalities, and tight heel cords.[129] Mutation of the potassium channel gene, *KCNA1*, on chromosome 12 is the culprit.

Longer episodes (lasting many hours) are seen in EA2, in association with nausea, vomiting, headache, dysarthria, and diplopia.[129] Nystagmus and mild gait difficulty can be present interictally. EA2 is related to mutations in a calcium channel gene, *CACNA1A*, on chromosome 19 and is allelic to familial hemiplegic migraines and SCA6.

EA3 presents with short spells of ataxia and vertigo accompanied by tinnitus, and is localized to chromosome 1q42.[130] EA4, whose chromosomal localization has not been determined, begins later in life with episodes of ataxia and vertigo lasting many hours.[131] EA5 is phenotypically similar to EA1 and is related to a mutation in *CACNB4* gene on chromosome 2q23.[132] Mutation in the *SLC1A3* gene on chromosome 5p13 is associated with EA6, which manifests with seizures, hemiplegia, and episodes of ataxia lasting 2 to 3 hours.[133] EA7 was reported in 7 members of a 4-generation family who experienced weakness, dysarthria, and vertigo beginning in the second decade.[134] Gene tests for many of the dominant and recessive ataxias are available[135] (see GeneTests, www.genetests.org), including SCA1, 2, 3, 5, 6, 7, 10, 12, 13, 14, and 17, and DRPLA. This list is likely to expand.

OTHER INHERITED ATAXIAS

Mutations in the mtDNA can cause progressive ataxia associated with myopathy, external ophthalmoplegia, endocrine deficiencies, short stature, and retinal pigmentary degeneration. Syndromes with ataxia associated with mitochondrial mutations include myoclonic epilepsy with ragged red fibers and neuropathy, ataxia, and retinitis pigmentosa. Less commonly, it is associated with progressive external ophthalmoplegia,

Table 2
Autosomal-dominant spinocerebellar ataxias (SCAs)

Name	Gene/Protein	Locus	Mechanism	Major Clinical Features
SCA1	*ATXN1*/Ataxin-1	6p22	CAG repeat expansion; gain- and loss-of-function; transcription dysregulation; alteration of neuronal Ca channel signaling; poor degradation of and accumulation in Purkinje cells. [B]	Age of onset varies early childhood to late adulthood (mean age, 30s). Cerebellar ataxia, dysarthria and UMN signs early. Later, dysphagia, ophthalmoparesis, sensory neuropathy, amyotrophy, slow saccades, cognitive decline. Chorea and dystonia possible. Diagnosis to death: 15–20 y. Anticipation is present.
SCA2	*ATXN2*/Ataxin-2	12q24	CAG repeat expansion; dysfunction of cellular RNA metabolism and endocytosis processes; possibly abnormal neuronal Ca channel signaling; [B60]	Similar to SCA1; very slow saccades, neuropathy, areflexia. Dystonia, DOPA-responsive parkinsonism, myoclonus, tremor and cognitive decline possible. Infantile form reported. Association with ALS. Anticipation is present.
SCA3 (Machado-Joseph disease)	*ATXN3*/Ataxin-3	14q32	CAG repeat expansion; de-ubiquitination and dysfunctional interaction with transcriptional factors leading to destabilization and neuronal cell death	Most common SCA worldwide. SCA1-like phenotype: Ataxia, brainstem signs (facial and tongue atrophy and fasciculations, dysphagia, poor cough), neuropathy, areflexia. Ophthalmoparesis, slow saccades, blepharospasm, eyelid retraction, cognitive decline, sleep and autonomic disturbances possible. DOPA-responsive parkinsonism and dystonia may predominate. Anticipation is present.

(*continued on next page*)

Table 2
(continued)

Name	Gene/Protein	Locus	Mechanism	Major Clinical Features
SCA4		16q24	Unknown	Late adulthood onset ataxia and sensory axonal motor neuropathy.
SCA5 (Lincoln ataxia)	*SPTBN2*/β-III Spectrin	11q13	Defect in neuronal membrane skeleton	Slowly progressive, early-onset bulbar signs and cerebellar syndrome.
SCA6	CACNA1A	19p13	CAG repeat expansion; cytoplasmic aggregations of the alpha-1A calcium channel protein	Late adulthood onset cerebellar syndrome with saccadic abnormalities and nystagmus. Anticipation is present.
SCA7	*ATXN7*/Ataxin-7	3p14	CAG repeat expansion; transcription dysregulation	Onset during first decade, Huntington disease–like phenotype with deafness and pigmentary retinopathy. Prominent anticipation is present.
SCA8	*ATXN8OS*/*ATXN8*/ Ataxin-8	13q21	RNA gain-of-function; repeat associated non-ATG (RAN) translation	Cerebellar syndrome with sensory neuropathy, spasticity, cognitive and psychiatric abnormalities. Reduced penetrance.
SCA10	*ATXN10*/Ataxin-10	22q13	ATTCT repeat expansion; gain-of-function causing RNA toxicity	Cerebellar syndrome with epilepsy. Anticipation is present.
SCA11	*TTBK2*/Tau tubulin kinase 2	15q15	Tau phosphorylation dysregulation	Cerebellar syndrome with hyperreflexia.
SCA12	*PPP2R2B*/Protein phosphorylase 2A	5q32	CAG repeat expansion; protein phosphatase (PP2A) and transcription regulation	Cerebellar syndrome including upper extremity tremor, hyperreflexia, axonal neuropathy, cognitive decline. Atrophy of cerebral cortex and cerebellum. Anticipation is present.
SCA13	*KCNC3*/KCNC3	19q13	Potassium channel dysfunction	Variable phenotype depending on the mutation. Early-onset cerebellar syndrome with cognitive dysfunction vs later onset cerebellar ataxia with normal ocular movements.

SCA14	*PRKCG*/Protein kinase C-gamma	19q13	Alterations of neuronal Ca channel signaling, synaptic transmission, proteasome degradation and neurites	Cerebellar syndrome, myoclonus in early-onset, dystonia and cognitive decline in some.
SCA15	*ITPR1*/ITPR1	3p26	Insufficiency in the smooth endoplasmic reticulum calcium channel IP3R1	Slowly progressive cerebellar syndrome.
SCA16	*ITPR1*/ITPR1	3p26	Insufficiency in the smooth endoplasmic reticulum calcium channel IP3R1	Slowly progressive cerebellar syndrome with head tremor.
SCA17 (HDL4)	*TBP*/TATA binding protein	6q27	CAG repeat expansion; Transcription dysregulation; reduced levels of chaperones	Cerebellar syndrome with UMN signs, extrapyramidal signs, epilepsy. Occasional hypogonadism. Anticipation is present.
SCA18	Unknown	7q22-q32	Unknown	Cerebellar syndrome with sensory neuropathy, muscle weakness and atrophy. Occasional deafness.
SCA19	*KCND3*/KCND3	1p21-q21	Potassium channel dysfunction	Cerebellar syndrome with variable reflexes, myoclonus, tremor. Occasional deafness, spasticity.
SCA20		11q12	Chromosomal duplication	Ataxia, dysphonia, palatal tremor. Dentate calcifications on imaging.
SCA21		7p21	Unknown	Slowly progressive cerebellar syndrome, hyperreflexia, parkinsonism unresponsive to L-DOPA.
SCA22	*KCND3*/KCND3	1p21	Potassium channel dysfunction;	Slowly progressive gait ataxia and nystagmus. Anticipation is reported.
SCA23	*PDYN*/Prodynorphin	20p13	Upregulation of dynorphin A leading to cerebellar toxicity	Ataxia with sensory loss and pyramidal signs.
SCA24				Now called SCAR4.
SCA25	Unknown	2p21-p15	Unknown	Cerebellar syndrome with sensory neuropathy and gastrointestinal features. Severe cerebellar atrophy.

(*continued on next page*)

Table 2
(*continued*)

Name	Gene/Protein	Locus	Mechanism	Major Clinical Features
SCA26	*EEF2*/EEF2	19p13	RNA metabolism, proteostatic dysruption	Slowly progressive cerebellar syndrome
SCA27	*FGF14*/fibroblast growth factor 14	13q33	Signal transduction; dysregulation of sodium channels	Cerebellar syndrome with psychiatric features, tremor, dyskinesia.
SCA28	*AFG3L2*/AFG3L2	18p11	Mitochondrial membrane protease dysfunction	Cerebellar syndrome with ophthalmoparesis and UMN signs. Myoclonic epilepsy rare.
SCA29	*ITPR1*/ITPR1	3p26	Unknown	Congenital, nonprogressive, variant of SCA15.
SCA30	Unknown	4q34	Unknown	Slowly progressive, late-onset cerebellar syndrome
SCA31	*BEAN*/BEAN	16q21	TGGAA repeat expansion; unknown mechanism but RNA toxicity is suspected	Late-adulthood onset.
SCA32	Unknown	7q32	Unknown	Cerebellar syndrome with azospermia and cognitive impairment.
SCA34	Unknown	6p12	Unknown	Skin lesions soon after birth resolving by adulthood when ataxia, dysarthria, nystagmus, and areflexia appear. Cognition and sensation unaffected.
SCA35	*TGM6*/Transglutaminase 6	20p13	Impaired cross-linking of proteins	Cerebellar syndrome with UMN signs, sensory loss, and spasmodic torticollis.
SCA36	NOP56/NOP56 ribonucleoprotein	20p13	GGCCTG repeat expansion; toxic RNA gain of function	Slowly progressive, late-onset cerebellar syndrome, UMN and LMN signs.
SCA37	Unknown	1p32	Unknown	Slowly progressive, late-onset cerebellar syndrome with abnormal vertical eye movements.

Abbreviations: ALS, amyotrophic lateral sclerosis; LMN, lower motor neuron; SCA, spinocerebellar ataxia; UMN, upper motor neuron.

Kearns-Sayre syndrome, and mitochondrial encephalopathy, lactic acidosis, and stroke-like episodes.

Fragile X tremor–ataxia syndrome is an X-linked disorder with ataxia described in the grandfathers of patients with fragile X mental retardation associated with mutation of the FMR1 gene.[136] A full mutation has an expansion of more than 200 CGG repeats, whereas normal chromosomes have fewer than 54 repeats. Other features of the syndrome include executive dysfunction, global brain atrophy, mild parkinsonism, dysautonomia, and psychiatric disturbances. Brain MRI classically shows T2 hyperintensity in the middle cerebellar peduncle and subcortical white matter changes. Testing for a premutation in patients with ataxia, tremor, or both, and family history of mental retardation may be worthwhile.

REFERENCES

1. Barnard RO, Campbell MJ, McDonald WI. Pathological findings in a case of hypothyroidism with ataxia. J Neurol Neurosurg Psychiatr 1971;34(6):755–60.
2. Jellinek EH, Kelly RE. Cerebellar syndrome in myxoedema. Lancet 1960; 2(7144):225–7.
3. Diener HC, Dichgans J, Bacher M, et al. Improvement of ataxia in alcoholic cerebellar atrophy through alcohol abstinence. J Neurol 1984;231(5):258–62.
4. Gottlieb JA, Luce JK. Cerebellar ataxia with weekly 5-fluorouracil administration. Lancet 1971;1(7690):138–9.
5. Sirven JI, Fife TD, Wingerchuk DM, et al. Second-generation antiepileptic drugs' impact on balance: a meta-analysis. Mayo Clin Proc 2007;82(1):40–7.
6. Mani J, Chaudhary N, Kanjalkar M, et al. Cerebellar ataxia due to lead encephalopathy in an adult. J Neurol Neurosurg Psychiatr 1998;65(5):797.
7. Gordon MF, Abrams RI, Rubin DB, et al. Bismuth subsalicylate toxicity as a cause of prolonged encephalopathy with myoclonus. Mov Disord 1995;10(2):220–2.
8. Boor JW, Hurtig HI. Persistent cerebellar ataxia after exposure to toluene. Ann Neurol 1977;2(5):440–2.
9. Odaka M, Yuki N, Yamada M, et al. Bickerstaff's brainstem encephalitis: clinical features of 62 cases and a subgroup associated with Guillain-Barre syndrome. Brain 2003;126(Pt 10):2279–90.
10. Matthews BR, Jones LK, Saad DA, et al. Cerebellar ataxia and central nervous system Whipple disease. Arch Neurol 2005;62(4):618–20.
11. Hoffmann LA, Jarius S, Pellkofer HL, et al. Anti-Ma and anti-Ta associated paraneoplastic neurological syndromes: 22 newly diagnosed patients and review of previous cases. J Neurol Neurosurg Psychiatr 2008;79(7):767–73.
12. Hadjivassiliou M, Grunewald RA, Lawden M, et al. Headache and CNS white matter abnormalities associated with gluten sensitivity. Neurology 2001;56(3):385–8.
13. Bayreuther C, Hieronimus S, Ferrari P, et al. Auto-immune cerebellar ataxia with anti-GAD antibodies accompanied by de novo late-onset type 1 diabetes mellitus. Diabetes Metab 2008;34(4 Pt 1):386–8.
14. Markakis I, Alexiou E, Xifaras M, et al. Opsoclonus-myoclonus-ataxia syndrome with autoantibodies to glutamic acid decarboxylase. Clin Neurol Neurosurg 2008;110(6):619–21.
15. Nanri K, Okita M, Takeguchi M, et al. Intravenous immunoglobulin therapy for autoantibody-positive cerebellar ataxia. Intern Med 2009;48(10):783–90.
16. Nociti V, Frisullo G, Tartaglione T, et al. Refractory generalized seizures and cerebellar ataxia associated with anti-GAD antibodies responsive to immunosuppressive treatment. Eur J Neurol 2010;17(1):e5.

17. Vulliemoz S, Vanini G, Truffert A, et al. Epilepsy and cerebellar ataxia associated with anti-glutamic acid decarboxylase antibodies. J Neurol Neurosurg Psychiatr 2007;78(2):187–9.
18. Fearnley JM, Stevens JM, Rudge P. Superficial siderosis of the central nervous system. Brain 1995;118(Pt 4):1051–66.
19. Fearnley J, Rudge P. Treatment of superficial siderosis of the central nervous system. Mov Disord 1995;10(5):685.
20. Delatycki MB, Williamson R, Forrest SM. Friedreich ataxia: an overview. J Med Genet 2000;37(1):1–8.
21. Pandolfo M. Friedreich ataxia: the clinical picture. J Neurol 2009;256(Suppl 1):3–8.
22. Mascalchi M, Salvi F, Piacentini S, et al. Friedreich's ataxia: MR findings involving the cervical portion of the spinal cord. AJR Am J Roentgenol 1994; 163(1):187–91.
23. Campuzano V, Montermini L, Molto MD, et al. Friedreich's ataxia: autosomal recessive disease caused by an intronic GAA triplet repeat expansion. Science 1996;271(5254):1423–7.
24. Manto M, Marmolino D. Cerebellar ataxias. Curr Opin Neurol 2009;22(4):419–29.
25. Bhidayasiri R, Perlman SL, Pulst SM, et al. Late-onset Friedreich ataxia: phenotypic analysis, magnetic resonance imaging findings, and review of the literature. Arch Neurol 2005;62(12):1865–9.
26. Zhu D, Burke C, Leslie A, et al. Friedreich's ataxia with chorea and myoclonus caused by a compound heterozygosity for a novel deletion and the trinucleotide GAA expansion. Mov Disord 2002;17(3):585–9.
27. Leonard H, Forsyth R. Friedreich's ataxia presenting after cardiac transplantation. Arch Dis Child 2001;84(2):167–8.
28. Kearney M, Orrell RW, Fahey M, et al. Antioxidants and other pharmacological treatments for Friedreich ataxia. Cochrane Database Syst Rev 2012;(4):CD007791.
29. Lagedrost SJ, Sutton MS, Cohen MS, et al. Idebenone in Friedreich ataxia cardiomyopathy-results from a 6-month phase III study (IONIA). Am Heart J 2011;161(3):639–45.e1.
30. Lynch DR, Willi SM, Wilson RB, et al. A0001 in Friedreich ataxia: biochemical characterization and effects in a clinical trial. Mov Disord 2012;27(8):1026–33.
31. Mariotti C, Fancellu R, Caldarazzo S, et al. Erythropoietin in Friedreich ataxia: no effect on frataxin in a randomized controlled trial. Mov Disord 2012;27(3):446–9.
32. Velasco-Sanchez D, Aracil A, Montero R, et al. Combined therapy with idebenone and deferiprone in patients with Friedreich's ataxia. Cerebellum 2011; 10(1):1–8.
33. Eppie Yiu GT, Peverill R, Lee K, et al. An Open Label Clinical Pilot Study of Resveratrol as a treatment for Friedreich Ataxia (S43. 006). Neurology 2013. Available at: http://www.neurology.org/cgi/content/meeting_abstract/80/1_MeetingAbstracts/S43.006.
34. Ristori G, Romano S, Visconti A, et al. Riluzole in cerebellar ataxia: a randomized, double-blind, placebo-controlled pilot trial. Neurology 2010;74(10): 839–45.
35. Sacca F, Piro R, De Michele G, et al. Epoetin alfa increases frataxin production in Friedreich's ataxia without affecting hematocrit. Mov Disord 2011;26(4):739–42.
36. Libri V, Yandim C, Athanasopoulos S, et al. Epigenetic and neurological effects and safety of high-dose nicotinamide in patients with Friedreich's ataxia: an exploratory, open-label, dose-escalation study. Lancet 2014;384(9942): 504–13.

37. Soragni E, Miao W, Iudicello M, et al. Epigenetic therapy for Friedreich ataxia. Ann Neurol 2014;76(4):489–508.
38. Ouahchi K, Arita M, Kayden H, et al. Ataxia with isolated vitamin E deficiency is caused by mutations in the alpha-tocopherol transfer protein. Nat Genet 1995; 9(2):141–5.
39. Cavalier L, Ouahchi K, Kayden HJ, et al. Ataxia with isolated vitamin E deficiency: heterogeneity of mutations and phenotypic variability in a large number of families. Am J Hum Genet 1998;62(2):301–10.
40. Di Donato I, Bianchi S, Federico A. Ataxia with vitamin E deficiency: update of molecular diagnosis. Neurol Sci 2010;31(4):511–5.
41. Mariotti C, Gellera C, Rimoldi M, et al. Ataxia with isolated vitamin E deficiency: neurological phenotype, clinical follow-up and novel mutations in TTPA gene in Italian families. Neurol Sci 2004;25(3):130–7.
42. Fogel BL, Perlman S. Clinical features and molecular genetics of autosomal recessive cerebellar ataxias. Lancet Neurol 2007;6(3):245–57.
43. Bomar JM, Benke PJ, Slattery EL, et al. Mutations in a novel gene encoding a CRAL-TRIO domain cause human Cayman ataxia and ataxia/dystonia in the jittery mouse. Nat Genet 2003;35(3):264–9.
44. Swift M, Heim RA, Lench NJ. Genetic aspects of ataxia telangiectasia. Adv Neurol 1993;61:115–25.
45. Mandriota SJ, Buser R, Lesne L, et al. Ataxia telangiectasia mutated (ATM) inhibition transforms human mammary gland epithelial cells. J Biol Chem 2010;285(17):13092–106.
46. Kastan MB, Lim DS. The many substrates and functions of ATM. Nat Rev Mol Cell Biol 2000;1(3):179–86.
47. Tanaka H, Mendonca MS, Bradshaw PS, et al. DNA damage-induced phosphorylation of the human telomere-associated protein TRF2. Proc Natl Acad Sci U S A 2005;102(43):15539–44.
48. D'Souza AD, Parish IA, Krause DS, et al. Reducing mitochondrial ROS improves disease-related pathology in a mouse model of ataxia-telangiectasia. Mol Ther 2013;21(1):42–8.
49. Lavin MF, Gueven N, Bottle S, et al. Current and potential therapeutic strategies for the treatment of ataxia-telangiectasia. Br Med Bull 2007;81–82:129–47.
50. Reliene R, Schiestl RH. Experimental antioxidant therapy in ataxia telangiectasia. Clin Med Oncol 2008;2:431–6.
51. Gatti RA, Perlman S. A proposed bailout for A-T patients? Eur J Neurol 2009; 16(6):653–5.
52. Menotta M, Biagiotti S, Bianchi M, et al. Dexamethasone partially rescues ataxia telangiectasia-mutated (ATM) deficiency in ataxia telangiectasia by promoting a shortened protein variant retaining kinase activity. J Biol Chem 2012;287(49): 41352–63.
53. Schiller CB, Lammens K, Guerini I, et al. Structure of Mre11-Nbs1 complex yields insights into ataxia-telangiectasia-like disease mutations and DNA damage signaling. Nat Struct Mol Biol 2012;19(7):693–700.
54. Embirucu EK, Martyn ML, Schlesinger D, et al. Autosomal recessive ataxias: 20 types, and counting. Arq Neuropsiquiatr 2009;67(4):1143–56.
55. Palmeri S, Rufa A, Pucci B, et al. Clinical course of two Italian siblings with ataxia-telangiectasia-like disorder. Cerebellum 2013;12(4):596–9.
56. Anheim M, Monga B, Fleury M, et al. Ataxia with oculomotor apraxia type 2: clinical, biological and genotype/phenotype correlation study of a cohort of 90 patients. Brain 2009;132(Pt 10):2688–98.

57. Silva MC, Coutinho P, Pinheiro CD, et al. Hereditary ataxias and spastic paraplegias: methodological aspects of a prevalence study in Portugal. J Clin Epidemiol 1997;50(12):1377–84.
58. Le Ber I, Moreira MC, Rivaud-Pechoux S, et al. Cerebellar ataxia with oculomotor apraxia type 1: clinical and genetic studies. Brain 2003;126(Pt 12):2761–72.
59. Mosesso P, Piane M, Palitti F, et al. The novel human gene aprataxin is directly involved in DNA single-strand-break repair. Cell Mol Life Sci 2005; 62(4):485–91.
60. Becherel OJ, Yeo AJ, Stellati A, et al. Senataxin plays an essential role with DNA damage response proteins in meiotic recombination and gene silencing. PLoS Genet 2013;9(4):e1003435.
61. Bassuk AG, Chen YZ, Batish SD, et al. In cis autosomal dominant mutation of Senataxin associated with tremor/ataxia syndrome. Neurogenetics 2007;8(1): 45–9.
62. Al Tassan N, Khalil D, Shinwari J, et al. A missense mutation in PIK3R5 gene in a family with ataxia and oculomotor apraxia. Hum Mutat 2012;33(2):351–4.
63. Baets J, Deconinck T, Smets K, et al. Mutations in SACS cause atypical and late-onset forms of ARSACS. Neurology 2010;75(13):1181–8.
64. Breckpot J, Takiyama Y, Thienpont B, et al. A novel genomic disorder: a deletion of the SACS gene leading to spastic ataxia of Charlevoix-Saguenay. Eur J Hum Genet 2008;16(9):1050–4.
65. Vermeer S, Meijer RP, Pijl BJ, et al. ARSACS in the Dutch population: a frequent cause of early-onset cerebellar ataxia. Neurogenetics 2008;9(3):207–14.
66. Takiyama Y. Sacsinopathies: sacsin-related ataxia. Cerebellum 2007;6(4): 353–9.
67. Parfitt DA, Michael GJ, Vermeulen EG, et al. The ataxia protein sacsin is a functional co-chaperone that protects against polyglutamine-expanded ataxin-1. Hum Mol Genet 2009;18(9):1556–65.
68. Girard M, Lariviere R, Parfitt DA, et al. Mitochondrial dysfunction and Purkinje cell loss in autosomal recessive spastic ataxia of Charlevoix-Saguenay (ARSACS). Proc Natl Acad Sci U S A 2012;109(5):1661–6.
69. Tzoulis C, Johansson S, Haukanes BI, et al. Novel SACS mutations identified by whole exome sequencing in a Norwegian family with autosomal recessive spastic ataxia of Charlevoix-Saguenay. PLoS One 2013;8(6):e66145.
70. Stevens JC, Murphy SM, Davagnanam I, et al. The ARSACS phenotype can include supranuclear gaze palsy and skin lipofuscin deposits. J Neurol Neurosurg Psychiatr 2013;84(1):114–6.
71. Miyatake S, Miyake N, Doi H, et al. A novel SACS mutation in an atypical case with autosomal recessive spastic ataxia of Charlevoix-Saguenay (ARSACS). Intern Med 2012;51(16):2221–6.
72. Gazulla J, Benavente I, Vela AC, et al. New findings in the ataxia of Charlevoix-Saguenay. J Neurol 2012;259(5):869–78.
73. Verhoeven WM, Egger JI, Ahmed AI, et al. Cerebellar cognitive affective syndrome and autosomal recessive spastic ataxia of charlevoix-saguenay: a report of two male sibs. Psychopathology 2012;45(3):193–9.
74. Synofzik M, Soehn AS, Gburek-Augustat J, et al. Autosomal recessive spastic ataxia of Charlevoix Saguenay (ARSACS): expanding the genetic, clinical and imaging spectrum. Orphanet J Rare Dis 2013;8:41.
75. Oguz KK, Haliloglu G, Temucin C, et al. Assessment of whole-brain white matter by DTI in autosomal recessive spastic ataxia of Charlevoix-Saguenay. AJNR Am J Neuroradiol 2013;34(10):1952–7.

76. Goh V, Helbling D, Biank V, et al. Next-generation sequencing facilitates the diagnosis in a child with twinkle mutations causing cholestatic liver failure. J Pediatr Gastroenterol Nutr 2012;54(2):291–4.
77. Hakonen AH, Isohanni P, Paetau A, et al. Recessive Twinkle mutations in early onset encephalopathy with mtDNA depletion. Brain 2007;130(Pt 11):3032–40.
78. Nikali K, Suomalainen A, Saharinen J, et al. Infantile onset spinocerebellar ataxia is caused by recessive mutations in mitochondrial proteins Twinkle and Twinky. Hum Mol Genet 2005;14(20):2981–90.
79. Korhonen JA, Gaspari M, Falkenberg M. TWINKLE Has 5' -> 3' DNA helicase activity and is specifically stimulated by mitochondrial single-stranded DNA-binding protein. J Biol Chem 2003;278(49):48627–32.
80. Korhonen JA, Pham XH, Pellegrini M, et al. Reconstitution of a minimal mtDNA replisome in vitro. EMBO J 2004;23(12):2423–9.
81. Matsushima Y, Farr CL, Fan L, et al. Physiological and biochemical defects in carboxyl-terminal mutants of mitochondrial DNA helicase. J Biol Chem 2008; 283(35):23964–71.
82. Farge G, Holmlund T, Khvorostova J, et al. The N-terminal domain of TWINKLE contributes to single-stranded DNA binding and DNA helicase activities. Nucleic Acids Res 2008;36(2):393–403.
83. Spelbrink JN, Li FY, Tiranti V, et al. Human mitochondrial DNA deletions associated with mutations in the gene encoding Twinkle, a phage T7 gene 4-like protein localized in mitochondria. Nat Genet 2001;28(3):223–31.
84. Hudson G, Deschauer M, Busse K, et al. Sensory ataxic neuropathy due to a novel C10Orf2 mutation with probable germline mosaicism. Neurology 2005; 64(2):371–3.
85. Wanders RJ, Jansen GA, Skjeldal OH. Refsum disease, peroxisomes and phytanic acid oxidation: a review. J Neuropathol Exp Neurol 2001;60(11): 1021–31.
86. Jansen GA, Waterham HR, Wanders RJ. Molecular basis of Refsum disease: sequence variations in phytanoyl-CoA hydroxylase (PHYH) and the PTS2 receptor (PEX7). Hum Mutat 2004;23(3):209–18.
87. Weinstein R. Phytanic acid storage disease (Refsum's disease): clinical characteristics, pathophysiology and the role of therapeutic apheresis in its management. J Clin Apheresis 1999;14(4):181–4.
88. Baldwin EJ, Gibberd FB, Harley C, et al. The effectiveness of long-term dietary therapy in the treatment of adult Refsum disease. J Neurol Neurosurg Psychiatr 2010;81(9):954–7.
89. Pilo B, de Blas G, Sobrido MJ, et al. Neurophysiological study in cerebrotendinous xanthomatosis. Muscle Nerve 2011;43(4):531–6.
90. Verrips A, Hoefsloot LH, Steenbergen GC, et al. Clinical and molecular genetic characteristics of patients with cerebrotendinous xanthomatosis. Brain 2000; 123(Pt 5):908–19.
91. Grandas F, Martin-Moro M, Garcia-Munozguren S, et al. Early-onset parkinsonism in cerebrotendinous xanthomatosis. Mov Disord 2002;17(6):1396–7.
92. Lagarde J, Roze E, Apartis E, et al. Myoclonus and dystonia in cerebrotendinous xanthomatosis. Mov Disord 2012;27(14):1805–10.
93. Su CS, Chang WN, Huang SH, et al. Cerebrotendinous xanthomatosis patients with and without parkinsonism: clinical characteristics and neuroimaging findings. Mov Disord 2010;25(4):452–8.
94. Federico A, Dotti MT, Gallus GN. Cerebrotendinous xanthomatosis. In: Pagon RA, Adam MP, Ardinger HH, et al, editors. GeneReviews(R). Seattle (WA): 1993.

95. Lange MC, Zetola VF, Teive HA, et al. Cerebrotendinous xanthomatosis: report of two Brazilian brothers. Arq Neuropsiquiatr 2004;62(4):1085–9.
96. Federico A, Dotti MT. Cerebrotendinous xanthomatosis: clinical manifestations, diagnostic criteria, pathogenesis, and therapy. J Child Neurol 2003; 18(9):633–8.
97. Ostrowska M, Banaszkiewicz K, Kilawiec A, et al. Cerebrotendinous xanthomatosis: a rare cause of spinocerebellar syndrome. Neurol Neurochir Pol 2011; 45(6):600–3.
98. Horvers M, Anttonen AK, Lehesjoki AE, et al. Marinesco-Sjogren syndrome due to SIL1 mutations with a comment on the clinical phenotype. Europ J Paediatr Neurol 2013;17(2):199–203.
99. Alter M, Talbert OR, Croffead G. Cerebellar ataxia, congenital cataracts, and retarded somatic and mental maturation. Report of cases of Marinesco-Sjogren syndrome. Neurology 1962;12:836–47.
100. Anttonen AK, Siintola E, Tranebjaerg L, et al. Novel SIL1 mutations and exclusion of functional candidate genes in Marinesco-Sjogren syndrome. Eur J Hum Genet 2008;16(8):961–9.
101. Van Raamsdonk JM. Loss of function mutations in SIL1 cause Marinesco-Sjogren syndrome. Clin Genet 2006;69(5):399–400.
102. Yis U, Cirak S, Hiz S, et al. Heterogeneity of Marinesco-Sjogren syndrome: report of two cases. Pediatr Neurol 2011;45(6):409–11.
103. Merlini L, Gooding R, Lochmuller H, et al. Genetic identity of Marinesco-Sjogren/myoglobinuria and CCFDN syndromes. Neurology 2002;58(2):231–6.
104. Anttonen AK, Mahjneh I, Hamalainen RH, et al. The gene disrupted in Marinesco-Sjogren syndrome encodes SIL1, an HSPA5 cochaperone. Nat Genet 2005;37(12):1309–11.
105. Harting I, Blaschek A, Wolf NI, et al. T2-hyperintense cerebellar cortex in Marinesco-Sjogren syndrome. Neurology 2004;63(12):2448–9.
106. Herva R, von Wendt L, von Wendt G, et al. A syndrome with juvenile cataract, cerebellar atrophy, mental retardation and myopathy. Neuropediatrics 1987; 18(3):164–9.
107. Sasaki K, Suga K, Tsugawa S, et al. Muscle pathology in Marinesco-Sjogren syndrome: a unique ultrastructural feature. Brain Dev 1996;18(1):64–7.
108. Sewry CA, Voit T, Dubowitz V. Myopathy with unique ultrastructural feature in Marinesco-Sjogren syndrome. Ann Neurol 1988;24(4):576–80.
109. Scholl UI, Dave HB, Lu M, et al. SeSAME/EAST syndrome–phenotypic variability and delayed activity of the distal convoluted tubule. Pediatr Nephrol 2012; 27(11):2081–90.
110. Scholl UI, Choi M, Liu T, et al. Seizures, sensorineural deafness, ataxia, mental retardation, and electrolyte imbalance (SeSAME syndrome) caused by mutations in KCNJ10. Proc Natl Acad Sci U S A 2009;106(14):5842–7.
111. Gros-Louis F, Dupre N, Dion P, et al. Mutations in SYNE1 lead to a newly discovered form of autosomal recessive cerebellar ataxia. Nat Genet 2007; 39(1):80–5.
112. Izumi Y, Miyamoto R, Morino H, et al. Cerebellar ataxia with SYNE1 mutation accompanying motor neuron disease. Neurology 2013;80(6):600–1.
113. Montero R, Pineda M, Aracil A, et al. Clinical, biochemical and molecular aspects of cerebellar ataxia and Coenzyme Q10 deficiency. Cerebellum 2007; 6(2):118–22.
114. Gironi M, Lamperti C, Nemni R, et al. Late-onset cerebellar ataxia with hypogonadism and muscle coenzyme Q10 deficiency. Neurology 2004;62(5):818–20.

115. Lamperti C, Naini A, Hirano M, et al. Cerebellar ataxia and coenzyme Q10 deficiency. Neurology 2003;60(7):1206–8.
116. Quinzii CM, Kattah AG, Naini A, et al. Coenzyme Q deficiency and cerebellar ataxia associated with an aprataxin mutation. Neurology 2005;64(3):539–41.
117. Horvath R. Update on clinical aspects and treatment of selected vitamin-responsive disorders II (riboflavin and CoQ 10). J Inherit Metab Dis 2012; 35(4):679–87.
118. Ishiura H, Fukuda Y, Mitsui J, et al. Posterior column ataxia with retinitis pigmentosa in a Japanese family with a novel mutation in FLVCR1. Neurogenetics 2011; 12(2):117–21.
119. Berciano J, Polo JM. Autosomal recessive posterior column ataxia and retinitis pigmentosa. Neurology 1998;51(6):1772–3.
120. Rajadhyaksha AM, Elemento O, Puffenberger EG, et al. Mutations in FLVCR1 cause posterior column ataxia and retinitis pigmentosa. Am J Hum Genet 2010;87(5):643–54.
121. Yanatori I, Yasui Y, Miura K, et al. Mutations of FLVCR1 in posterior column ataxia and retinitis pigmentosa result in the loss of heme export activity. Blood Cells Mol Dis 2012;49(1):60–6.
122. Montalvo AL, Filocamo M, Vlahovicek K, et al. Molecular analysis of the HEXA gene in Italian patients with infantile and late onset Tay-Sachs disease: detection of fourteen novel alleles. Hum Mutat 2005;26(3):282.
123. Suzuki K. Neuropathology of late onset gangliosidoses. A review. Dev Neurosci 1991;13(4–5):205–10.
124. Koide R, Ikeuchi T, Onodera O, et al. Unstable expansion of CAG repeat in hereditary dentatorubral-pallidoluysian atrophy (DRPLA). Nat Genet 1994;6(1): 9–13.
125. Rossi M, Perez-Lloret S, Doldan L, et al. Autosomal dominant cerebellar ataxias: a systematic review of clinical features. Eur J Neurol 2014;21(4):607–15.
126. Almeida-Silva UC, Hallak JE, Junior WM, et al. Association between spinocerebellar ataxias caused by glutamine expansion and psychiatric and neuropsychological signals - a literature review. Am J Neurodegener Dis 2013;2(2): 57–69.
127. Trott A, Houenou LJ. Mini-review: spinocerebellar ataxias: an update of SCA genes. Recent Pat DNA Gene Seq 2012;6(2):115–21.
128. Matilla-Duenas A, Ashizawa T, Brice A, et al. Consensus paper: pathological mechanisms underlying neurodegeneration in spinocerebellar ataxias. Cerebellum 2014;13(2):269–302.
129. Jen JC, Graves TD, Hess EJ, et al. Primary episodic ataxias: diagnosis, pathogenesis and treatment. Brain 2007;130(Pt 10):2484–93.
130. Steckley JL, Ebers GC, Cader MZ, et al. An autosomal dominant disorder with episodic ataxia, vertigo, and tinnitus. Neurology 2001;57(8):1499–502.
131. Farmer TW, Mustian VM. Vestibulocerebellar ataxia. A newly defined hereditary syndrome with periodic manifestations. Arch Neurol 1963;8:471–80.
132. Escayg A, De Waard M, Lee DD, et al. Coding and noncoding variation of the human calcium-channel beta4-subunit gene CACNB4 in patients with idiopathic generalized epilepsy and episodic ataxia. Am J Hum Genet 2000;66(5):1531–9.
133. de Vries B, Mamsa H, Stam AH, et al. Episodic ataxia associated with EAAT1 mutation C186S affecting glutamate reuptake. Arch Neurol 2009;66(1):97–101.
134. Kerber KA, Jen JC, Lee H, et al. A new episodic ataxia syndrome with linkage to chromosome 19q13. Arch Neurol 2007;64(5):749–52.

135. Pagon RA. Genetests: an online genetic information resource for health care providers. J Med Libr Assoc 2006;94(3):343–8.
136. Leehey MA. Fragile X-associated tremor/ataxia syndrome: clinical phenotype, diagnosis, and treatment. J Investig Med 2009;57(8):830–6.

Gait Disorders

Joseph Jankovic, MD

KEYWORDS

• Gait • Bradykinesia • Ataxia • Parkinsonism • Freezing of gait • Parkinson disease • Progressive supranuclear palsy • Basal ganglia

KEY POINTS

- Slowness of gait is a normal consequence of aging but can be accelerated in the setting of Parkinson disease and other parkinsonian disorders.
- Lower-body parkinsonism usually indicates the presence of a vascular cause.
- Most gait disorders in the elderly are of multifactorial origin, including prior strokes, orthopedic or arthritic problems, peripheral neuropathy, and a fear of falling.

Videos of typical Parkinson's Disease (1), Parkinson's Disease (2), progressive supranuclear palsy, progressive gait difficulty, and psychogenic tremor and gait accompany this article at http://www.neurologic.theclinics.com/

INTRODUCTION

Gait, the act and manner of walking, is a learned complex motor skill that facilitates locomotion. Although it can be performed automatically and without conscious effort, gait requires the integration of mechanisms of locomotion with those of balance, motor control, cognition, and musculoskeletal function.[1,2] Bipedal gait, along with language and speech, are the abilities that differentiate humans from their ancestors. Normal gait is critical to an individual's quality of life and, therefore, disorders of gait, often associated with postural instability, are a source of considerable handicap and distress. Because of reduced reserves to support balance and gait, the elderly are more prone to falls.[3] Although particularly common among the elderly, gait disorders can affect people of any age. Several studies of healthy elderly individuals have shown reduced velocity of gait and length of stride, increased double-limb support interval, decreased push-off power, and a more flat-footed landing. These changes indicate adaptation by the elderly toward a safer, more stable gait pattern because of deterioration in strength and motor responses for an efficient control of balance during walking. With aging, body sway increases, whereas dynamic balance becomes

Department of Neurology, Parkinson's Disease Center and Movement Disorders Clinic, Baylor College of Medicine, 6550 Fannin, Suite 1801, Houston, TX 77030, USA
E-mail address: josephj@bcm.edu

Neurol Clin 33 (2015) 249–268
http://dx.doi.org/10.1016/j.ncl.2014.09.007 neurologic.theclinics.com
0733-8619/15/$ – see front matter

compromised, and leg strength, particularly ankle dorsiflexion strength, declines. Slow gait speed is one of the hallmarks of frailty of the elderly.[4,5]

Although walking tends to slow with normal aging, this abnormality does not seem to correlate with white matter changes.[6] A pooled analysis from 9 selected cohorts has provided evidence that the speed of gait may correlate with longer survival in older adults.[7]

Gait disturbances must have been recognized and treated throughout history, but cases with primary gait disturbance have been documented in the literature only in the last hundred years.[8] During that time, different terms have been used to describe various gait abnormalities, such as Bruns frontal ataxia, a form of severe disequilibrium caused by mass lesions in the frontal lobe; trepidant abasia, manifested by start hesitation, freezing, and turning pauses; and marche á petits pas, a small-stepped gait in patients with frontal lobe disorders.[9,10]

CLINICAL MANIFESTATIONS

Patients with gait or walking disability may have trouble characterizing their gait difficulties. They often complain of weakness, unsteadiness, slowness, shuffling, stiffness, heaviness, stumbling, staggering and falling, numbness, heaviness, fatigability, and pain. Slow and cautious gait may be accompanied by muscle stiffness (rigidity), postural instability, and fear of falling. Parkinsonian gaits are characterized chiefly by the combination of shuffling steps, start hesitation, and freezing (as if the feet were glued to the floor) associated with stooped posture, flexed knees, narrow base, and turning en bloc (Videos 1 and 2). Recognition of freezing is important because it denotes poor prognosis; most patients have to use a wheelchair within 5 years after onset of freezing.[11] In a cross-sectional survey of 672 patients with idiopathic Parkinson disease (PD), 257 (38.2%) reported freezing of gait (FOG) during the on state, which correlated with longer duration of PD duration, higher scores on the Unified Parkinson Disease Rating Scale (UPDRS), the presence of apathy, higher levodopa equivalent daily dose, and more frequent exposure to antimuscarinics.[12] Gait and balance are particularly problematic in the postural-instability–gait-difficulty (PIGD) subtype of PD.[13] In some patients with PD or other movement disorders, such as dystonia, gait may be impaired by marked flexion of the neck and trunk; so-called bent spine or camptocormia.[14]

In the assessment of gait and posture, the examiner should observe the pattern of movement of the whole body when the patient walks and turns.[15] The various gait disorders are differentiated by typical manifestations and physical signs into the following categories: hemiparetic, paraparetic, spastic, and sensory. Sensory ataxia causes uncoordinated gait, whereas bilateral footdrop indicates severe neuropathy; other gaits include waddling gait (indicates proximal myopathy), dystonic, choreic, antalgic, vertiginous, and psychogenic (**Table 1**). Although there are limitations to this categorization, including phenomenologic overlap, this classification is useful to facilitate communication among clinicians. Also, this classification may be helpful in localizing the responsible lesion or lesions and in finding the most likely cause of the gait disorder.

CAUSES

Gait disorders often result from lesions or dysfunctions at different levels of the central and peripheral nervous system and the musculoskeletal system. However, it may not always be possible to identify a single cause for the impaired gait. Multiple factors may contribute to a patient's ambulatory abnormality.

Table 1
Physical signs of gait disorders

Physical Signs	Description	Associated Signs
Hemiparetic gait	Extension and circumduction of 1 leg	Weakness on the affected side; hyperreflexia; extensor plantar response; flexed arm
Paraparetic gait	Stiffness, extension, adduction, and scissoring of both legs	Bilateral leg weakness, hyperreflexia, spasticity, and extensor plantar responses
Sensory gait	Unsteadiness of walking when visual input is withdrawn	Positive Romberg sign; decreased position sense
Steppage gait	Weakness of foot dorsiflexors; footdrop; excessive flexion of hips and knees when walking; short strides; unilateral or bilateral	Atrophy of distal leg muscles; decreased ankle reflex; possible sensory loss
Cautious gait	Wide-based, careful, slow steps; reaching for support; as in walking on ice; better at home than in open spaces	Associated often with anxiety, fear of open spaces, and fear of falling
Apraxic gait	Difficulty initiating a step; freezing; feet almost stuck to floor; turn hesitation; shuffling gait	Hypokinesia; muscular rigidity; grasp reflexes; possible resting tremor, dementia, or urinary incontinence
Propulsive or retropulsive gait	Body's center of gravity appears to be either in front of or behind the patient, who is struggling to keep the feet up to center of gravity; festination	Hypokinesia; muscular rigidity; postural instability
Ataxic gait	Wide-based gait; incoordination; staggering; decomposition of movements	Dysmetria; dysdiadochokinesia; tremor; postural instability
Astasia	Primary balance disorder	Postural instability
Waddling gait	Wide-based gait; swaying; toe-walk; lumbar lordosis; symmetric	Proximal muscle weakness of lower extremities
Dystonic gait	Sustained abnormal posture of the foot or leg; distorted gait; hyperflexion of hips	Action-related gait disturbance; atypical presentations
Choreic gait	Irregular, dancelike gait; slow and wide-based; spontaneous knee flexion and leg raising	Athetotic and choreic movements of the upper extremities
Antalgic gait	Limping; avoidance of bearing full weight on the affected leg; limitation of range of movement	Pain in lower extremity aggravated by leg, hip, and thigh movement as well as weight bearing
Vertiginous gait	Unsteady gait; falling to one side; postural imbalance	Vertigo; nausea; nystagmus
Psychogenic (hysterical) gait	Bizarre and nonphysiologic gait; different varieties; rare fall or injury	Give-way weakness; Hoover sign; other signs of conversion

Gait disorders have been classified according to cause, clinical characteristics, or levels of function.[8] Gait disorders may be caused by cerebral lesions, either cortical, subcortical, or both, and these include (1) frontal gait disorders, (2) cortical-subcortical gait disorders, (3) subcortical gait disorders, (4) hyperkinetic gait disorders, and (5) subcortical astatic disorders (**Box 1**). Although there is some overlap among these 5 types of cerebral gait disorders, they can be differentiated in most cases based on the predominant phenotype.

Frontal gait disorders have been described by a variety of terms, including Bruns ataxia, marche à petits pas, gait apraxia, lower-body parkinsonism, and arteriosclerotic or vascular parkinsonism.[16] The prevalence of gait disturbance is considerably higher among the elderly, and the presence of abnormal gait in the elderly is a significant predictor of the risk of developing dementia.[17] Patients with Alzheimer disease often have a cautious gait. Frontal release signs (gegenhalten and other primitive reflexes) often accompany frontal gait disorder. Normal-pressure hydrocephalus should be considered in the differential diagnosis of all patients with progressive gait disturbance. One study found that patients with normal-pressure hydrocephalus can be differentiated from patients with PD by a broad-based gait and lack of influence of external clues on locomotion.[18]

Cortical-subcortical gait disorders have also been termed trepidant abasia, gait ignition failure, primary progressive freezing gait, or motor blocks.[19] Subcortical gait disorders, presumably resulting from thalamic lesions, have been also termed thalamic astasia, thalamic ataxia, and subcortical disequilibrium. Causes of this condition are frequently vascular or degenerative lesions in the cerebral white and gray matter causing disconnections between cortical, subcortical, and brainstem structures.[20] Early stages of progressive supranuclear palsy and other parkinsonian disorders can show this subcortical gait pattern. In contrast with the shuffling, narrow-based gait, bent knees, and tiptoeing typical of PD,[21] patients with progressive supranuclear palsy tend to have a more broad-based gait with knee extension, and instead of turning en bloc they tend to pivot on their toes and sometimes even cross their legs, which contributes to frequent falls (Video 3).[22] Focal epilepsy, presumably from cortical focus, may cause a paroxysmal gait disorder.[23]

Hyperkinetic gait disorders include choreic and dystonic gaits, and bouncy (myoclonic) gait. An abnormal gait, termed tardive gait, has been described in patients who showed other features of tardive dyskinesia and has been characterized as a dancing or ducklike gait.[24] Patients with orthostatic tremor have no trouble walking but they are usually unable to stand for more than a few minutes because of vibration, cramp, or other vaguely described discomfort caused by a high frequency (14–16 Hz) tremor in the legs.[25] This condition is in contrast with orthostatic myoclonus, which is manifested by jerking, shaking movements in the legs and bouncing stance, with difficulties in gait initiation and other gait problems.[26,27]

Pyramidal gait disorders present in a hemiparetic and spastic pattern. They are usually caused by stroke, demyelination, mass, or trauma to the motor cortex or the corticospinal tracts. These gaits are typically narrow based because of hyperadduction of the legs, often referred to as scissor gait.

Cerebellar gait disorders, characterized by broad-based, irregular, ataxic gait, can be produced by any insult to the cerebellum. The Scale for the Assessment and Rating of Ataxia, a simple, validated measurement tool, has been used to assess ataxia as well as gait and postural disorders and to measure their response to therapeutic interventions.[28] Brainstem and myelopathic gait disorders have distinct clinical characteristics and are produced by damage to the brainstem or spinal cord, and include a combination of cerebellar and sensory ataxia as well as spasticity.

Box 1
Anatomic clinical etiologic classification of gait disorders

1. Frontal gait disorders
   A. Clinical features
      I. Pure
         a. Short stride
         b. Abnormal stance (wide>narrow base, variable, crossing of legs)
         c. Freezing (motor blocks)
         d. Loss of balance (disequilibrium in response to perturbation, unable to stand or sit unsupported)
         e. Inappropriate postural adjustments when arising from chair (extending instead of flexing trunk and legs) or turning in bed
         f. Stiff trunk and legs (military gait)
         g. Leg apraxia (difficultly with stepping or bicycling movements)
         h. Minimal or no improvement with cues
      II. Associated findings
         a. Pseudobulbar palsy
         b. Cognitive impairment
         c. Pyramidal signs
         d. Urinary disturbance
         e. Foot grasp
         g. Frontal release signs
   B. Pathology and pathogenesis
      I. Bilateral frontal lobe white matter lesions
      II. Anterior cerebral artery infarction
      III. Periventricular multi-infarct state
      IV. Binswanger disease
      V. Pick disease
      VI. Frontal mass
      VII. Normal-pressure hydrocephalus
      VIII. Disconnection between motor, premotor, and supplementary motor cortex and subcortical motor areas such as the basal ganglia, brainstem, and cerebellum
2. Cortical-subcortical gait disorders
   A. Clinical features
      I. Pure
         a. Freezing (motor blocks)
         b. Start hesitation
         c. Turn hesitation
         d. Blocking in narrow spaces
         e. Shuffling
         f. Stride normal or lengthens with walking (no festination)

g. Normal stepping or bicycling movements (in sitting or supine position)
h. Normal postural responses
i. Normal arm swing
j. No improvement with cues

II. Associated findings
a. Cognitive impairment
b. Dysarthria
c. Loss of manual dexterity
d. Loss of balance and postural responses
e. Bradykinesia
f. Rigidity
g. Loss of associated movements

B. Pathology and pathogenesis
I. Nonspecific cortical and subcortical white matter lesions
II. Frontal cortical hypometabolism
III. Early stages of progressive supranuclear palsy and other parkinsonian disorders
IV. Cortical-brainstem disconnection

3. Subcortical hypokinetic gait disorders

A. Clinical features
I. Pure
a. Short stride
b. Slow
c. Shuffling
d. Narrow base
e. Festination
f. Freezing (motor blocks)
g. Start hesitation
h. Turns en block
i. Abnormal postural responses (retropulsion>propulsion) and falling
j. Motor blocks improve with cues

II. Associated findings
a. Parkinson disease
1. Rest tremor
2. Body bradykinesia
3. Hypomimia
4. Dysarthria
5. Flexed posture and knees
6. Other parkinsonian features

b. Parkinsonism plus
1. Parkinsonism-plus gait (stiff, knees extended, wide base, freezing, unsteady, frequent falls)

2. Ocular palsy (vertical>horizontal)
3. Neck extension or flexion
4. Pseudobulbar palsy
5. Dysautonomia
6. Crossing of feet and pivoting on turning, toe walking

B. Pathology and pathogenesis
I. Vascular (or other lesions) in the thalamus
II. Basal ganglia
III. Brainstem (pedunculopontine nucleus)
IV. Parkinson disease
V. Progressive supranuclear palsy
VI. Multiple system atrophy

4. Subcortical hyperkinetic gait disorders

A. Clinical features
I. Choreic
a. Random brief movements
b. Wide-based stance
c. Variable stride and timing
d. Disequilibrium in later stages

II. Dystonic
a. Inversion of foot or other foot/leg deformities
b. Bizarre gait pattern improved by walking backwards
c. Dystonic paraparesis in dopa-responsive dystonia

III. Athetotic
a. Slow
b. Often associated with dystonia and spasticity

IV. Stereotypic
a. Bizarre but patterned gait

V. Myoclonic
a. Wide based
b. Bouncing stance
c. Drop attacks

VI. Tremulous
a. Orthostatic tremor present while standing but disappear while walking

VII. Other

B. Pathology and pathogenesis
I. Huntington disease
II. Primary and secondary dystonia
III. Tardive dyskinesia
IV. Cerebral palsy

V. Other hyperkinetic movement disorders

5. Subcortical astasia
   - A. Clinical features
     - I. Marked disequilibrium
       - a. Unable to stand or sit
       - b. Falls like a falling log
     - II. Normal strength and sensation
   - B. Pathology and pathogenesis
     - I. Thalamotomy
     - II. Thalamic strokes
     - III. Thalamic arteriovenous malformation
     - IV. Putaminal or pallidal strokes
6. Pyramidal gait
   - A. Clinical features
     - I. Shoulder adducted
     - II. Elbow flexed
     - III. Forearm pronated and wrist flexed
     - IV. Hip slightly flexed and knee extended
     - V. Slow circumduction of affected leg with toe dragging
     - VI. Wide stance
     - VII. Spasticity on the affected side
   - B. Pathology and pathogenesis
     - I. Cerebral hemisphere (internal capsule) stroke
     - I. Demyelination
     - III. Tumor or other lesions
7. Cerebellar gait
   - A. Clinical features
     - I. Wide-based stance
     - II. Marked disequilibrium and particularly rapid postural adjustments
     - III. Dyssynergia of leg movements (irregular and variable)
     - IV. Dysmetria (erratic foot placement)
     - V. Titubation
     - VI. Bouncing gait when combined with spasticity (spastic ataxia)
   - B. Pathology and pathogenesis
     - I. Strokes
     - II. Demyelination
     - III. Cerebellar degenerations
     - IV. Other cerebellar disorders
8. Brainstem gait
   - A. Clinical features
     - I. Marked disequilibrium

II. Bouncing stance
III. Drop attacks (negative myoclonus)
IV. Hypertonia
V. Other brainstem signs

B. Pathology and pathogenesis
I. Strokes
II. Demyelination
III. Other brainstem disorders

9. Myelopathic gait
A. Clinical features
I. Stiff (spastic) legs
II. Narrow base with adduction of legs (scissors gait)
III. Slow and deliberate, dragging
V. Other myelopathic signs

B. Pathology and pathogenesis
I. Cervical spondylosis with compressive myelopathy
II. Multiple sclerosis
III. Spinal cord injury
IV. Infarct
V. And so forth

10. Neuromuscular-skeletal gait
A. Clinical features
I. Myopathic
a. Waddling
b. Proximal weakness
c. Lordosis
d. Toe walking
II. Neuropathic
a. Steppage
b. Distal weakness
c. Distal sensory loss
III. Orthopedic
a. Associated with arthritis or other joint or skeletal abnormalities
b. Slow and stiff gait

11. Sensory-deprivation gait
A. Clinical features
I. Sensory ataxia
a. Wide base
b. Slow
c. Slapping

d. Cautious
e. Improves with visual guidance
II. Vestibular ataxia
III. Visual ataxia
B. Pathology and pathogenesis
I. Peripheral neuropathy
III. Posterior column degeneration (tabes dorsalis or subacute combined degeneration)

12. Cautious gait
A. Clinical features
I. Short stride
II. Mildly widened base
III. Slow
IV. Turns en bloc
V. Arms abducted and flexed (anticipating loss of balance, reaching for support)
VI. Improves with minimal support (light touch)
VII. Mild postural instability
VIII. Guarded or restrained gait
IX. Associated anxiety or phobias
X. No motor blocks (freezing) or shuffling
B. Pathology and pathogenesis
I. Normal or exaggerated response to real or perceived disequilibrium
II. Impaired postural responses caused by abnormal sensory-motor-skeletal function

13. Psychogenic gait disorders
A. Clinical features
I. Bizarre gait and stance (astasia-abasia)
I. Widely lurching but without falls
III. Other positive criteria for hysteria and psychogenic disorders
B. Pathology and pathogenesis
I. Normal

Cautious gait disorders have been labeled with many different terms, including senile gait, space phobia, pseudoagoraphobia, postfall syndrome, adaptive gait, and walking-on-ice gait (Video 4).[22,29] This is one of the most common abnormal gait patterns in the elderly.[30] Although there is some overlap between cautious gait and senile gait, kinematics in older, healthy adults typically show slower speed, shorter stride, reduced arm swing, flexed knees, and reduced toe clearance.[30] In contrast with parkinsonian gait, patients with senile gait do not manifest other features of PD. In many cases, cautious gait first appears after a fall, even if the fall is not associated with any injury. As a result of the fall, some patients, particularly the elderly, lose confidence in their ability to walk and to maintain normal balance. They then suddenly or gradually adopt the wide-based, careful gait (as if walking on ice) with a need to hold to the wall, objects, or an attendant. They may be unable to walk in open spaces (pseudoagoraphobia), but are able to walk inside a house holding on to the walls and furniture. However, their balance may be well preserved because they are often able to walk barely touching the examiner's finger or hand. In some cases the patient becomes completely incapacitated by the severe fear of falling.

In addition to gait disorders of central origin, many different gait disorders are caused by damage to or dysfunction of the peripheral nervous system. Waddling gait is the characteristic feature of myopathic gait disorders, resulting from proximal muscle weakness. Causes include muscular dystrophies, myopathies, myasthenia gravis, and certain other neuromuscular diseases. Patients with neuropathic gait disorders have distal muscle weakness that may be unilateral or bilateral. In order to compensate for footdrop, the patients develop a high-steppage gait. If sensory alterations accompany weakness, the diagnosis of peripheral neuropathy is more assured. Sensory-deprivation gait disorders are commonly produced by the loss of proprioceptive input from the legs. Lesions that interrupt large-diameter sensory afferent fibers, such as peripheral neuropathies and posterior root, ganglion, or column damage, can cause this unsteady gait pattern. Vestibular dysfunction or deprivations of auditory and visual inputs can also evoke such conditions.

Many gait disorders are not of neurologic origin. For example, orthopedic gait disorders, associated with arthritis or other joint and skeletal abnormalities, are characterized by a slow, stiff, and painful (antalgic) pattern. Psychogenic gait disorders often produce a bizarre and almost acrobatic gait. They may present as a parkinsonian gait,[31] as lurching and markedly unsteady gait (but without falling; termed astasia-abasia), or the presentation may be varied and inconsistent, not congruous with any organic gait disorder (Video 5).[32,33]

PATHOGENESIS AND PATHOPHYSIOLOGY

Human walking is a skilled locomotor behavior in which the erect, moving body is supported stably by first one leg and then the other. Superimposed on the basic pattern of bipedal locomotion, there are personal modifications and characteristics that are unique to each individual. Although humans have used the bipedal form of locomotion for millions of years, a quadrupedal gait has been reported in rare individuals as a result of certain gene mutations,[34] thus indicating that bipedal gait is not only phylogenetically but also genetically programmed. Quadrupedal locomotion in these families alternatively may be caused by compensation for problems with balance caused by congenital cerebellar hypoplasia.

Gait has been classically studied in the forms of the walking cycle. It is the time interval between successive floor contacts of each foot and is divided into the stance and swing phases. The cycle begins when the heel of one foot touches the floor. Stance is the period during which the foot is on the ground. Swing applies to the time the foot is in the air for limb advancement. Stride is the actions of one limb during a walking cycle. The average normal time distribution of a cycle is 60% for stance and 40% for swing. The stance phases of the two limbs overlap, such that 20% of the cycle is with both feet on the ground (double-limb support). The duration of the gait cycle varies with a person's walking speed. Both stance and swing phases are shortened as walking speed increases. Also, walking faster proportionally lengthens single-limb support and shortens the double-limb support intervals.

Four fundamental requirements are essential for successful locomotion: (1) maintenance of balance and upright posture, (2) gait initiation, (3) generation of rhythmic locomotion, and (4) adaptation of movements to meet the environmental demands and the goals of the individual.[35] In order to maintain a normal gait, the musculoskeletal system must be able to keep the body in an upright posture, and a control system is also necessary to sustain this upright posture by supporting reflexes. To start walking, there has to be a mechanism for gait initiation or ignition. The body's center of gravity must be shifted laterally onto one foot to allow the other to be raised and step forward. Then, a stepping generator needs to be activated to produce rhythmic alternating movements of the legs and to propel the body in the intended direction of progression. An additional requirement for normal locomotion is the ability to adapt the body to changes in speed, turning, differences in the support surface, alterations in footwear, and unexpected body displacements.

The production of a stable gait requires a coordinated control of locomotion and balance that involves the interaction of a variety of afferent and efferent neural systems. The afferent system provides proprioceptive, vestibular, and visual inputs. The integrative system consists of components of the brainstem, cerebellum, subcortex, and frontal cortex. It interprets all available sensory inputs and selects appropriate motor programs and patterns of muscle activation for posture, balance, and gait. The efferent system is composed of the peripheral nerves and muscles that execute movement.

The pedunculopontine nucleus seems to play a role as a locomotion generator, and stimulation of the nucleus may improve gait in experimental primates.[36] The pedunculopontine nucleus, a collection of cholinergic neurons located in the caudal mesencephalic tegmentum, receives direct bilateral descending projections from the subthalamic nucleus, the dorsal and ventral striatum, the pallidum, and the substantia nigra reticulata. Descending projections from the pallidum and the substantia nigra reticulata are mediated by the inhibitory neurotransmitter gamma-aminobutyric acid, and the pedunculopontine nucleus in turn provides excitatory ascending projections to the striatal output nuclei via acetylcholine and glutamate. Although the functional role of these pedunculopontine nucleus projections is not well known, the pedunculopontine nucleus seems to mediate the influence of the basal ganglia on motor mechanisms of the brainstem and spinal cord, including gait, posture, and balance, and as such it constitutes a major component of the mesencephalic locomotor center.[37] We reported a patient with bilateral pedunculopontine nucleus infarcts whose dominant clinical feature was sudden onset of FOG, thus providing evidence that this nucleus is involved in human locomotion and that its damage may lead to abnormal gait, particularly freezing.[36]

Stimulation of the pedunculopontine nucleus in the cat produces stepping and other rhythmic events, whereas an inhibition of the pedunculopontine nucleus leads to a reduction of locomotor activity.[38] In one study, the presence of neurofibrillary tangles in substantia nigra correlated with gait impairment in the elderly but not with other parkinsonian features.[39] The most efficient way to objectively ascertain FOG is to ask patients to repeatedly make rapid 360° narrow turns from standstill, on the spot, and in both directions.[40] Patients often adopt a variety of cues or tricks to overcome the freezing attacks: marching to command (left, right, left, right), stepping over objects (eg, the end of a walking stick, a pavement stone, cracks in the floor), walking to music or a metronome, shifting body weight, rocking movements, and other alleviating maneuvers.[41] This behavior suggests that the motor program for gait is intact, but patients with FOG have difficulties accessing it. Neuroimaging studies have provided evidence that PD-related FOG is caused by impaired interactions between frontoparietal cortical regions and subcortical structures, such as the striatum, and that FOG is caused by decoupling between the cortical cognitive control network and the basal ganglia network.[42,43] FOG may be caused in large part by altered connectivity between the cortex, particularly the supplementary motor area, and the basal ganglia, particularly the subthalamic nucleus.[44] Furthermore, high-beta oscillations in the subthalamic nucleus suggest that this high oscillatory activity might interfere with the frontal cortex–basal ganglia networks, which contributes to the pathophysiology of FOG in PD.[45]

Although FOG is considered a typical sign of PD and has traditionally been attributed to dopaminergic deficiency, there is a growing body of evidence that nondopaminergic systems play an important role in mediating this parkinsonian gait disorder.[8,9] In addition to noradrenergic deficiency, the cholinergic system also seems to be involved in FOG. In a cross-sectional study involving 143 patients with PD and using PET imaging, patients with FOG had lower dopaminergic striatal activity, decreased neocortical cholinergic innervation, and greater neocortical deposition of β-amyloid compared with nonfreezers.[46]

EPIDEMIOLOGY

Gait disorders with a variety of neurologic and nonneurologic causes are common, especially in the elderly. In a cross-sectional, population-based study of 488 community-residing elderly aged 60 to 97 years who underwent a thorough neurologic assessment including a standardized gait evaluation, 32.2% had impaired gait.[47] Of the individuals with impaired gait, 24.0% had a neurologic gait disorder, 17.4% had nonneurologic gait problems, and 9.2% had a combination of both. Depressed mood and cognitive dysfunction increased the risk of gait disorders. About 40% of persons 80 years of age or older have at least 1 fall annually.[48] Accidental injury is the sixth leading cause of death among the elderly, and it most often results from a fall.[49] The nonfatal results from falls are also significant, including physical injury, fear, functional deterioration, and institutionalization.

DIFFERENTIAL DIAGNOSIS

In order to distinguish the various forms of gait disorders and to determine their specific causes, clinicians must start with a thorough medical history and a detailed physical and neurologic examination. Recognition of the key clinical characteristics of abnormal gait is critical to the diagnosis (see **Table 1**).[15,22] Some gait problems, particularly in the elderly, are multifactorial.

Acute or subacute gait disorders need to be separated from the chronic progressive disorders. Rapidly evolving gait difficulty, with a history measured in hours, days, or at most a few weeks, represents a higher order of urgency and a different differential diagnosis. Trauma, stroke, subdural hematoma, mass lesions of the brain and spinal cord, Guillain-Barré syndrome, as well as acute encephalopathy and intoxication are causes that must be considered in gait disorders that evolve acutely or subacutely. These conditions are mostly reversible and should be treated aggressively. The differential diagnosis of a chronic and slowly progressive gait disorder is broad. They can be divided into disorders affecting the afferent nervous system, disorders affecting the integrative nervous system, disorders affecting the efferent nervous system, and nonneurologic disorders (**Box 2**).

Box 2
Common causes for chronic gait disorders

Disorders affecting the afferent nervous system

- Sensory peripheral neuropathies
- Multiple sensory deficits
- Vestibular dysfunction

Disorders affecting the integrative nervous system

- Cerebrovascular disease
- Multi-infarct state
- Binswanger disease
- Chronic subdural hematoma
- Neoplasms
- Normal-pressure hydrocephalus
- Cerebral palsy
- Multiple sclerosis
- Metabolic encephalopathies
- Drugs and toxins
- Parkinson disease
- Progressive supranuclear palsy
- Multiple system atrophy
- Wilson disease
- Secondary parkinsonism
- Huntington disease
- Idiopathic torsion dystonia
- Other hyperkinetic movement disorders
- Spinocerebellar degenerations
- Paraneoplastic cerebellar degeneration

Disorders affecting the efferent nervous system

- Cervical spondylitic myelopathy
- Myopathies
- Peripheral motor neuropathies
- Other neuromuscular diseases

Nonneurologic causes

- Arthritis
- Musculoskeletal deformities
- Depression
- Psychogenic disorders

DIAGNOSTIC EVALUATION

The diagnostic work-up of a gait disorder must be thorough but thoughtful. Because the causes of gait disturbance are so diverse, the clinician cannot order laboratory studies arbitrarily. The search for diagnosis first needs to be narrowed by a careful history and examination. In addition, clinical characteristics of impaired gait (see **Table 1**) can be identified by watching the patient rise from a chair, stand, walk, turn while walking, balance on 1 foot, walk through open and narrow spaces, and respond to push-pull perturbation.[15] At present, clinical evaluation is still superior to quantitative gait analysis in deriving the correct diagnosis and treatment of gait disorders. A clinical rating scale, the Gait and Balance Scale, has been developed to assess severity of gait and balance problems and their response to treatment.[50] It consists of historical information and examination of 14 different gait and balance parameters designed to assess the severity of these functional domains. It was validated against 2 computerized gait analysis instruments: GAITRite and Pro Balance Master.

When a central nervous system lesion is suspected, computed tomography or MRI of the brain should be performed. For patients with myelopathic signs, the spinal cord, including the region of the foramen magnum, should be investigated by myelography or MRI. Evoked potential studies can be used to recognize brainstem or spinal cord disorders. Peripheral disorders such as myopathies and neuropathies are examined by electromyography and nerve conduction studies. Muscle or nerve biopsies are sometimes necessary in patients suspected of myopathy or neuropathy. Cerebrospinal fluid (CSF) analysis can be important to identify infectious, inflammatory, or demyelinating causes. Toxic and metabolic causes can be explored by drug screen and blood work. Vitamin B_{12} deficiency, thyroid dysfunction, and neurosyphilis should be ruled out. Hearing and ophthalmologic evaluation are obtained when appropriate. DNA testing is now available for an increasing number of genetic diseases, including Duchenne and Becker muscular dystrophies, Charcot-Marie-Tooth disease, and spinocerebellar degenerations.

MANAGEMENT

Treatment is directed principally at correcting the reversible causes of gait disorders. If this is not possible, the goals of management are to curb further progression of disability and to avoid recurrence of known causes. Other important aims are to improve ambulation, promote independence, and prevent falls. Improving functions of afferent sensory systems essential for gait and balance may be helpful. Identification and correction of remedial problems with visual acuity, hearing, vestibular function, and proprioception are important.

Patients with cautious gait may respond to intensive gait and psychological training. Because of frequent background of obsessive-compulsive disorder and anxiety, anxiolytic medications and serotonin reuptake inhibitors often provide additional important benefit. Gait disorders cause reduced mobility and independence, and can be disabling. Prevention is designed to avoid all injuries and diseases to the musculoskeletal and nervous systems. In one study a decrease of risk for falling by 57% was noted among those patients with PD who practiced regular physical activity before the onset of their disease.[51]

Gait training with rhythmic auditory stimulation improves gait velocity, stride length, and step cadence in patients with PD. Slow and shuffling gait in these patients can also be helped by attentional strategies and visual or auditory cues.[41,52,53] The administration of auditory stimulation at a frequency matching the preferred walking cadence led to a decrease in stride time in patients with PD and to an increase in step amplitude compared with controls.[53]

Symptomatic measures to help patients with gait disorders improve ambulation include gait analysis and evaluation by a physiatrist, appropriate gait and balance training, and other adjunct physical therapy.[54] Aerobic walking has also been found to improve fitness, motor function, fatigue, mood, executive control, and quality of life in patients with mild to moderate PD.[55] Proper footwear, bracing, or various other assistive devices (eg, canes, walkers) are useful in preventing falls. Survey of the home by a professional to eliminate obstacles and safety hazards increases mobility at home and makes ambulation safer. In addition, increasing patients' and family members' awareness of the consequences of falls and techniques to reduce the risks of fall decreases the frequency of falling.

Medications for patients, especially the elderly, need to be monitored closely to avoid overuse and interactions that may produce side effects such as somnolence, dizziness, or imbalance that compromise normal gait. Although levodopa is not considered highly effective for the treatment of FOG, a 4-year follow-up of patients with PD initially treated either with levodopa or pramipexole showed that levodopa treatment resulted in a significant reduction in the risk of freezing (25.3% vs 37.1%; hazard ratio, 1.70; $P = .01$).[56] Another study of patients with PD treated with levodopa who had been taking deprenyl, a monoamine oxidase inhibitor, for 7 years, compared with those changed to placebo after only 5 years, showed significantly less freezing in patients treated with deprenyl for a longer period.[57] This finding is consistent with another study of the same patient population, which showed that patients randomized to deprenyl had a lower risk of freezing than those assigned to placebo.[58] Although a minority of patients with freezing as the dominant parkinsonian symptom improve with L-threo-3,4-dihydroxyphenylserine, tricyclic antidepressants, or atomoxetine,[59] suggesting underlying noradrenergic deficiency, most such patients do not improve with any pharmacologic therapy. Functional electrical stimulation of the peroneal or tibial nerve may help in overcoming freezing, but this technique has not been formally evaluated.[60]

Normal-pressure hydrocephalus, typically manifested by shuffling (so-called magnetic gait), urinary incontinence, and cognitive decline, is often associated with other neurodegenerative disorder and, therefore, the diagnosis is often missed.[61] In a retrospective study of 41 patients at the Mayo Clinic who underwent an invasive diagnostic procedure for evaluation of suspected normal-pressure hydrocephalus between 1995 and 2003, 13 ultimately received shunts.[62] Definite gait improvement was documented in 75% at 3 to 6 months after shunt placement, but it decreased to 33% at 3 years. Patients with cognitive impairment, urinary incontinence, or postural instability experienced little or no sustained benefit. The complications rate was 33% and 1 patient died during the perioperative period. In addition, 5 of 12 patients were later found to have an alternate diagnosis. External lumbar drainage of CSF (about 25 mL every 3 hours except at night over 72 hours) was investigated in 15 patients, 7 of whom improved in gait and 6 in attention.[63] Despite a median drain volume of 470 mL (range, 160–510 mL), the mean ventricular size was reduced by only 4.2% and the ratio of volume contraction to drain volume was only 0.9%. The investigators concluded that the clinical improvement in patients with normal-pressure hydrocephalus is related to the continued CSF drainage rather than the reduction in ventricular volume. Thus a 20-mL extraction is easily replaced in about 3 hours, consistent with the accepted CSF production of 15 to 20 mL/h.

Another potential treatment of gait disorders associated with PD is deep brain stimulation (DBS). Although subthalamic or pallidal DBS may provide some improvement in gait and balance, low-frequency stimulation of the pedunculopontine nucleus, which has been implicated in locomotion, has been reported to have variable, mostly disappointing, results in 6 patients.[64] Another study involving 6 patients suggested that unilateral pedunculopontine nucleus DBS reduces the frequency of PD-related falls.[65] In a double-blind study using objective spatiotemporal gait analysis, parkinsonian patients with severe FOG who underwent caudal pedunculopontine tegmental nucleus DBS improved objective measures of gait freezing, with bilateral stimulation being more effective than unilateral stimulation.[66] Concomitant low-frequency stimulation of pedunculopontine nucleus and caudal zona incerta improves motor symptoms in patients with PD.[67] A study of 12 patients with PD who underwent a combined subthalamic nucleus (STN) and substantia nigra pars compacta (SNpc) DBS suggests that this approach might be useful in the treatment of FOG.[68]

SUMMARY

Gait disorders are frequently accompanied by loss of balance and falls, and are a common cause of disability, particularly among the elderly. Although a specific cause for the gait and balance disorder can often be identified, in many cases the cause is multifactorial, involving both neurologic and nonneurologic systems. Gait disorders are often difficult to treat, but physical therapy and training, coupled with pharmacologic and surgical therapy, can usually provide some improvement in ambulation, which translates into better quality of life. More research is needed on the mechanisms of gait and its disorders as well as on symptomatic therapies. Dalfampridine, known as 4-aminopyridine, is a broad-spectrum potassium channel blocking drug that is the only drug currently approved for the treatment of gait disorder, but only in multiple sclerosis.[69] It is not known whether this drug would also be helpful in ataxia and other gait abnormalities, including parkinsonian gait disorders. Better understanding of the pathophysiology of gait disorders should lead to more specific, pathogenesis-targeted therapies.

SUPPLEMENTARY DATA

Supplementary data related to this article can be found online at http://dx.doi.org/10.1016/j.ncl.2014.09.007.

REFERENCES

1. Nutt JG. Higher-level gait disorders: an open frontier. Mov Disord 2013;28(11):1560–5.
2. Zitser J, Jankovic J, Giladi N. Disorders of gait. In: Jankovic J, Tolosa E, editors. Parkinson's disease and movement disorders. 6th edition. Philadelphia: Lippincott Williams & Wilkins; 2015.
3. Tinetti ME. Clinical practice: preventing falls in elderly persons. N Engl J Med 2003;348:42–9.
4. Clegg A, Young J, Iliffe S, et al. Frailty in elderly people. Lancet 2013;381(9868):752–62.
5. Tung EE, Chen CY, Takahashi PY. Common curbsides and conundrums in geriatric medicine. Mayo Clin Proc 2013;88(6):630–5.
6. Elbaz A, Vicente-Vytopilova P, Tavernier B, et al. Motor function in the elderly: evidence for the reserve hypothesis. Neurology 2013;81(5):417–26.
7. Studenski S, Perera S, Patel K, et al. Gait speed and survival in older adults. JAMA 2011;305(1):50–8.
8. Nutt JG, Marsden CD, Thompson PD. Human walking and higher-level gait disorders, particularly in the elderly. Neurology 1993;43:268–79.

9. Nutt JG, Bloem BR, Giladi N, et al. Freezing of gait: moving forward on a mysterious clinical phenomenon. Lancet Neurol 2011;10(8):734–44.
10. Cohen RG, Klein KA, Nomura M, et al. Inhibition, executive function, and freezing of gait. J Parkinsons Dis 2014;4(1):111–22.
11. Factor SA, Higgins DS, Qian J. Primary progressive freezing gait: a syndrome with many causes. Neurology 2006;66(3):411–4.
12. Perez-Lloret S, Negre-Pages L, Damier P, et al. Prevalence, determinants, and effect on quality of life of freezing of gait in Parkinson disease. JAMA Neurol 2014;71(7):884–90.
13. Thenganatt MA, Jankovic J. Parkinson disease subtypes. JAMA Neurol 2014; 71(4):499–504.
14. Jankovic J. Camptocormia, head drop and other bent spine syndromes: heterogeneous etiology and pathogenesis of Parkinsonian deformities. Mov Disord 2010;25(5):527–8.
15. Morris J, Jankovic J. Neurological clinical examination. London: Hodder Arnold; 2012. p. 1–128.
16. Mehanna R, Jankovic J. Movement disorders in cerebrovascular disease. Lancet Neurol 2013;12(6):597–608.
17. Verghese J, Lipton RB, Hall CB, et al. Abnormality of gait as a predictor of non-Alzheimer's dementia. N Engl J Med 2002;347(22):1761–8.
18. Stolze H, Kuhtz-Buschbeck JP, Drucke H, et al. Comparative analysis of the gait disorder of normal pressure hydrocephalus and Parkinson's disease. J Neurol Neurosurg Psychiatry 2001;70:289–97.
19. Schaafsma JD, Balash Y, Gurevich T, et al. Characterization of freezing of gait subtypes and the response of each to levodopa in Parkinson's disease. Eur J Neurol 2003;10(4):391–8.
20. Masdeu JC, Wolfson L, Lantos G. Brain white-matter changes in the elderly prone to falling. Arch Neurol 1989;46:1292–6.
21. Djaldetti R, Hellmann M, Melamed E. Bent knees and tiptoeing: late manifestations of end-stage Parkinson's disease. Mov Disord 2004;19:1325–8.
22. Fahn S, Jankovic J, Hallett M. Principles and practice of movement disorders, Churchill Livingstone. Philadelphia: Elsevier; 2011. p. 1–548.
23. Neville BG, Boyd SG. Selective epileptic gait disorder. J Neurol Neurosurg Psychiatry 1995;58:371–3.
24. Kuo SH, Jankovic J. Tardive gait. Clin Neurol Neurosurg 2008;110:198–201.
25. Yaltho TC, Ondo WG. Orthostatic tremor: A review of 45 cases. Parkinsonism Relat Disord 2014;20(7):723–5.
26. Glass GA, Ahlskog JE, Matsumoto JY. Orthostatic myoclonus: a contributor to gait decline in selected elderly. Neurology 2007;68(21):1826–30.
27. van Gerpen JA. A retrospective study of the clinical and electrophysiological characteristics of 32 patients with orthostatic myoclonus. Parkinsonism Relat Disord 2014;20(8):889–93.
28. Marquer A, Barbieri G, Pérennou D. The assessment and treatment of postural disorders in cerebellar ataxia: a systematic review. Ann Phys Rehabil Med 2014;57(2):67–78.
29. Schniepp R, Wuehr M, Huth S, et al. Gait characteristics of patients with phobic postural vertigo: effects of fear of falling, attention, and visual input. J Neurol 2014;261(4):738–46.
30. Snijders AH, van de Warrenburg BP, Giladi N, et al. Neurological gait disorders in elderly people: clinical approach and classification. Lancet Neurol 2007;6: 63–74.

31. Jankovic J. Diagnosis and treatment of psychogenic parkinsonism. J Neurol Neurosurg Psychiatry 2011;82:1300–3.
32. Ferrara J, Jankovic J. Psychogenic movement disorders in children. Mov Disord 2008;23:1875–81.
33. Thenganatt MA, Jankovic J. Psychogenic movement disorders. Neurol Clin, in press.
34. Türkmen S, Hoffmann K, Demirhan O, et al. Cerebellar hypoplasia, with quadrupedal locomotion, caused by mutations in the very low-density lipoprotein receptor gene. Eur J Hum Genet 2008;16(9):1070–4.
35. Horak FB, Diener HC, Nashner LM. Influence of central set on human postural responses. J Neurophysiol 1989;62:841–53.
36. Kuo SH, Kenney C, Jankovic J. Bilateral pedunculopontine nuclei stroke presenting as freezing of gait. Mov Disord 2008;23(4):616–9.
37. Mena-Segovia J, Bolam JP, Magill PJ. Pedunculopontine nucleus and basal ganglia: distant relatives or part of the same family? Trends Neurosci 2004;27:585–8.
38. Munro-Davies LE, Winter J, Aziz TZ, et al. The role of the pedunculopontine region in basal-ganglia mechanisms of akinesia. Exp Brain Res 1999;129(4):511–7.
39. Schneider JA, Li JL, Li Y, et al. Substantia nigra tangles are related to gait impairment in older persons. Ann Neurol 2006;59(1):166–73.
40. Snijders AH, Haaxma CA, Hagen YJ, et al. Freezer or non-freezer: clinical assessment of freezing of gait. Parkinsonism Relat Disord 2012;18(2):149–54.
41. Patel N, Jankovic J, Hallett M. Sensory aspects of movement disorders. Lancet Neurol 2014;13(1):100–12.
42. Filippi M, van den Heuvel MP, Fornito A, et al. Assessment of system dysfunction in the brain through MRI-based connectomics. Lancet Neurol 2013;12(12):1189–99.
43. Shine JM, Matar E, Ward PB, et al. Freezing of gait in Parkinson's disease is associated with functional decoupling between the cognitive control network and the basal ganglia. Brain 2013;136(Pt 12):3671–81.
44. Fling BW, Cohen RG, Mancini M, et al. Functional reorganization of the locomotor network in Parkinson patients with freezing of gait. PLoS One 2014;9(6):e100291.
45. Toledo JB, López-Azcárate J, Garcia-Garcia D, et al. High beta activity in the subthalamic nucleus and freezing of gait in Parkinson's disease. Neurobiol Dis 2013;64C:60–5.
46. Bohnen NI, Frey KA, Studenski S, et al. Extra-nigral pathological conditions are common in Parkinson's disease with freezing of gait: An in vivo positron emission tomography study. Mov Disord 2014;29(9):1118–24.
47. Mahlknecht P, Kiechl S, Bloem BR, et al. Prevalence and burden of gait disorders in elderly men and women aged 60-97 years: a population-based study. PLoS One 2013;8(7):e69627.
48. Tinetti ME, Speechley M, Ginter SF. Risk factors for falls among elderly persons living in the community. N Engl J Med 1988;319:1701–7.
49. Sattin RW. Falls among older persons: a public health perspective. Annu Rev Public Health 1992;13:489–508.
50. Thomas M, Jankovic J, Suteerawattananon M, et al. Clinical gait and balance scale (GABS): validation and utilization. J Neurol Sci 2004;217(1):89–99.
51. Gazibara T, Pekmezovic T, Kisic Tepavcevic D, et al. Fall frequency and risk factors in patients with Parkinson's disease in Belgrade, Serbia: A cross-sectional study. Geriatr Gerontol Int 2014. [Epub ahead of print].

52. Suteerawattananon M, Morris GS, Etnyre BR, et al. Effects of visual and auditory cues on gait in individuals with Parkinson's disease. J Neurol Sci 2004;219(1–2): 63–9.
53. Arias P, Cudeiro J. Effects of rhythmic sensory stimulation (auditory, visual) on gait in Parkinson's disease patients. Exp Brain Res 2008;186(4):589–601.
54. Gobbi LT, Oliveira-Ferreira MD, Caetano MJ, et al. Exercise programs improve mobility and balance in people with Parkinson's disease. Parkinsonism Relat Disord 2009;15(Suppl 3):S49–52.
55. Uc EY, Doerschug KC, Magnotta V, et al. Phase I/II randomized trial of aerobic exercise in Parkinson disease in a community setting. Neurology 2014;83: 413–25.
56. Holloway RG, Shoulson I, Fahn S, et al. Pramipexole vs levodopa as initial treatment for Parkinson disease: a 4-year randomized controlled trial. Arch Neurol 2004;61(7):1044–53.
57. Shoulson I, Oakes D, Fahn S, et al. Impact of sustained deprenyl (selegiline) in levodopa-treated Parkinson's disease: a randomized placebo-controlled extension of the deprenyl and tocopherol antioxidative therapy of parkinsonism trial. Ann Neurol 2002;51(5):604–12.
58. Giladi N, McDermott MP, Fahn S, et al. Freezing of gait in PD. Prospective assessment of the DATATOP cohort. Neurology 2001;56:1712–21.
59. Jankovic J. Atomoxetine for freezing of gait in Parkinson disease. J Neurol Sci 2009;284(1–2):177–8.
60. Sujith OK. Functional electrical stimulation in neurological disorders. Eur J Neurol 2008;15(5):437–44.
61. Kiefer M, Unterberg A. The differential diagnosis and treatment of normal-pressure hydrocephalus. Dtsch Arztebl Int 2012;109(1–2):15–25.
62. Klassen BT, Ahlskog JE. Normal pressure hydrocephalus: how often does the diagnosis hold water? Neurology 2011;77(12):1119–25.
63. Lenfeldt N, Hansson W, Larsson A, et al. Three-day CSF drainage barely reduces ventricular size in normal pressure hydrocephalus. Neurology 2012;79(3): 237–42.
64. Ferraye MU, Debû B, Fraix V, et al. Effects of pedunculopontine nucleus area stimulation on gait disorders in Parkinson's disease. Brain 2010;133(Pt 1):205–14.
65. Moro E, Hamani C, Poon YY, et al. Unilateral pedunculopontine stimulation improves falls in Parkinson's disease. Brain 2010;133(Pt 1):215–24.
66. Thevathasan W, Cole MH, Graepel CL, et al. A spatiotemporal analysis of gait freezing and the impact of pedunculopontine nucleus stimulation. Brain 2012; 135(Pt 5):1446–54.
67. Khan S, Gill SS, Mooney L, et al. Combined pedunculopontine-subthalamic stimulation in Parkinson disease. Neurology 2012;78(14):1090–5.
68. Weiss D, Walach M, Meisner C, et al. Nigral stimulation for resistant axial motor impairment in Parkinson's disease? A randomized controlled trial. Brain 2013; 136(Pt 7):2098–108.
69. Egeberg MD, Oh CY, Bainbridge JL. Clinical overview of dalfampridine: an agent with a novel mechanism of action to help with gait disturbances. Clin Ther 2012; 34(11):2185–94.

Movement Disorders in Systemic Diseases

Werner Poewe, MD*, Atbin Djamshidian-Tehrani, MD

KEYWORDS

- Movement disorders • Systemic disease • Basal ganglia • Autoimmune disorders
- Metabolic disorders • Endocrine disorders • Paraneoplastic disorders
- Intoxications

KEY POINTS

- Movement disorders may be the harbinger of an underlying systemic disease.
- Careful neurologic examination, considering associated systemic features in combination with neuroimaging and laboratory tests, will help narrow down the differential diagnosis and may lead to the final diagnosis.
- Management will often involve a multidisciplinary team including neurologists and the primary care physician, but also allied health professionals, such as physical, occupational, and speech and language therapists.
- Unlike neurodegenerative movement disorders, those occurring in the setting of systemic diseases are frequently amenable to causal treatment of the underlying condition, thus making early correct diagnostic classification a key priority.

Videos of Parkinsonism in cerebral toxoplasmosis and typical orofacial dyskinesias accompany this article http://www.neurologic.theclinics.com/

INTRODUCTION

The term *movement disorders* includes a variety of different neurologic diseases that classically involve dysfunction of the basal ganglia. Prototypic movement disorders, such as parkinsonism, chorea, or dystonia, commonly result from a variety of neurodegenerative or structural brain diseases, but movement disorders also can be presenting signs of cerebral involvement in a broad spectrum of systemic diseases, such as infectious, metabolic, endocrine, paraneoplastic, and autoimmune disorders (**Table 1**). A comprehensive review of all systemic conditions that may cause symptomatic movement disorders is beyond the scope of this article, and we refer the

Department of Neurology, Innsbruck Medical University, Anichstraße 35, Innsbruck A-6020, Austria
* Corresponding author.
E-mail address: werner.poewe@i-med.ac.at

Neurol Clin 33 (2015) 269–297
http://dx.doi.org/10.1016/j.ncl.2014.09.015

Table 1
Overview of common causes of movement disorders in systemic diseases

Etiology	Movement Disorders
Infectious diseases	
Whipple disease	Oculo-masticatory myorhythmia
Neurosyphilis	Parkinsonism, chorea
CNS-tuberculosis	Tremor, chorea, myoclonus, dystonia, and parkinsonism
HIV	Hemichorea, tremor, parkinsonism, dystonia
Toxoplasmosis	Hemichorea-hemiballism
Neurocysticercosis	Generally rare: parkinsonism, hemichorea
Lyme disease	Parkinsonism
Streptococcus infection	Parkinsonism, Sydenham -chorea (children)
Autoimmune disorders	
Systemic lupus erythematosus	Chorea. Parkinsonism rare
Sjögren syndrome	Parkinsonism
Antiphospholipid antibody syndrome	Rare: Parkinsonism, chorea
Stiff person syndrome	Hyperlordosis, ataxia
Neuro- Behçet	Chorea, ataxia
Celiac disease	Ataxia, parkinsonism, chorea
Paraneoplastic disorders	
Anti-Yo/APCA	Ataxia, tremor
Anti-NMDAR encephalitis	Dystonia, orofacial dyskinesias, ballism, myorhythmia
Amphiphysin	Stiff person syndrome (hyperlordosis, rigidity, ataxia)
Anti-Hu/ANNA-1	Dystonia, chorea, tremor, parkinsonism
CV2/CRMP5	Chorea, dystonia, ataxia
Ma1/Ma2	Parkinsonism
Hu/ANNA-2/VGKC	Myoclonus
Tr	Ataxia
Ri/ANNA-2	Dystonia, parkinsonism (PSP-like), opsoclonus-myoclonus
VGCC	Ataxia
Metabolic	
Wilson disease	Dystonia, parkinsonism, "wing-beating" tremor
Acquired hepatocerebral degeneration	Orobuccolingual dyskinesias, parkinsonism
Hemochromatosis	Ataxia, tremor, parkinsonism
Renal failure	Asterixis, restless legs syndrome. Parkinsonism rare
Endocrine	
Nonketotic hyperglycemia	Hemichorea- hemiballism, asterixis
Hypoglycemia	Paroxysmal chorea
Hyperthyroidism	Tremor, chorea
Hypothyroidism	Parkinsonism
Hypoparathyroidism	Parkinsonism, ataxia, tremor
Hematological	
Polycythemia rubra vera	Chorea

Chorea acanthocytosis	Chorea, feeding dystonia
McLeod syndrome	Chorea
Lysosomal storage disease	
Gaucher	Parkinsonism, dystonia
Niemann-Pick C	Parkinsonism, supranuclear vertical gaze palsy, dystonia
Metal and nonmetal systemic intoxication	
Carbon monoxide	Parkinsonism
Manganese	Parkinsonism
MPTP	Parkinsonism
Ephedrone	Parkinsonism
Carbon monoxide	Parkinsonism
Carbon disulfide	Parkinsonism
Cyanide	Parkinsonism, dystonia, apraxia of eyelid opening
Toluene	Parkinsonism
Ethanol	Ataxia, parkinsonism
Thallium	Chorea

Abbreviations: ANNA, antineuronal nuclear antibody; APCA, anti–Purkinje cell antibody; CNS, central nervous system; HIV, human immunodeficiency virus; MPTP, 1-methyl-4-phenyl-1,2,3,6-tetrahydropyridine; NMDAR, N-methyl-D-aspartate receptor; PSP, progressive supranuclear gaze palsy.

reader to recent monographs on the subject.[1] Here we mainly focus on those clinical settings in which systemic diseases can lead to movement disorders in adults.

INFECTIOUS DISEASES

Infectious diseases can induce movement disorders in the acute, subacute, and chronic stages, either via direct infection of the central nervous system (CNS), or by inducing parainfectious autoimmune processes, such as the acute onset of chorea in children with rheumatic fever due to streptococcus infection. Here we focus on those infectious etiologies that are commonly associated with movement disorders or should be borne in mind as differential diagnoses when there is a suspicion of a symptomatic movement disorder. These clinical scenarios include viral, bacterial, fungal, and protozoic infections, the latter 2 mainly in the setting of immunocompromised patients, and in some parts of the world also helminthic CNS infestations.

Whipple Disease

Whipple disease (WD) is a rare systemic infection caused by the anaerobic, gram-positive bacterium *Tropheryma whipplei*. It can affect multiple organs, including the brain, and is more common in men than women (87% vs 13%). The estimated annual incidence is fewer than 1 per 1,000,000 population.[2] Nevertheless, it is extremely important not to miss the diagnosis, as it is a curable condition that is potentially fatal if left untreated.

The prodromal stage lasts for approximately 6 years and is characterized by unspecific symptoms, such as arthralgia and arthritis. In the steady-state phase, patients may complain of abdominal cramping, weight loss, and diarrhea.[3] Neurologic complications occur in up to 60% of patients[3] and may even present in isolation without any signs of a systemic infection. Approximately 50% of patients develop a supranuclear gaze palsy, which may resemble progressive supranuclear gaze palsy (PSP).[3] Hypophonia, reduced postural stability, and parkinsonism may occur. In approximately 20% of cases, convergence-divergence pendular oscillations, which are in synchrony with a 1-Hz oculo-masticatory myorhythmia, are seen.[4] Cognitive decline, which may progress to dementia, also is common.

The diagnosis is challenging and in some it may not be possible to obtain diagnostic proof in life. The classical findings in biopsies of the duodenum or the jejunum are periodic acid-Schiff (PAS)-positive macrophages in the lamina propria containing the bacteria. Polymerase chain reaction (PCR) of the cerebrospinal fluid (CSF) is confirmatory in patients with isolated CNS-WD.[5] MRI of the brain can show tumorlike or multifocal lesions in the midbrain, thalamus, and temporal lobe,[5] or signal abnormalities in the middle cerebellar peduncle (**Fig. 1**).

Patients require long-term antibiotic therapy. Initially, parenteral administration of ceftriaxone 2 g in combination with intramuscular injection of streptomycin 1 g per day for 14 days is recommended followed by oral administration of high doses of trimethoprim-sulfamethoxazole (160 mg/800 mg) three times a day (tds) for 1 to 2 years. Parkinsonism can improve under antibiotic therapy[6]; however, relapses can occur even several years after cessation of therapy.

Key points: Whipple disease	
Prevalence	Estimated annual incidence is <1 per 1,000,000 More common in men than women
Clinical presentation	50% supranuclear gaze palsy, 20% convergence-divergence pendular oscillations, 1-Hz oculo-masticatory myorhythmia
Diagnosis	Presence of PAS-positive macrophages in duodenal or jejunal biopsies; positive *Tropheryma whipplei* PCR in CSF
Therapy	Parenteral antibiotic therapy followed by oral antibiotics for 2 years

Tuberculosis

The frequency of movement disorders in tuberculous meningitis is approximately 17%.[7] Although dystonia, chorea, myoclonus, and parkinsonism also have been reported, tremor is the most common movement disorder and occurred in two-thirds of the cases in one study.[7,8] Neuroimaging in patients with tuberculous meningitis can be normal, but in 50% may show secondary vascular lesions in the basal ganglia or thalamus.[8]

Intracranial tuberculomas can cause movement disorders in up to 30% of cases.[7] Chorea and dystonia has been associated with deep intracranial tuberculomas, whereas tremor was observed in patients with surface lesions.[7] Apart from cerebral lesions, spinal tuberculomas also have been reported to cause tremor and myoclonus.[7] The therapy usually consists of isoniazid (plus pyridoxal phosphate), rifampin, pyrazinamide, ethambutol, and steroids.

Key points: Tuberculosis	
Etiology	Occurs in 1% of patients with systemic tuberculosis
Clinical presentation	All types of movement disorders, including tremor, chorea, myoclonus, dystonia, and parkinsonism
Diagnosis	CSF or culture isolating *Mycobacterium tuberculosis*
Therapy	Isoniazid (plus pyridoxal phosphate), rifampin, pyrazinamide, ethambutol, and steroids

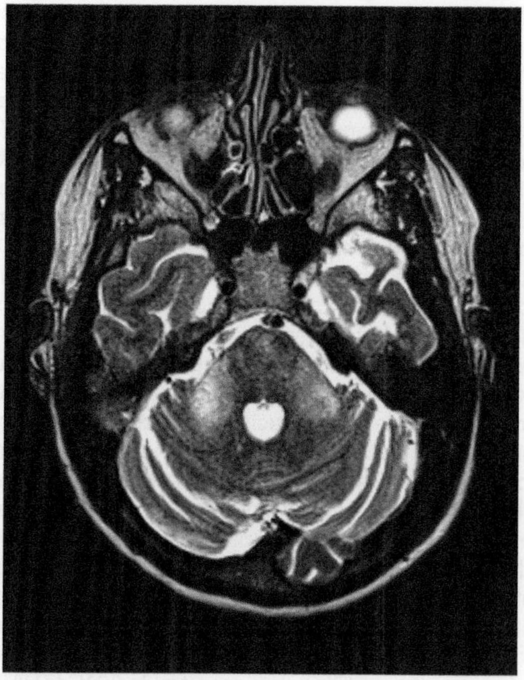

Fig. 1. T2-weighted MRI demonstrating signal abnormalities in the middle cerebellar peduncles bilaterally in a patient with WD.

Neurosyphilis

Although movement disorders are rare in patients with neurosyphilis, *Treponema pallidum* infections can cause symptoms mimicking corticobasal syndrome, with arm levitation, asymmetric bradykinesia, and myoclonus.[9] Parkinsonism, generalized chorea mimicking Huntington disease, hemichorea, ataxia, laryngeal dystonia, and myoclonus also have been described. Furthermore, neurosyphilis can cause PSP-like symptoms.[10] MRI findings may show infarction or inflammation of the midbrain and basal ganglia. Antibiotic use with parenteral penicillin G (3–4 million units tds for 14 days) remains gold standard therapy. Rigorous follow-up tests are necessary to assess whether the infection has vanished.

Key points: Neurosyphilis	
Etiology	Caused by *Treponema pallidum* infections
Clinical presentation	Movement disorder presentations (rare): parkinsonism, chorea, ataxia, corticobasal syndrome
Diagnosis	CSF and serum antibody test
Therapy	Antibiotic therapy with penicillin G

Human Immunodeficiency Virus–Related and AIDS-Related Movement Disorders

In 2012, the global prevalence of human immunodeficiency virus (HIV) infection was approximately 34 million with approximately 2.2 million new HIV infections.[11] The prevalence of movement disorders in patients with AIDS or HIV varies between 2%

and up to 44%.[7] Movement disorders may sometimes be the initial manifestation of AIDS,[12] of an HIV infection during serum conversion, or of an opportunistic infection[13] and generally increase with disease duration.

Hemichorea-hemiballism may be the most frequently seen movement disorders, although the prevalence is unclear. One study reported that 5 (1.4%) of 345 patients with AIDS suffered from hemichorea-hemiballism.[14] Onset of symptoms is generally subacute and unilateral.[12] Cerebral MRI commonly reveals multiple lesions, often caused by cerebral toxoplasmosis, affecting the contralateral striatum or subthalamic nucleus.[13] Pyrimethamine and sulfadiazine were effective in improving or resolving symptoms in some,[12,14] but not all, studies.[15]

Tremor can occur at all stages of the disease and increases up to 44% in patients with dementia.[16] Typically, patients exhibit a bilateral postural tremor but a rest tremor or a Holmes tremor also may occur.[13] Depending on the size of the study, estimates suggest that parkinsonism is seen in between 5% and up to 50% of patients with AIDS.[17] Often some atypical features, such as symmetric bradykinesia and rigidity and early postural instability occur. A classical resting tremor also may be absent.[13] Parkinsonism is commonly a result of HIV encephalopathy,[18] although it also may occur as a complication of opportunistic infections, such as cerebral toxoplasmosis, WD, progressive multifocal leukoencephalopathy, and CNS tuberculosis.[13] The therapeutic value of dopamine replacement therapy in HIV/AIDS parkinsonism is unclear and combined antiretroviral therapy (cART) is more likely to alleviate symptoms.

Dystonia, myoclonus, opsoclonus-myoclonus, and paroxysmal dyskinesias are rare complications and can be a complication of opportunistic infections.[13]

Finally, restless legs syndrome (RLS) was reported in 30% of HIV-positive patients in one series and was inversely correlated with the CD4+ cell count.[19] Ten of these patients were treated with levodopa and reported a significant alleviation of symptoms.[19]

Key points: HIV-related and AIDS-related movement disorders	
Etiology	Global estimated prevalence of HIV: 34 million Estimates of movement disorders in patients with HIV/AIDS vary between 2% and 44%
Clinical presentation	Common: hemichorea-hemiballism, parkinsonism, tremor, RLS Rare: dystonia, myoclonus, and paroxysmal dyskinesias
Diagnosis	HIV test, MRI imaging to screen for vascular and opportunistic infections
Therapy	cART Chorea induced by toxoplasmosis: pyrimethamine and sulfadiazine, dopamine receptor blockers Role of dopamine replacement therapy in patients with parkinsonism conflicting

Sydenham Chorea

Sydenham chorea (SC) is the most common cause of chorea in children.[20] It is caused by Group A beta-hemolytic *Streptococcus* and occurs in 25% of patients with acute rheumatic fever. Typical age of onset is 8 to 9 years, and girls are more commonly affected. Onset is abrupt and consists of orofacial movements, tics, chorea, and dysarthria. Chorea is generalized but may at times also be asymmetric or unilateral. Hypotonia is seen in most patients and, when severe, 2% of patients develop a flaccid quadriparesis often labeled as "chorea paralytica."[21] Neuropsychiatric symptoms, such as obsessive compulsive disorder, are common. Despite strong indicators that

SC is an autoimmune process, a definitive autoantibody has not been found. Sixty percent to 80% of patients have cardiac involvement[22] and half of the patients still have chorea 2 years after onset of symptoms.[23]

Steroids alone or in combination with intravenous immunoglobulin are used in cases with severe chorea. Valproic acid or carbamazepine, rather than neuroleptic therapy, are preferred for symptomatic treatment.[21] Antibiotic prophylaxis following the acute rheumatic fever guidelines until the age of 21 is recommended to avoid rheumatic heart disease.[21]

Key points: Sydenham chorea	
Etiology	SC is the commonest cause of acute chorea in children
Clinical presentation	Orofacial movements, tics, chorea, and dysarthria are common Psychiatric side effects, such as obsessive compulsive behavior, may occur
Diagnosis	
Therapy	Antibiotic therapy Chorea: steroids, immunoglobulins, valproic acid or carbamazepine

Other Viral Infections Causing Movement Disorders

A variety of different viruses can cause movement disorders as a symptom of viral encephalitis. The most important are summarized in **Table 2**; a comprehensive review of these viral encephalitides is beyond the scope of this review.

Table 2
Common causes of viral infections causing movement disorders

Virus	Species	Movement Disorder
DNA		
Herpesviridae	Herpesvirus	Chorea, athetosis, tics, parkinsonism
	Epstein Barr	Chorea, opsoclonus-myoclonus, parkinsonism
	Cytomegalovirus	Chorea, parkinsonism
	Varicella zoster	Myoclonus, hemichorea, ataxia, parkinsonism
RNA		
Flaviviridae	West Nile	Opsoclonus-myoclonus, parkinsonism
	Japanese encephalitis	Parkinsonism, chorea, dystonia
	Tick-borne encephalitis	Chorea, tremor
Paramyxoviridae	Measles	Myoclonus, chorea, parkinsonism
Picornaviridae	Coxsackie virus	Parkinsonism
	Echo virus	Parkinsonism
	Polio virus	Parkinsonism
Orthomyxoviridae	Influenza virus	Chorea, parkinsonism
Bornaviridae	Borna disease virus	Parkinsonism
Togaviridae	Rubella virus	Chorea
Retrovirus	Human immunodeficiency virus (HIV)	Hemichorea/Hemiballism, parkinsonism, tremor (dystonia, myoclonus, opsoclonus, paroxysmal dyskinesias rare)

Adapted from Jang H, Boltz DA, Webster RG, et al. Viral parkinsonism. Biochim Biophys Acta 2009;1792(7):714–21. http://dx.doi.org/10.1016/j.bbadis.2008.08.001; with permission.

Fungal and Protozoal Infections

Cerebral toxoplasmosis almost always affects immunocompromised subjects, including those with HIV infections (see earlier in this article), and toxoplasmic abscesses commonly involve the basal ganglia, thalamus, and upper brain stem (**Fig. 2**), giving rise to a variety of movement disorders depending on anatomic location. Hemichorea-hemiballism is probably the most common and often relates to contralateral basal-ganglia or, rarely, thalamic lesions, but similar lesions also may produce focal or hemidystonia.[24] Parkinsonism can occur both with unilateral and bilateral basal ganglia abscesses, and generalized chorea also has been observed in patients with bilateral basal ganglia or thalamic lesions (Video 1).[14] Holmes tremor has been associated with toxoplasmic abscesses in the midbrain but also thalamus.

Movement disorders in CNS toxoplasmosis may respond to specific antitoxoplasmic therapy with sulfadiazine and pyrimethamine, but symptoms may persist even after resolution of abscesses, such that additional symptomatic therapy is required, including antidopaminergic agents to control chorea, levodopa or dopamine agonists to treat parkinsonism, or anticholinergics and focal botulinum toxin injections for dystonia.

Movement disorders in CNS toxoplasmosis at a glance

- Cerebral toxoplasmosis is almost exclusively seen in immunocompromised patients
- Clinical presentation: hemichorea-hemiballism, parkinsonism, focal dystonia
- Diagnosis: Neuroimaging may reveal contralateral basal ganglia lesion
- Therapy: Antitoxoplasmic treatment
- Dopamine blocking agents for hemichorea
- Dopamine replacement therapy for patients with parkinsonism

Similar to CNS toxoplasmosis, *fungal encephalitis* is usually associated with immunocompromised states and fungal abscesses may give rise to movement disorders depending on anatomic site. Parkinsonism has been observed in patients with *cryptococcal abscesses* in the basal ganglia[25,26] and hemichorea was associated with lesions in the contralateral head of the caudate.[27]

Helminthic Brain Infections

The most common parasitic worm infection invading the central nervous system is neurocysticercosis, which is endemic in Asia, Eastern Europe, and South America.[7] Neurocysticercosis is caused by the pork tape worm *Taenia solium*. Although neurocysticercosis is the most common cause for seizures in developing countries and the parasitic cysts affect the basal ganglia in 25%, movement disorders occur in only 3.5% of cases.[7,28] A few case reports have described levodopa-responsive akinetic-rigid parkinsonism[29,30]; however, in most cases, parkinsonism is secondary to hydrocephalus.[7] Further, dystonia, hemichorea, myoclonus, and hemifacial spasms have been described.[7,28] The proposed underlying mechanisms for movement disorders include a direct mass effect due to the cyst itself, ischemia in the basal ganglia due to vasculitis, and inflammatory processes.[7,28] In most cases, albendazole at 15 mg/kg per day for 3 days or 30 mg/kg per day for ventricular and subarachnoid cysts is effective. However, in some patients, surgical removal of the cyst or other drugs, such as praziquantel, phenobarbital, or primidone, are indicated.[7]

Key points: Helminthic brain infections	
Etiology	Neurocysticercosis is the most common helminthic infection
Clinical presentation	Movement disorders are rare, parkinsonism is mainly caused by hydrocephalus; case reports of dystonia, hemichorea, myoclonus, and hemifacial spasms
Diagnosis	MRI, serologic detection of antibodies to *Taenia solium*
Therapy	Antihelminthic therapy with albendazole or praziquantel

AUTOIMMUNE-MEDIATED MOVEMENT DISORDERS

Movement disorders occasionally may occur as presenting symptoms in patients with systemic autoimmune disease or may associate with antibodies directed to neuronal antigens, including neurotransmitter receptors. The latter is the case in patients with paraneoplastic movement disorders (see later in this article).

Systemic Lupus Erythematosus

Systemic lupus erythematosus (SLE) usually affects middle-aged women and has a prevalence that ranges between 20 and 150 cases per 100,000.[31] The disease, often called the "great imitator," affects various different organs. Antinuclear antibodies and anti–double-stranded DNA are diagnostic serologic markers.[31] Antiphospholipid syndrome (APS) is closely related and is characterized by recurrent vascular thrombosis (venous, small vessel, or arterial) associated with persistently positive antiphospholipid antibodies (lupus anticoagulant, cardiolipin antibodies, and β_2 glycoprotein antibodies).[32]

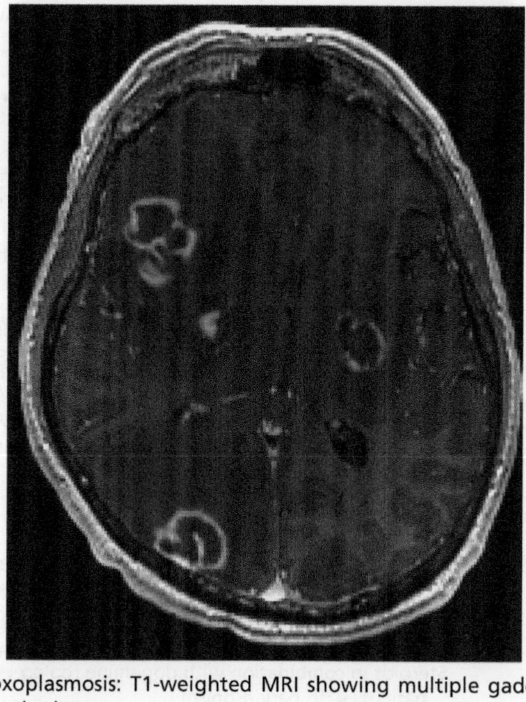

Fig. 2. Cerebral toxoplasmosis: T1-weighted MRI showing multiple gadolinium-enhancing lesions with perifocal edema.

Neurologic complications, which also are part of the diagnostic criteria, include seizures and psychosis,[31] but movement disorders also may occasionally dominate the clinical presentation. Chorea has been reported with a prevalence of 2% to 3%.[33] These patients are usually younger (mean age 20.6 years), of female predominance (84%–96%), and have a high prevalence of antiphospholipid antibodies.[33–35]

Parkinsonism is a rare complication of SLE and fewer than 40 cases have been reported since 1930, 10 with juvenile onset of parkinsonism.[36] Tremor was less frequently observed than bradykinesia and rigidity.[37] Patients may develop rapidly progressive apathy and bilateral bradykinesia.[38] Parkinsonism, probably triggered by thrombo-occlusive vasculopathy and white matter changes, also can be seen in patients with APS. In these patients, response to dopamine replacement therapy is generally poor.[37]

The diagnosis of movement disorders as a result of SLE is challenging. The presence of serologic markers typical for SLE or APS and exclusion of other causes, such as vascular chorea and Huntington disease, points toward an autoimmune process.

Most patients with chorea respond to either steroids or neuroleptic therapy. In some cases, intravenous immunoglobulin or plasma exchange has been described to alleviate symptoms.[34] All patients with SLE and parkinsonism improved either with dopamine replacement therapy alone or in combination with prednisolone, plasma exchange, and cyclophosphamide.[38]

Key points: Systemic lupus erythematosus	
Prevalence	Ranges between 20 and 150 cases per 100,000
Clinical presentation	Chorea either generalized or hemichorea occurs in 3%; parkinsonism rare
Diagnosis	Apart from neurologic signs, presence of 4 of 11 symptoms (malar rash, discoid rash, photosensitivity, oral ulcers, arthritis, serositis, kidney-blood and immunologic disorder, positive antinuclear antibodies
Therapy	Steroids, neuroleptics, immunotherapy Parkinsonism: dopamine replacement therapy, steroids

Sjögren Syndrome

Sjögren syndrome is characterized by lymphocytic infiltration of the lacrimal and salivary gland. Patients complain of xerostomia (dry mouth) and xerophthalmia (dry eyes). Antinuclear antibodies, such as SSA/Ro and SSB/La, may be positive.[39] Movement disorders, particularly parkinsonism, have been described in 2 distinct groups of patients: one group has abnormal white matter lesions on the T2-weighted cranial MRI scans and presents with an akinetic rigid form. Typically, these patients do not respond to dopamine replacement therapy.[40] The other group resembles idiopathic Parkinson disease (PD). These patients have a normal MRI scan, a good response to dopamine replacement therapy, and have motor fluctuations.[41] Other rarely seen movement disorders include chorea, dystonia, and dystonic tremor.

Key points: Sjögren syndrome	
Clinical presentation	Parkinsonism; chorea, dystonia, tremor rare
Diagnosis	Antinuclear antibodies, such as SSA/Ro and SSB/La; salivary gland and labial biopsy; T2-weighted abnormalities in basal ganglia in patients with parkinsonism
Therapy	Steroids in combination with dopamine replacement therapy in patients with parkinsonism

A variety of other autoimmune disorders can cause movement disorders, the most common are listed in **Table 3**.

PARANEOPLASTIC MOVEMENT DISORDERS

Paraneoplastic movement disorders are very rare autoimmune complications that occur in patients with cancer, where the symptoms cannot be attributed to a direct invasion of the tumor, a metastasis, or side effects of the oncological therapy.[42] Often paraneoplastic symptoms may precede the diagnosis of the underlying tumor.[43] Usually immunologic cross reactions between the protein expressed by the tumor and the neuronal cells cause these symptoms. Clinically, symptoms progress more rapidly than in neurodegenerative disorders, CSF examination often shows pleocytosis, elevated protein levels, high immunoglobulin G index, and oligoclonal bands. Presence of antineuronal antibodies can point toward the underlying cancer.

Anti–N-Methyl-D-Aspartate Receptor Encephalitis

This rapidly progressive encephalitis, which predominantly affects women, was first described in 2005 in 4 young women with ovarian teratoma.[44] The underlying cause of this disease is an antibody against *N*-methyl-D-aspartate (NMDA) receptor, which affects children and young adults with and without teratoma.[45] In a case series of 100 patients, 91% were female with a mean age of 23 years (range 5–76 years).[46] Although an underlying tumor is rare in children and male patients, more than 50% of female patients aged 18 and older had an ovarian teratoma.[47,48] In contrast, only 5% of adult male patients with anti-NMDA receptor encephalitis had an underlying tumor.

Movement disorders are a prominent part of the clinical presentation of this condition. Characteristically, patients develop orofacial dyskinesias,[49,50] which can involve jaw opening and closing,[50] facial grimacing[49] or tongue protrusion, kissing, and frowning (Video 2).[48] In addition to stereotypies, many patients also have slow rest and postural rhythmic movements (myorhythmia). Psychiatric symptoms, such as psychosis, hallucinations, agitation, insomnia, and catatonia, are frequently seen[51–53] and epileptic seizures occur more commonly in children than adults.[45,48]

Table 3
Other common systemic autoimmune disorders causing movement disorders

Syndrome	Movement Disorder	Diagnostic Test
Steroid-responsive autoimmune encephalitis (Hashimoto)	Tremor (80%) Ataxia and gait disorder (66%) Myoclonus (37%) Cognitive impairment (36%) Psychiatric problems (30%) Strokelike episodes	Antithyroglobulin antibodies Antithyroperoxidase antibodies MRI brain scan
Celiac disease	Cerebellar ataxia Polyneuropathy Myelopathy Chorea Parkinsonism	Antigliadin antibodies Anti-TG2 antibodies Anti-TG6 antibodies
Behçet disease	Chorea Ataxia	MRI brain scan (basal ganglia hyperintensities) Cerebrospinal fluid

In 50% of patients, brain MRI shows hyperintensities in T2 or fluid attenuated inversion recovery signal in multiple brain areas, including the hippocampus, the cortex, the brainstem, the basal ganglia, and the cerebellum, and sometimes the spinal cord is involved as well.[47] CSF may reveal pleocytosis, elevated protein levels, and in some oligoclonal bands. In women, gynecological screening for an underlying ovarian teratoma is necessary.

In one large multicenter study with 577 patients (37% children younger than 18), immunotherapy with steroids, immunoglobulins, and plasma exchange, in combination with removal of tumor (if present), resulted in neurologic improvement in 81% of patients after a follow-up period of 2 years. In patients who did not respond to first-line immunotherapy, rituximab, cyclophosphamide, or both improved outcome compared with those who did not receive any therapy. Factors for good outcome included early initiation of therapy and lack of intensive care unit admission.[45]

Key points: Antibody against *N*-methyl-D-aspartate (NMDA) receptor encephalitis	
Prevalence	NMDA receptor encephalitis affects female more than male patients
	More than 50% of adult female patients had an ovarian teratoma
Clinical presentation	Orofacial dyskinesias and psychiatric complications
Diagnosis	Anti-NMDA receptor antibodies; detection of underlying teratoma; 50% of patients have brain MRI hyperintensities in multiple brain areas
Therapy	Immunotherapy in combination with removal of tumor

Paraneoplastic Cerebellar Degeneration

Paraneoplastic cerebellar degeneration is one of the most common paraneoplastic syndromes. Unspecific symptoms, such as vertigo, nausea, and flulike symptoms, are typical harbingers of the disease. Patients then develop rapidly progressing ataxia, dysarthria, and diplopia.[54] A high-amplitude tremor that can in some cases resemble essential tremor is often seen. In the early stages of the disease, cranial MRI imaging can be normal and PET scans may show hypermetabolism, but as the disease progresses, MRI scans reveal cerebellar atrophy and PET scans show hypometabolism.[54]

The most common underlying tumors are breast and gynecologic cancer,[55] small-cell lung cancer,[56] and Hodgkin lymphoma.[57] The corresponding antibodies for breast and gynecologic cancer are anti-Yo antibodies and anti-Tr antibodies associated with Hodgkin lymphoma, which both have a high specificity.[54] Forty-one percent of patients with small-cell lung cancer develop antibodies to voltage-gated calcium channels (with or without Lambert-Eaton myasthenic syndrome) and 23% develop anti-Hu antibodies.[54]

There is no standard treatment guideline for these patients. Treatment of the underlying tumor is necessary to stabilize the symptoms. The evidence for immune therapy, such as corticosteroids, plasma exchange, and administration of immunoglobulins, is conflicting.

Opsoclonus-Myoclonus Syndrome

This is a rare condition that was first described in 1962 in 6 children with ataxia, myoclonus, and opsoclonus.[58] Coexisting mild behavioral, cognitive, and mood changes may occur.

Although a neuroblastoma is found in 50% of children with opsoclonus myoclonus,[54] various types of other cancers, particularly breast and lung cell cancer, but also testicular and ovarian tumors, have been associated with opsoclonus myoclonus in adults.[59] Older age, a more severe clinical presentation, and a higher frequency of encephalopathy may point toward paraneoplastic causes.[60] Although anti-Ri antibodies may occur in patients with breast and ovarian cancer, most patients are antibody negative.[54]

A subgroup of patients with opsoclonus-myoclonus also develop truncal titubation and ataxia, termed opsoclonus-myoclonus ataxia (OMA) syndrome. Truncal ataxia and gait difficulties are common, and limb ataxia, tremor, and dysarthria are rarely seen. Typically, symptoms progress rapidly and, within a few weeks, may result in severe disability. Patients with OMA with paraneoplastic cause are older than patients with idiopathic OMA (mean age 66 vs 47 years).[60]

Cranial MRI with gadolinium enhancement is necessary to exclude structural abnormalities, such as thalamic infarction, multiple sclerosis, hydrocephalus, or metastasis. Most MRI scans are, however, normal. High-resolution chest and abdominal computed tomography (CT), as well as gynecologic screening and mammography in women, should be performed. If negative, a whole-body PET scan should be considered.[61]

Although in children with neuroblastoma, immunotherapies, such as corticosteroids, intravenous immunoglobulin, plasma exchange, cyclophosphamide, or rituximab, may be useful, in adults, immunotherapy is less effective and tumor therapy is more efficacious.[54]

Stiff Person Syndrome

Stiff person syndrome is a rare disorder presenting with thoracolumbar muscle stiffness, rigidity, and spasms triggered by emotional stimuli and stress. The estimated prevalence is 1 to 2 cases per million.[62] Although most patients have the classical autoimmune variant, approximately 15% of patients have an underlying cancer. The most common tumors are breast cancer and small cell lung cancer,[32] although cases with colon cancer, thymoma, and Hodgkin lymphoma have been described.[62]

Onset is typically an insidious, with painful spams and ataxia. Hyperlordosis because of abdominal and paraspinal muscular co-contraction is frequently seen.[62] Female gender and older age of disease onset are more commonly observed in paraneoplastic stiff person syndrome.[63] Type 1 diabetes can occur in 35% of patients with the autoimmune form.[64]

Stiff person syndrome is a clinical diagnosis based on the Dalakas criteria (**Box 1**).[64] Elevated antibodies against glutamic acid decarboxylase in serum and liquor can be detected in most cases.[62] Antiamphiphysin antibodies in serum or liquor can be found in 5% of patients with paraneoplastic stiff person syndrome. A CT chest scan, as well as gynecologic investigations and mammography is necessary and if negative then a whole-body PET scan is recommended.[63]

Muscle relaxants, such as benzodiazepines, gabapentin, baclofen, or immunotherapy, such as steroids, intravenous immunoglobulin, plasma exchange, or rituximab may alleviate symptoms.[62]

In patients with paraneoplastic stiff person syndrome, tumor extinction in combination with chemotherapy and steroids may be beneficial.[63] Typically, these patients respond poorly to diazepam.

A variety of different tumors are associated with onconeuronal antibodies causing movement disorders (**Table 4**). These paraneoplastic symptoms precede the cancer diagnosis in most cases.[65]

Box 1
Clinical diagnosis criteria of stiff person syndrome

- Stiffness in the axial muscles, prominently in the abdominal and thoracolumbar paraspinal muscle leading to a fixed deformity (hyperlordosis)
- Superimposed painful spasms precipitated by unexpected noises, emotional stress, tactile stimuli
- Confirmation of the continuous motor unit activity in agonist and antagonist muscles by electromyography
- Absence of neurologic or cognitive impairments that could explain the stiffness
- Positive serology for GAD65 (or amphiphysin) autoantibodies, assessed by immunocytochemistry, Western blot, or radioimmunoassay

Response to diazepam[a]

[a] Not part of the original criteria.

Adapted from Dalakas MC. Stiff person syndrome: advances in pathogenesis and therapeutic interventions. Curr Treat Options Neurol 2009;11(2):102–10; with permission.

Table 4
Common paraneoplastic movement disorders

Tumor	Associated Antibodies	Movement Disorder
Ovarian teratoma	NMDAR	Chorea
Small-cell lung cancer	CV2/CRMP5	
Small-cell lung cancer	Hu/ANNA-1	
Ovarian teratoma	NMDAR	Dystonia
Small-cell lung cancer	CV2/CRMP5	
Small-cell lung cancer	Hu/ANNA-1	
Small-cell lung cancer, breast, gyn	Ri/ANNA-2	
Testis, non–small-cell lung cancer	Ma1/Ma2	Atypical parkinsonism
Small-cell lung cancer, breast, gyn	Ri/ANNA-2	
B-cell lymphoma	Hu/ANNA-1	
Small-cell lung cancer, breast	Amphiphysin	Stiff person syndrome
Ovarian teratoma	NMDAR	Orofacial dyskinesia
Small-cell lung cancer, breast	Ri/ANNA-2	Opsoclonus-myoclonus
Breast	Hu/ANNA-2	Myoclonus
Various different tumors	VGKC	
Breast, gyn	Yo/APCA	Ataxia
Hodgkin lymphoma	Tr	
Small-cell lung cancer	VGCC	
Small-cell lung cancer	Amphiphysin	
Small-cell lung cancer	CV2/CRMP5	
Small-cell lung cancer	Hu/ANNA-1	Tremor
Ovarian, breast	Yo/APCA	

Abbreviations: ANNA, antineuronal nuclear antibody; APCA, anti–Purkinje cell antibody; gyn, gynecological tumors; NMDAR, N-methyl-D-aspartate receptor.

Adapted from Poewe W, Jankovic J. Movement disorders in neurologic and systemic disease. New York: Cambridge University Press; 2014. p. 39–51.

MOVEMENT DISORDERS IN METABOLIC DISORDERS

Most metabolic disorders may eventually affect brain function and thus also give rise to different types of movement disorders. Classical examples in adult neurology are movement disorders in the context of liver and renal disease, as well as late-onset types of lysosomal storage disorders.

Wilson Disease

Wilson disease is an autosomal recessive disorder of copper metabolism causing accumulation of copper chiefly in hepatocytes and other tissues, including the brain. Wilson disease has a prevalence of 1:30,000[66] and is caused by mutations in the ATP7B gene.[67]

Between 50% and up to 70% of patients with Wilson disease have neurologic or neuropsychiatric symptoms, such as anxiety, cognitive impairment, impulsivity, or apathy.[68] Patients who present with movement disorders are usually older than those with hepatic presentation and younger than those with psychiatric symptoms.[68] Two forms of neurologic Wilson disease have been described. The juvenile form is characterized by dystonia and rigidity, whereas the other pseudosclerotic form presents usually after the age of 20, with mainly ataxia and tremor. Parkinsonism, cranial involvement such as dysarthria, dysphagia, drooling, and a risus sardonicus are typical.[66] In some patients, the tremor can be of low frequency, when arms are raised with elbows bent, giving it a characteristic "wing beating" appearance.[66] Other movement disorders, such as myoclonus, tics, and oculogyric crisis are rare.

Patients with Wilson disease have a typical triad of a Kayser-Fleischer ring, low serum ceruloplasmin, and elevated 24-hour urinary copper levels. However, the absence of a Kayser-Fleischer ring does not exclude the diagnosis. MRI of the brain may reveal the "face of the giant panda" sign (**Fig. 3**), signal changes in the basal ganglia, thalamus, and brainstem.[69]

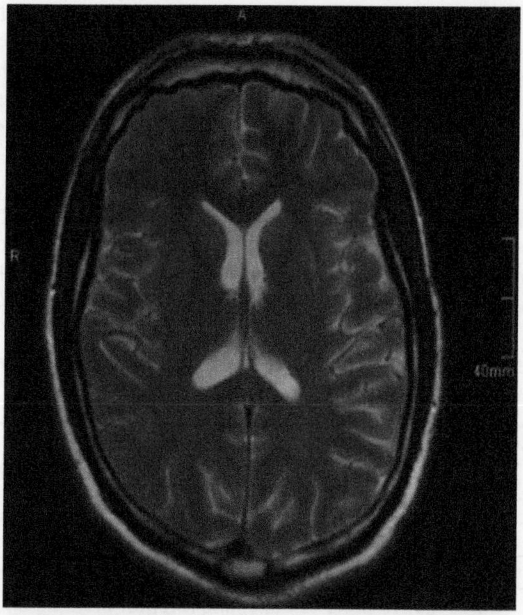

Fig. 3. T2-weighted MRI shows bilateral basal ganglia lesions in a patient with carbon monoxide poisoning.

Left untreated, Wilson disease leads to anarthria, liver failure, and inevitably to death. Treatment is targeted to reduce copper load. Increased copper secretion is achieved with the chelating agents trientine and D-penicillamine, which should be taken in combination with vitamin B6. Initially, both drugs (more common in D-penicillamine than with trientine) can cause worsening of symptoms, which may be due to a transient increase in free serum copper.[70] Zinc salt blocks absorption of copper but is less potent and sometimes used as a maintenance therapy. In patients with liver failure or decompensated cirrhosis, liver transplantation is indicated but bares the risk of operation, immunosuppression, and graft-versus-host reaction.

Key points: Wilson disease	
Prevalence	Prevalence of Wilson disease is 1:30,000
Etiology	Autosomal recessive disorder due to mutations in the *ATP7B* gene on chromosome 13
Clinical presentation	Dystonia (including risus sardonicus), tremor, ataxia, and parkinsonism; myoclonus, tics, and oculogyric crisis rare
Diagnosis	Triad of a Kayser-Fleischer ring, low serum ceruloplasmin, and elevated 24-hour urinary copper levels
Therapy	Chelating agents in combination with vitamin B6 Initial worsening may occur, less frequently seen with trientine Liver transplantation in patients with liver failure

Chronic Acquired Hepatolenticular Degeneration

This symptom may develop subacutely or insidiously, either within a few weeks or up to a decade. It is caused by portal-systemic shunting leading to excessive concentration of manganese in CSF and serum. The clinical course is usually progressive, although spontaneous remissions have been described. The prevalence rate is unknown. Survival after onset of symptoms ranges between a few weeks and up to 30 years.[71]

The most characteristic clinical features are orobuccolingual dyskinesias. Dystonia, apathy, dysarthria, bradyphrenia, chorea, ataxia, myelopathy, and parkinsonism also are common.[7,71] Although parkinsonism can closely resemble idiopathic PD, there are some atypical features, such as early postural instability, cognitive impairment, a bilateral tremor (more pronounced on action than at rest), and a faster disease progression.[72]

The diagnosis is challenging, as there are no reliable markers.[71] Cranial MRI, particularly in patients with cirrhosis, typically shows T1-weighted pallidal hyperintensities.[71]

No treatment guidelines have been established so far. Patients with orofacial dyskinesias or chorea may benefit from dopamine receptor blocking agents, such as tetrabenazine. The evidence for dopamine replacement therapies in patients with parkinsonism is conflicting, with some studies reporting improvement[72,73] and others reporting no benefit.[74,75]

Liver transplantation can improve all aspects of neurologic symptoms[71,75] but bares the risk of graft-versus-host reaction.[71]

Key points: Chronic acquired hepatolenticular degeneration	
Prevalence	Prevalence of chronic acquired hepatolenticular degeneration is unknown
Clinical presentation	Orobuccolingual dyskinesias, dystonia, dysarthria, and parkinsonism
Diagnosis	Pallidal hyperintensities on cranial MRI due to manganese deposition
Therapy	Chorea may respond to dopamine receptor blocking agents; evidence for dopamine replacement therapy in patients with parkinsonism is conflicting; liver transplantation is indicated in patients with liver failure

Hypermanganesemia with Dystonia, Polycythemia, and Cirrhosis

Hypermanganesemia with dystonia, polycythemia, and cirrhosis (HMDPC) is a rare syndrome of increased serum manganese, hepatomegaly, and polycythemia that predominantly presents during childhood but adult patients have been reported as well. Movement disorders are a prominent part of the syndrome because of manganese accumulation affecting the caudate and lentiform nuclei and dentate nuclei. The most common types of movement disorders described are parkinsonism and various forms of tremor.[76] A recently discovered mutation in the *SLC30A10* gene causes the syndrome, which is potentially treatable with oral chelation treatment and inhibitors of manganese absorption, leading to improvement of both movement disorders and hepatopathy.

Key points: Hypermanganesemia with dystonia, polycythemia, and cirrhosis (HMDPC)	
Prevalence	Rare multisystemic disease
Clinical presentation	Parkinsonism, dystonia, and tremor
Diagnosis	Mutation in *SLC30A10* gene; manganese accumulation in basal ganglia on MRI
Therapy	Chelation therapy to normalize manganese and iron levels

Renal Failure

Uremic encephalopathy is a manifestation of acute or chronic renal failure. Approximately 20% of patients with acute kidney failure who are admitted to the intensive care unit develop neurologic symptoms. In contrast, those with chronic renal failure often develop only subtle signs.[77] The spectrum of uremic encephalopathy ranges from mild inattention to severe confusion and coma. Asterixis and multifocal myoclonus, often found in acute liver failure and hepatic encephalopathy, are common.[7] Other movement disorders, such as parkinsonism[78] and chorea, are rare.

The prevalence of uremia-induced RLS in patients with renal failure is approximately 22% and increases to 38% in those who have concomitant polyneuropathy.[79] Dopamine replacement therapy has shown to be efficacious in alleviating symptoms.[77]

Another rare autosomal recessive disease is *action myoclonus renal failure syndrome*, which is a form of progressive myoclonus epilepsy. In contrast to uremic encephalopathy, these patients do not improve after kidney transplantation or dialysis. Clinically, patients present initially with a tremor at rest and on action. With disease progression, multifocal myoclonic jerks dominate the clinical picture.[80] The disease is caused by a loss-of-function mutation of the *SCARB2* gene encoding the lysosomal integral membrane protein type 2 (*LIMP-2*) gene.[81]

Key points: Renal failure	
Clinical presentation	Renal failure can cause a variety of movement disorders, typically asterixis, multifocal myoclonus, and RLS; parkinsonism is rare
Diagnosis	Patients with uremic encephalopathy can improve after dialysis or kidney transplantation

MOVEMENT DISORDERS IN IRON DYSREGULATION

Hereditary hemochromatosis is an autosomal recessive disorder and the most common cause of systemic iron overload. Excessive iron accumulates in many organs, including the brain.[82] Movement disorders are generally rare, among these, parkinsonism and ataxia are the most common. Neuroimaging studies have shown iron deposition in the basal ganglia, although none of these patients had movement disorders.[83] The diagnosis is usually made by assessing serum iron levels, transferrin, and ferritin saturation. Iron overload should be removed by regular phlebotomy. Those few patients reported with parkinsonism responded well to dopamine replacement therapy.

Key points: Hereditary hemochromatosis	
Etiology	Iron overload is usually caused by hereditary hemochromatosis
Clinical presentation	Clinical presentation: rare: parkinsonism and ataxia
Diagnosis	Serum iron, transferrin levels, ferritin; basal ganglia lesions on MRI or CT
Therapy	Phlebotomy Parkinsonism: dopamine replacement therapy

A large group of heterogeneous disorders collectively termed neurodegeneration of brain iron accumulation (NBIA) can cause movement disorders. Accumulation of brain iron within the basal ganglia is usually seen on T2-weighted MRI images. Movement disorders usually present in childhood; however, adult-onset cases can exist (**Table 5**).[84]

MOVEMENT DISORDERS IN ENDOCRINE DISORDERS

Similar to metabolic disorders, the spectrum of endocrine conditions causing movement disorders is broad. Those with classical movement disorder presentations are summarized in the following paragraphs.

Nonketotic Hyperglycemia

Onset of symptoms is usually acute in adults with type 2 diabetes. Chorea and hemichorea-hemiballismus are the presenting movement disorders. Other movement

Table 5
Most common neurodegeneration of brain iron accumulation (NBIA) causing movement disorders

NBIA	MRI Sign	Movement Disorder	Genetics
Pantothenate kinase associated neurodegeneration (*PKAN*)	Eye of the tiger	Oromandibular dystonia, dysarthria, parkinsonism, ataxia, spasticity	Recessive (*PANK2* gene)
PLA2G6	Iron deposition in globus pallidus and substantia nigra	Dystonia-parkinsonism	Recessive (*PLA2G6*)
Neuroferritinopathy	Cystic changes and iron accumulation in basal ganglia	Chorea, dystonia, parkinsonism	Dominant (*FTL*)
Aceruloplasminemia	Iron accumulation in basal ganglia	Craniofacial dyskinesias, ataxia	Recessive (ceruloplasmin gene)
Kufor-Rakeb disease	Iron accumulation in basal ganglia may occur	Parkinsonism, supranuclear gaze palsy, mini-myoclonus	Recessive (*ATP13A2*)

disorders include asterixis, seizures, and altered levels of consciousness. T1-weighted MRI brain scans reveal hyperintensities in the contralateral putamen.[85] These signal abnormalities usually resolve within months after clinical improvement. The mechanisms of hemichorea-hemiballism in this syndrome are likely microvascular lesions,[86] and depletion of gamma-aminobutyric acid and acetylcholine in the putamen.

Treatment involves correction of glucose levels. Dopamine blocking agents, such as neuroleptics, sodium valproate, and benzodiazepines, may be useful.[85]

Key points: Nonketotic hyperglycemia	
Clinical presentation	Acute hemichorea-hemiballism in older adults with type 2 diabetes [asterixis, reduced level of consciousness, and seizures may occur]
Diagnosis	Hyperglycemia, T1-weighted hyperintensity of contralateral putamen
Therapy	Correction of glucose levels, dopamine-blocking agents
Prognosis	Chorea usually resolves within days

Hyperthyroidism

Tremor is the most common movement disorder in patients with hyperthyroidism and can resemble essential tremor. Clinically, tremor occurs on action and affects the upper limbs, but cases of orthostatic tremor have been reported.[87] Other movement disorders, such as chorea, athetosis, and ballism, have been reported in fewer than 2% of patients.[88] Chorea usually affects young woman with Graves disease. Other rare movement disorders include myoclonus, task-specific dystonia, and cervical dystonia.[89] The pathophysiology is unknown, but may involve an influence of thyroid hormone on motor excitability. Symptoms usually respond to correction of elevated thyroid levels. Beta-blockers also are effective in reducing tremor.

Key points: Hyperthyroidism	
Prevalence	Rare, no epidemiologic studies
Clinical presentation	Action-tremor common; chorea, athetosis, paroxysmal dyskinesias, and dystonia are rare
Diagnosis	Elevated thyroid function tests
Therapy	Correction of hormonal levels; beta-blockers

Other causes of movement disorders in endocrine diseases are listed in **Table 6**.

MOVEMENT DISORDERS IN HEMATOLOGICAL DISEASE

Neuro-Acanthocytosis

This heterogeneous disorder presents with chorea, psychiatric complications, such as compulsive behavior and a frontosubcortical type of dementia, and erythrocyte acanthocytosis.

Chorea-Acanthocytosis

Chorea-acanthocytosis is a rare autosomal recessive disease caused by mutation of the *VPS13A* gene.[90] The age of onset is typically between 25 and 45 years and manifests with buccolingual dyskinesias, tongue protrusions ("feeding dystonia"), mutilations of tongue and lips, generalized chorea, and peripheral

Table 6
Common causes of endocrine disorders causing movement disorders

Etiology	Movement Disorder
Hypothyroidism	Parkinsonism
Addison disease	Parkinsonism
Hypoparathyroidism	Parkinsonism, ataxia, tremor, chorea, myoclonus
Hyperparathyroidism	Parkinsonism
Hypoglycemia	Paroxysmal chorea

neuropathy.[91] Blood smears may show acanthocytes and elevation of CK levels is seen in most cases. Western blot is more specific and shows reduced chorein expression.

The disease is chronically progressive. Dopamine-blocking agents, such as neuroleptics, can reduce chorea.

Key points: Chorea-acanthocytosis	
Prevalence	Rare, no epidemiologic studies
Etiology	Autosomal-recessive mutations of *VPS13A* gene on chromosome 9q21 (coding for chorein)
Age on onset	Mid adulthood (age ~25–45 years)
Clinical presentation	Progressive chorea, cognitive decline, buccolingual dyskinesias with tongue protrusion, mutilations of tongue and lips, peripheral neuropathies, psychiatric symptoms, epileptic seizures (rare)
Diagnosis	Acanthocytes in blood smears (>4%), CK elevation, reduced chorein expression
Therapy	Dopamine-blocking agents
Prognosis	Relentlessly progressive, reduced life-expectancy

McLeod Syndrome

McLeod syndrome is an X-linked disorder typically manifesting between 30 and 40 years. Cardiomyopathy (in 67%), myopathy, orofacial dyskinesias, and neuropathy are typically seen. In contrast to chorea-acanthocytosis, self-mutilation and the "feeding dystonia" are rare. Neuropsychiatric complications, such as obsessive compulsive disorders and psychosis, are common.[92] Therapy is symptomatic to reduce chorea.

Key points: McLeod syndrome	
Prevalence	Prevalence of McLeod syndrome unknown
Etiology	X-linked disorder
Age on onset	Mid adulthood (age ~30–40 years)
Clinical presentation	Progressive chorea, cognitive decline with psychiatric symptoms, cardiomyopathy; self-mutilation and feeding dystonia rare
Diagnosis	Acanthocytes in blood smear, mutation in *XK* gene
Therapy	Dopamine-blocking agents
Prognosis	Progressive with reduced life-expectancy

Polycythemia Vera

Polycythemia vera is a sporadic myeloproliferative disorder of the hematopoietic stem cells. The annual incidence is 2 to 10 cases per million population.[93] Movement disorders are generally rare. Chorea is the most common and occurs in 0.5% and up to 5% of cases. Chorea can be unilateral or generalized with orofaciolingual involvement.[94] Mutation in the janus kinase 2 (*JAK2*) gene, which is necessary for apoptosis,[95] may be responsible for chorea. Excess of erythrocytes, which in turn lead to hyperviscosity, may lead to reduced cerebral flow in the basal ganglia, although this theory could not be confirmed in a case report.[96] Chorea usually respond to dopamine-blocking agents and benzodiazepines. Phlebotomy also has been also shown to improve chorea.[97]

Key points: Polycythemia vera	
Prevalence	Chorea occurs in up to 5% of patients with polycythemia vera
Clinical presentation	Chorea can be unilateral or generalized with orofaciolingual involvement
Diagnosis	Elevated red blood cell mass, splenomegaly, and arterial oxygen saturation ≥92%
Therapy	Dopamine-blocking agents, benzodiazepines, and phlebotomy

MOVEMENT DISORDERS IN SYSTEMIC INTOXICATIONS

Manganese

Manganese toxicity can cause an extrapyramidal syndrome with symmetric bradykinesia, a dystonic "cock" gait, postural instability, and dysarthria. These neurologic symptoms are collectively termed as manganism and are often seen ephedrone abusers[98,99] and have been also described in welders who work poorly ventilated places.[100] Symptoms are usually progressive despite cessation of manganese exposure. Diagnosis can be made by measuring manganese levels in pubic hair.[101] Furthermore, T1-weighted MRI brain imaging shows typical pallidal lesions, whereas dopamine transporter (DAT) scans are normal.[98,101] There is currently no effective treatment. Some cases responded to chelation therapy,[102] but in most cases there was no improvement of clinical symptoms.[101]

Key points: Manganese toxicity	
Prevalence	Typically seen in welders and ephedrone abusers
Clinical presentation	Dystonia, parkinsonism, "cock gait," and severe dysarthria ("pallidal speech"); usually progressive despite cessation of exposure
Diagnosis	High concentration of manganese in pubic hair; T1-weighted pallidal lesions on MRI
Therapy	Chelation therapy may alleviate symptoms in a minority of patients

Methanol

Methanol is widely used, for example as a fuel additive or for the production of plastic. Once ingested, it is metabolized in the liver to formic acid, which is neurotoxic.[103] Lethargy, nausea, and, in some, coma or death can occur. Movement disorders include parkinsonism, ataxia, and dystonia.[103,104] CT and MRI brain imaging typically show bilateral putaminal lesions with or without hemorrhage and subcortical white matter lesions.[105] Symptoms are usually progressive and unresponsive to therapy such as anticholinergic drugs. However, dopamine-replacement therapy may be effective in alleviating motor handicaps.[106]

Key points: Methanol toxicity	
Toxicity	Methanol becomes toxic after being metabolized in the liver
Clinical presentation	Parkinsonism, ataxia and dystonia; symptoms usually progressive
Diagnosis	Bilateral putaminal lesion with or without hemorrhage on neuroimaging
Therapy	Usually progressive, dopamine-replacement therapy may alleviate symptoms

Carbon Monoxide

Carbon monoxide poisoning is common, causing more than 50,000 emergency department visits in the United States each year.[107] Carbon monoxide is a fragrance-free, tasteless gas that has greater affinity to hemoglobin than oxygen. Acute intoxication can lead to movement disorders such as rigidity, tremor, chorea, and generalized dystonia.[108] Chronic low-dose exposure, seen in firefighters, has been suggested to cause parkinsonism in later life.[109] T2-weighted MRI brain imaging may show basal ganglia lesions (see **Fig. 3**).[107] Administration of normobaric 100% oxygen is recommended. The use of hyperbaric oxygen is still conflicting[107] and is not readily available everywhere.

Key points: Carbon monoxide poisoning	
Toxicity	Usually occurs in poorly ventilated rooms with fuel-burning heaters or gas stoves and in suicide attempts inhaling car exhaust fumes
Clinical presentation	Altered consciousness, seizures, and cardiac arrest are frequently seen; movement disorders include chorea, dystonia, tremor, and rigidity
Diagnosis	Clinical history, T2-weighted MRI brain scan may reveal lesions in the basal ganglia and the hippocampus
Therapy	Inhalation of normobaric 100% oxygen

Cyanide

Cyanide is a lethal mitochondrial toxin resulting in respiratory arrest. Once indigested in a dose above 3 mg per kg of body weight, it leads to coma and rapid death.[108] Chronic exposure in miners can lead to parkinsonism, dystonia, and apraxia of eye lid opening.[110,111] Parkinsonism is caused by lesions in the basal ganglia, particularly the globus pallidus and the putamen.[110] Anticholinergic therapy can improve apraxia of eyelid opening, and parkinsonism may respond to amantadine in combination with levodopa.[111]

Key points: cyanide toxicity	
Toxicity	Cyanide is one of the most lethal toxins
Clinical presentation	Death follows within minutes; chronic exposure: parkinsonism, dystonia, and apraxia of eyelid opening
Diagnosis	History; neuroimaging may reveal lesions in the globus pallidus and the putamen
Therapy	Anticholinergics and dopamine-replacement therapy may improve apraxia of eyelid opening and parkinsonism; botulinum toxin should be considered for dystonia

Table 7
Summary of common movement disorders in metal and nonmetal intoxications

Chorea	Dystonia	Parkinsonism
Psychostimulants	Manganese	Carbon monoxide
Ethanol	Ephedrone	Manganese
Thallium	Carbon monoxide	MPTP
	Cyanide	Ephedrone
		Carbon monoxide
		Carbon disulfide
		Cyanide
		Toluene
		Ethanol

Abbreviation: MPTP, 1-methyl-4-phenyl-1,2,3,6-tetrahydropyridine.

An overview of the most common systemic intoxications can be found in **Table 7**.

SUMMARY

- Movement disorders are a common but still underrecognized complication of a wide spectrum of systemic diseases.
- A careful medical history and judicious use of laboratory tests are required to recognize or rule out symptomatic causes of movement disorders.
- In many conditions, MRI of the brain may provide important clues to movement disorder etiologies in the setting of systemic diseases.
- Recognizing the underlying medical cause has important therapeutic implications. Commonly, specific treatment of the underlying condition will improve the secondary movement disorder, but often additional symptomatic therapy is also necessary.

SUPPLEMENTARY DATA

Supplementary data related to this article can be found online at http://dx.doi.org/10.1016/j.ncl.2014.09.015.

REFERENCES

1. Poewe W, Jankovic J. Movement disorders in neurological and systemic disease. New York: Cambridge University Press; 2014.
2. Schneider T, Moos V, Loddenkemper C, et al. Whipple's disease: new aspects of pathogenesis and treatment. Lancet Infect Dis 2008;8(3):179–90. http://dx.doi.org/10.1016/S1473-3099(08)70042-2.
3. Fenollar F, Puechal X, Raoult D. Whipple's disease. N Engl J Med 2007;356(1):55–66. http://dx.doi.org/10.1056/NEJMra062477.
4. Schwartz MA, Selhorst JB, Ochs AL, et al. Oculomasticatory myorhythmia: a unique movement disorder occurring in Whipple's disease. Ann Neurol 1986;20(6):677–83. http://dx.doi.org/10.1002/ana.410200605.
5. Compain C, Sacre K, Puechal X, et al. Central nervous system involvement in Whipple disease: clinical study of 18 patients and long-term follow-up. Medicine 2013;92(6):324–30. http://dx.doi.org/10.1097/MD.0000000000000010.
6. Uldry PA, Bogousslavsky J. Partially reversible parkinsonism in Whipple's disease with antibiotherapy. Eur Neurol 1992;32(3):151–3.

7. Alarcon F, Gimenez-Roldan S. Systemic diseases that cause movement disorders. Parkinsonism Relat Disord 2005;11(1):1–18. http://dx.doi.org/10.1016/j.parkreldis.2004.10.003.
8. Alarcon F, Duenas G, Cevallos N, et al. Movement disorders in 30 patients with tuberculous meningitis. Mov Disord 2000;15(3):561–9.
9. Benito-Leon J, Alvarez-Linera J, Louis ED. Neurosyphilis masquerading as corticobasal degeneration. Mov Disord 2004;19(11):1367–70. http://dx.doi.org/10.1002/mds.20221.
10. Shah BB, Lang AE. Acquired neurosyphilis presenting as movement disorders. Mov Disord 2012;27(6):690–5. http://dx.doi.org/10.1002/mds.24950.
11. Fauci AS, Folkers GKJ. Toward an AIDS-free generation. Am Med Assoc 2012;344:343–4. Available at: http://jama.jamanetwork.com/article.aspx?articleID=1221711.
12. Sanchez-Ramos JR, Factor SA, Weiner WJ, et al. Hemichorea-hemiballismus associated with acquired immune deficiency syndrome and cerebral toxoplasmosis. Mov Disord 1989;4(3):266–73. http://dx.doi.org/10.1002/mds.870040308.
13. Tse W, Cersosimo MG, Gracies JM, et al. Movement disorders and AIDS: a review. Parkinsonism Relat Disord 2004;10(6):323–34. http://dx.doi.org/10.1016/j.parkreldis.2004.03.001.
14. Piccolo I, Causarano R, Sterzi R, et al. Chorea in patients with AIDS. Acta Neurol Scand 1999;100(5):332–6.
15. Krauss JK, Pohle T, Borremans JJ. Hemichorea and hemiballism associated with contralateral hemiparesis and ipsilateral basal ganglia lesions. Mov Disord 1999;14(3):497–501.
16. Navia BA, Jordan BD, Price RW. The AIDS dementia complex: I. Clinical features. Ann Neurol 1986;19(6):517–24. http://dx.doi.org/10.1002/ana.410190602.
17. Jang H, Boltz DA, Webster RG, et al. Viral parkinsonism. Biochim Biophys Acta 2009;1792(7):714–21. http://dx.doi.org/10.1016/j.bbadis.2008.08.001.
18. Mirsattari SM, Power C, Nath A. Parkinsonism with HIV infection. Mov Disord 1998;13(4):684–9. http://dx.doi.org/10.1002/mds.870130413.
19. Happe S, Kundmuller L, Reichelt D, et al. Comorbidity of restless legs syndrome and HIV infection. J Neurol 2007;254(10):1401–6. http://dx.doi.org/10.1007/s00415-007-0563-2.
20. Smith MT, Lester-Smith D, Zurynski Y, et al. Persistence of acute rheumatic fever in a tertiary children's hospital. J Paediatr Child Health 2011;47(4):198–203. http://dx.doi.org/10.1111/j.1440-1754.2010.01935.x.
21. Mohammad SS, Ramanathan S, Brilot F, et al. Autoantibody-associated movement disorders. Neuropediatrics 2013;44(6):336–45. http://dx.doi.org/10.1055/s-0033-1358603.
22. Cardoso F, Eduardo C, Silva AP, et al. Chorea in fifty consecutive patients with rheumatic fever. Mov Disord 1997;12(5):701–3. http://dx.doi.org/10.1002/mds.870120512.
23. Cardoso F, Vargas AP, Oliveira LD, et al. Persistent Sydenham's chorea. Mov Disord 1999;14(5):805–7.
24. Nath A, Hobson DE, Russell A. Movement disorders with cerebral toxoplasmosis and AIDS. Mov Disord 1993;8(1):107–12. http://dx.doi.org/10.1002/mds.870080119.
25. Camargos ST, Teixeira AL Jr, Cardoso F. Parkinsonism associated with basal ganglia cryptococcal abscesses in an immunocompetent patient. Mov Disord 2006;21(5):714–5. http://dx.doi.org/10.1002/mds.20789.

26. Wszolek Z, Monsour H, Smith P, et al. Cryptococcal meningoencephalitis with parkinsonian features. Mov Disord 1988;3(3):271–3. http://dx.doi.org/10.1002/mds.870030312.
27. Namer IJ, Tan E, Akalin E, et al. A case of hemiballismus during cryptococcal meningitis. Rev Neurol (Paris) 1990;146(2):153–4 [in French].
28. Cosentino C, Velez M, Torres L, et al. Neurocysticercosis-induced hemichorea. Mov Disord 2006;21(2):286–7. http://dx.doi.org/10.1002/mds.20759.
29. Sa DS, Teive HA, Troiano AR, et al. Parkinsonism associated with neurocysticercosis. Parkinsonism Relat Disord 2005;11(1):69–72. http://dx.doi.org/10.1016/j.parkreldis.2004.07.009.
30. Lima PM, Munhoz RP, Teive HA. Reversible parkinsonism associated with neurocysticercosis. Arq Neuropsiquiatr 2012;70(12):965–6.
31. Tsokos GC. Systemic lupus erythematosus. N Engl J Med 2011;365(22):2110–21. http://dx.doi.org/10.1056/NEJMra1100359.
32. Panzer J, Dalmau J. Movement disorders in paraneoplastic and autoimmune disease. Curr Opin Neurol 2011;24(4):346–53. http://dx.doi.org/10.1097/WCO.0b013e328347b307.
33. Cervera R, Asherson RA, Font J, et al. Chorea in the antiphospholipid syndrome. Clinical, radiologic, and immunologic characteristics of 50 patients from our clinics and the recent literature. Medicine 1997;76(3):203–12.
34. Reiner P, Galanaud D, Leroux G, et al. Long-term outcome of 32 patients with chorea and systemic lupus erythematosus or antiphospholipid antibodies. Mov Disord 2011;26(13):2422–7. http://dx.doi.org/10.1002/mds.23863.
35. Baizabal-Carvallo JF, Bonnet C, Jankovic J. Movement disorders in systemic lupus erythematosus and the antiphospholipid syndrome. J Neural Transm 2013;120(11):1579–89.
36. Khubchandani RP, Viswanathan V, Desai J. Unusual neurologic manifestations (I): parkinsonism in juvenile SLE. Lupus 2007;16(8):572–5. http://dx.doi.org/10.1177/0961203307081421.
37. Barton B, Zauber SE, Goetz CG. Movement disorders caused by medical disease. Semin Neurol 2009;29(2):97–110. http://dx.doi.org/10.1055/s-0029-1213731.
38. Tan EK, Chan LL, Auchus AP. Reversible parkinsonism in systemic lupus erythematosus. J Neurol Sci 2001;193(1):53–7.
39. Jonsson R, Brun J. Sjögren's syndrome. Oxford (United Kingdom): John Wiley & Sons, Ltd; 2010. p. 202–21.
40. Walker RH, Spiera H, Brin MF, et al. Parkinsonism associated with Sjogren's syndrome: three cases and a review of the literature. Mov Disord 1999;14(2):262–8.
41. Hassin-Baer S, Levy Y, Langevitz P, et al. Anti-beta2-glycoprotein I in Sjogren's syndrome is associated with parkinsonism. Clin Rheumatol 2007;26(5):743–7. http://dx.doi.org/10.1007/s10067-006-0398-8.
42. Poser J. Paraneoplastic syndromes. Rev Neurol (Paris) 2002;158:899–906.
43. Darnell RB, Posner JB. Paraneoplastic syndromes affecting the nervous system. Semin Oncol 2006;33(3):270–98. http://dx.doi.org/10.1053/j.seminoncol.2006.03.008.
44. Vitaliani R, Mason W, Ances B, et al. Paraneoplastic encephalitis, psychiatric symptoms, and hypoventilation in ovarian teratoma. Ann Neurol 2005;58(4):594–604. http://dx.doi.org/10.1002/ana.20614.
45. Titulaer MJ, McCracken L, Gabilondo I, et al. Treatment and prognostic factors for long-term outcome in patients with anti-NMDA receptor encephalitis: an observational cohort study. Lancet Neurol 2013;12(2):157–65. http://dx.doi.org/10.1016/S1474-4422(12)70310-1.

46. Dalmau J, Gleichman AJ, Hughes EG, et al. Anti-NMDA-receptor encephalitis: case series and analysis of the effects of antibodies. Lancet Neurol 2008; 7(12):1091–8. http://dx.doi.org/10.1016/S1474-4422(08)70224-2.
47. Dalmau J, Lancaster E, Martinez-Hernandez E, et al. Clinical experience and laboratory investigations in patients with anti-NMDAR encephalitis. Lancet Neurol 2011;10(1):63–74. http://dx.doi.org/10.1016/S1474-4422(10)70253-2.
48. Florance NR, Davis RL, Lam C, et al. Anti-N-methyl-D-aspartate receptor (NMDAR) encephalitis in children and adolescents. Ann Neurol 2009;66(1): 11–8. http://dx.doi.org/10.1002/ana.21756.
49. Sansing LH, Tuzun E, Ko MW, et al. A patient with encephalitis associated with NMDA receptor antibodies. Nat Clin Pract Neurol 2007;3(5):291–6. http://dx.doi.org/10.1038/ncpneuro0493.
50. Iizuka T, Sakai F, Ide T, et al. Anti-NMDA receptor encephalitis in Japan: long-term outcome without tumor removal. Neurology 2008;70(7):504–11. http://dx.doi.org/10.1212/01.wnl.0000278388.90370.c3.
51. Kruse JL, Jeffrey JK, Davis MC, et al. Anti-N-methyl-D-aspartate receptor encephalitis: a targeted review of clinical presentation, diagnosis, and approaches to psychopharmacologic management. Ann Clin Psychiatry 2014;26(2):111–9.
52. Baizabal-Carvallo JF, Jankovic J. Movement disorders in autoimmune diseases. Mov Disord 2012;27(8):935–46. http://dx.doi.org/10.1002/mds.25011.
53. Baizabal-Carvallo JF, Stocco A, Muscal E, et al. The spectrum of movement disorders in children with anti-NMDA receptor encephalitis. Mov Disord 2013; 28(4):543–7.
54. Dalmau J, Rosenfeld MR. Paraneoplastic syndromes of the CNS. Lancet Neurol 2008;7(4):327–40. http://dx.doi.org/10.1016/S1474-4422(08)70060-7.
55. Peterson K, Rosenblum MK, Kotanides H, et al. Paraneoplastic cerebellar degeneration. I. A clinical analysis of 55 anti-Yo antibody-positive patients. Neurology 1992;42(10):1931–7.
56. Mason WP, Graus F, Lang B, et al. Small-cell lung cancer, paraneoplastic cerebellar degeneration and the Lambert-Eaton myasthenic syndrome. Brain 1997; 120(Pt 8):1279–300.
57. Shams'ili S, Grefkens J, de Leeuw B, et al. Paraneoplastic cerebellar degeneration associated with antineuronal antibodies: analysis of 50 patients. Brain 2003;126(Pt 6):1409–18.
58. Kinsbourne M. Myoclonic encephalopathy of infants. J Neurol Neurosurg Psychiatry 1962;25(3):271–6.
59. Hero B, Schleiermacher G. Update on pediatric opsoclonus myoclonus syndrome. Neuropediatrics 2013;44(6):324–9. http://dx.doi.org/10.1055/s-0033-1358604.
60. Bataller L, Graus F, Saiz A, et al. Spanish Opsoclonus-Myoclonus Study G. Clinical outcome in adult onset idiopathic or paraneoplastic opsoclonus-myoclonus. Brain 2001;124(Pt 2):437–43.
61. Wong A. An update on opsoclonus. Curr Opin Neurol 2007;20(1):25–31. http://dx.doi.org/10.1097/WCO.0b013e3280126b51.
62. Hadavi S, Noyce AJ, Leslie RD, et al. Stiff person syndrome. Pract Neurol 2011; 11(5):272–82. http://dx.doi.org/10.1136/practneurol-2011-000071.
63. Murinson BB, Guarnaccia JB. Stiff-person syndrome with amphiphysin antibodies: distinctive features of a rare disease. Neurology 2008;71(24):1955–8. http://dx.doi.org/10.1212/01.wnl.0000327342.58936.e0.
64. Dalakas MC. Stiff person syndrome: advances in pathogenesis and therapeutic interventions. Curr Treat Options Neurol 2009;11(2):102–10.

65. Grant R, Graus F. Paraneoplastic movement disorders. Mov Disord 2009;24(12): 1715–24. http://dx.doi.org/10.1002/mds.22658.
66. Machado A, Chien HF, Deguti MM, et al. Neurological manifestations in Wilson's disease: report of 119 cases. Mov Disord 2006;21(12):2192–6. http://dx.doi.org/10.1002/mds.21170.
67. Tanzi RE, Petrukhin K, Chernov I, et al. The Wilson disease gene is a copper transporting ATPase with homology to the Menkes disease gene. Nat Genet 1993;5(4):344–50. http://dx.doi.org/10.1038/ng1293-344.
68. Taly AB, Meenakshi-Sundaram S, Sinha S, et al. Wilson disease: description of 282 patients evaluated over 3 decades. Medicine 2007;86(2):112–21. http://dx.doi.org/10.1097/MD.0b013e318045a00e.
69. Prashanth LK, Sinha S, Taly AB, et al. Do MRI features distinguish Wilson's disease from other early onset extrapyramidal disorders? An analysis of 100 cases. Mov Disord 2010;25(6):672–8. http://dx.doi.org/10.1002/mds.22689.
70. Brewer GJ, Askari F, Dick RB, et al. Treatment of Wilson's disease with tetrathiomolybdate: V. Control of free copper by tetrathiomolybdate and a comparison with trientine. Transl Res 2009;154(2):70–7. http://dx.doi.org/10.1016/j.trsl.2009.05.002.
71. Ferrara J, Jankovic J. Acquired hepatocerebral degeneration. J Neurol 2009; 256(3):320–32. http://dx.doi.org/10.1007/s00415-009-0144-7.
72. Burkhard PR, Delavelle J, Du Pasquier R, et al. Chronic parkinsonism associated with cirrhosis: a distinct subset of acquired hepatocerebral degeneration. Arch Neurol 2003;60(4):521–8. http://dx.doi.org/10.1001/archneur.60.4.521.
73. Klos KJ, Ahlskog JE, Josephs KA, et al. Neurologic spectrum of chronic liver failure and basal ganglia T1 hyperintensity on magnetic resonance imaging: probable manganese neurotoxicity. Arch Neurol 2005;62(9):1385–90. http://dx.doi.org/10.1001/archneur.62.9.1385.
74. Park HK, Kim SM, Choi CG, et al. Effect of trientine on manganese intoxication in a patient with acquired hepatocerebral degeneration. Mov Disord 2008;23(5): 768–70. http://dx.doi.org/10.1002/mds.21957.
75. Shulman LM, Minagar A, Weiner WJ. Reversal of parkinsonism following liver transplantation. Neurology 2003;60(3):519.
76. Quadri M, Federico A, Zhao T, et al. Mutations in SLC30A10 cause parkinsonism and dystonia with hypermanganesemia, polycythemia, and chronic liver disease. Am J Hum Genet 2012;90(3):467–77. http://dx.doi.org/10.1016/j.ajhg.2012.01.017.
77. Seifter JL, Samuels MA. Uremic encephalopathy and other brain disorders associated with renal failure. Semin Neurol 2011;31(2):139–43. http://dx.doi.org/10.1055/s-0031-1277984.
78. Lee PH, Shin DH, Kim JW, et al. Parkinsonism with basal ganglia lesions in a patient with uremia: evidence of vasogenic edema. Parkinsonism Relat Disord 2006;12(2):93–6. http://dx.doi.org/10.1016/j.parkreldis.2005.07.009.
79. Walters AS. Toward a better definition of the restless legs syndrome. The International Restless Legs Syndrome Study Group. Mov Disord 1995;10(5):634–42. http://dx.doi.org/10.1002/mds.870100517.
80. Badhwar A, Berkovic SF, Dowling JP, et al. Action myoclonus-renal failure syndrome: characterization of a unique cerebro-renal disorder. Brain 2004; 127(Pt 10):2173–82. http://dx.doi.org/10.1093/brain/awh263.
81. Berkovic SF, Dibbens LM, Oshlack A, et al. Array-based gene discovery with three unrelated subjects shows SCARB2/LIMP-2 deficiency causes myoclonus

epilepsy and glomerulosclerosis. Am J Hum Genet 2008;82(3):673–84. http://dx.doi.org/10.1016/j.ajhg.2007.12.019.

82. Dusek P, Jankovic J, Le W. Iron dysregulation in movement disorders. Neurobiol Dis 2012;46(1):1–18. http://dx.doi.org/10.1016/j.nbd.2011.12.054.
83. Berg D, Hoggenmuller U, Hofmann E, et al. The basal ganglia in haemochromatosis. Neuroradiology 2000;42(1):9–13.
84. Schneider SA, Hardy J, Bhatia KP. Syndromes of neurodegeneration with brain iron accumulation (NBIA): an update on clinical presentations, histological and genetic underpinnings, and treatment considerations. Mov Disord 2012;27(1):42–53. http://dx.doi.org/10.1002/mds.23971.
85. Oh SH, Lee KY, Im JH, et al. Chorea associated with non-ketotic hyperglycemia and hyperintensity basal ganglia lesion on T1-weighted brain MRI study: a meta-analysis of 53 cases including four present cases. J Neurol Sci 2002;200(1–2):57–62.
86. Mestre T, Ferreira J, Pimentel J. Putaminal petechial haemorrhage as the cause of non-ketotic hyperglycaemic chorea: a neuropathological case correlated with MRI findings. BMJ Case Rep 2009;2009. http://dx.doi.org/10.1136/bcr.08.2008.0785.
87. Tan EK, Lo YL, Chan LL. Graves disease and isolated orthostatic tremor. Neurology 2008;70(16 Pt 2):1497–8. http://dx.doi.org/10.1212/01.wnl.0000310405.36026.92.
88. Yu JH, Weng YM. Acute chorea as a presentation of Graves disease: case report and review. Am J Emerg Med 2009;27(3):369.e1–3. http://dx.doi.org/10.1016/j.ajem.2008.05.031.
89. Tan EK, Chan LL. Movement disorders associated with hyperthyroidism: expanding the phenotype. Mov Disord 2006;21(7):1054–5. http://dx.doi.org/10.1002/mds.20883.
90. Walker RH, Danek A, Dobson-Stone C, et al. Developments in neuroacanthocytosis: expanding the spectrum of choreatic syndromes. Mov Disord 2006;21(11):1794–805. http://dx.doi.org/10.1002/mds.21108.
91. Sokolov E, Schneider SA, Bain PG. Chorea-acanthocytosis. Pract Neurol 2012;12(1):40–3. http://dx.doi.org/10.1136/practneurol-2011-000045.
92. Walker RH, Jung HH, Danek A. Neuroacanthocytosis. Handb Clin Neurol 2011;100:141–51. http://dx.doi.org/10.1016/B978-0-444-52014-2.00007-0.
93. Cao M, Olsen RJ, Zu Y. Polycythemia vera: new clinicopathologic perspectives. Arch Pathol Lab Med 2006;130(8):1126–32. http://dx.doi.org/10.1043/1543-2165(2006)130[1126:PV]2.0.CO;2.
94. Marvi MM, Lew MF. Polycythemia and chorea. Handb Clin Neurol 2011;100:271–6. http://dx.doi.org/10.1016/B978-0-444-52014-2.00019-7.
95. Staerk J, Kallin A, Demoulin JB, et al. JAK1 and Tyk2 activation by the homologous polycythemia vera JAK2 V617F mutation: cross-talk with IGF1 receptor. J Biol Chem 2005;280(51):41893–9. http://dx.doi.org/10.1074/jbc.C500358200.
96. Kim W, Kim JS, Lee KS, et al. No evidence of perfusion abnormalities in the basal ganglia of a patient with generalized chorea-ballism and polycythaemia vera: analysis using subtraction SPECT co-registered to MRI. Neurol Sci 2008;29(5):351–4. http://dx.doi.org/10.1007/s10072-008-0994-2.
97. Midi I, Dib H, Koseoglu M, et al. Hemichorea associated with polycythaemia vera. Neurol Sci 2006;27(6):439–41. http://dx.doi.org/10.1007/s10072-006-0727-3.
98. Sanotsky Y, Lesyk R, Fedoryshyn L, et al. Manganic encephalopathy due to "ephedrone" abuse. Mov Disord 2007;22(9):1337–43. http://dx.doi.org/10.1002/mds.21378.

99. Sikk K, Haldre S, Aquilonius SM, et al. Manganese-induced parkinsonism due to ephedrone abuse. Parkinsons Dis 2011;2011:865319. http://dx.doi.org/10.4061/2011/865319.
100. Bowler RM, Gocheva V, Harris M, et al. Prospective study on neurotoxic effects in manganese-exposed bridge construction welders. Neurotoxicology 2011; 32(5):596–605. http://dx.doi.org/10.1016/j.neuro.2011.06.004.
101. Selikhova M, Fedoryshyn L, Matviyenko Y, et al. Parkinsonism and dystonia caused by the illicit use of ephedrone–a longitudinal study. Mov Disord 2008; 23(15):2224–31. http://dx.doi.org/10.1002/mds.22290.
102. Jiang YM, Mo XA, Du FQ, et al. Effective treatment of manganese-induced occupational Parkinsonism with p-aminosalicylic acid: a case of 17-year follow-up study. J Occup Environ Med 2006;48(6):644–9. http://dx.doi.org/10.1097/01.jom.0000204114.01893.3e.
103. Carcaba V, Garcia Amorin Z, Rodriguez Junquera R, et al. Parkinsonism and putaminal lesion from methanol intoxication. An Med Interna 2002;19(8):438–9.
104. Finkelstein Y, Vardi J. Progressive parkinsonism in a young experimental physicist following long-term exposure to methanol. Neurotoxicology 2002;23(4–5): 521–5.
105. Blanco M, Casado R, Vazquez F, et al. CT and MR imaging findings in methanol intoxication. AJNR Am J Neuroradiol 2006;27(2):452–4.
106. LeWitt PA, Martin SD. Dystonia and hypokinesis with putaminal necrosis after methanol intoxication. Clin Neuropharmacol 1988;11(2):161–7.
107. Weaver LK. Clinical practice. Carbon monoxide poisoning. N Engl J Med 2009; 360(12):1217–25. http://dx.doi.org/10.1056/NEJMcp0808891.
108. Pappert EJ. Toxin-induced movement disorders. Neurol Clin 2005;23(2):429–59. http://dx.doi.org/10.1016/j.ncl.2004.12.007.
109. Minerbo G, Jankovic J. Prevalence of Parkinson's disease among firefighters. Neurology 1990;40(Suppl):348.
110. Uitti RJ, Rajput AH, Ashenhurst EM, et al. Cyanide-induced parkinsonism: a clinicopathologic report. Neurology 1985;35(6):921–5.
111. Carella F, Grassi MP, Savoiardo M, et al. Dystonic-parkinsonian syndrome after cyanide poisoning: clinical and MRI findings. J Neurol Neurosurg Psychiatry 1988;51(10):1345–8.

Index

Note: Page numbers of article titles are in **boldface** type.

Neurol Clin 33 (2015) 299–313
http://dx.doi.org/10.1016/S0733-8619(14)00105-4 neurologic.theclinics.com
0733-8619/15/$ – see front matter

G

H

P

Printed and bound by CPI Group (UK) Ltd, Croydon, CR0 4YY
08/06/2025
01896875-0006